Developmental Aspects of Health Compliance Behavior

DEVELOPMENTAL ASPECTS OF HEALTH COMPLIANCE BEHAVIOR

Edited by

NORMAN A. KRASNEGOR
National Institute of Child Health and
Human Development

LEONARD EPSTEIN
University of Pittsburgh

SUZANNE BENNETT JOHNSON
J. Hillis Miller Health Center,
Gainesville, Florida

SUMNER J. YAFFE
National Institute of Child Health and
Human Development

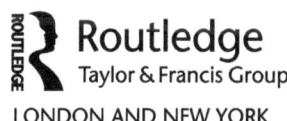

LONDON AND NEW YORK

First published by 1993
Lawrence Erlbaum Associates, Inc.
365 Broadway
Hillsdale, New Jersey 07642

This edition published 2013 by Routledge
2 Park Square, Milton Park, Abingdon, Oxfordshire OX14 4RN
711 Third Avenue, New York, NY 10017

First issued in paperback 2016

Routledge is an imprint of the Taylor and Francis Group, an informa business

Copyright © 1993 by Lawrence Erlbaum Associates, Inc.

All rights reserved. No part of this book may be reprinted or reproduced or utilised in any form or by any electronic, mechanical, or other means, now known or hereafter invented, including photocopying and recording, or in any information storage or retrieval system, without permission in writing from the publishers.

Notice:
Product or corporate names may be trademarks or registered trademarks, and are used only for identification and explanation without intent to infringe.

Library of Congress Cataloging in Publication Data
Developmental aspects of health compliance behavior / edited by Norman
   A. Krasnegor . . . [et al.].
      p.   cm.
   Includes bibliographical references and indexes.
   ISBN 0-8058-1112-5
   1. Health behavior.   2. Health behavior in children.   3. Patient
compliance.   4. Medicine, Preventive.   I. Krasnegor, Norman A.
   [DNLM: 1. Health Behavior—in adolescence—congresses. 2. Health
Behavior—in infancy & childhood—congresses. 3. Patient
Compliance—in adolescence—congresses. 4. Patient Compliance—in
infancy & childhood—congresses.   W 85 D489]
RA776.9.D48   1992
616'.0019—dc20
DNLM/DLC
for Library of Congress   92-23023
                                                                     CIP

ISBN 13: 978-1-138-99069-2 (pbk)
ISBN 13: 978-0-8058-1112-4 (hbk)

Contents

Preface ix

Introduction   1
   Norman A. Krasnegor

**PART I: DEFINITION OF COMPLIANCE AND OVERVIEW
OF HEALTH COMPLIANCE RESEARCH**   7
   Norman A. Krasnegor

  1. **Enlarging the Scope of the Compliance Construct: Toward Developmental and Motivational Relevance**   11
     Paul Karoly

  2. **Compliance Research in Pediatric and Adolescent Populations: Two Decades of Research**   29
     Jacqueline Dunbar-Jacob, E. Jean Dunning, and Kathleen Dwyer

PART II: THEORIES OF HEALTH COMPLIANCE BEHAVIOR   53
   Norman A. Krasnegor

  3. **Toward a Developmental Theory of Compliance**   59
     Ronald J. Iannotti and Patricia J. Bush

4. **Family Context and Compliance Behavior in Chronically Ill Children** 77
   Barbara J. Anderson and James C. Coyne

5. **Theories of Compliance, and Turning Necessities Into Preferences: Application to Adolescent Health Action** 91
   Howard Leventhal

6. **Why Do Adolescents Have Difficulty Adhering to Health Regimes?** 125
   Jeanne Brooks-Gunn

PART III: MEASUREMENT 153
Norman A. Krasnegor

7. **Chronic Diseases of Childhood: Assessing Compliance With Complex Medical Regimens** 157
   Suzanne Bennett Johnson

8. **The Measurement of Compliance: Medication Taking** 185
   Peter Rudd

PART IV: PREVENTION 215
Norman A. Krasnegor

9. **Improving Compliance in Childhood Injury Control** 219
   Edward R. Christophersen

10. **Compliance and Long-Term Follow-Up for Childhood Obesity: Retrospective Analysis** 233
    Leonard H. Epstein, Alice Valoski, and James McCurley

11. **Health Promotion and Disease Prevention: A Social Action Conception of Compliance Behavior** 251
    Craig K. Ewart

PART V: INTERVENTION 281
Norman A. Krasnegor

12. **Adherence Intervention Research: The Need for a Multilevel Approach** 285
    W. Stewart Agras

13. **Medication Compliance and Childhood Asthma** 303
    Thomas L. Creer

14. **Compliance Interventions for Children With Diabetes and Other Chronic Diseases** 335
    Alan M. Delamater

Epilogue: Future Research Directions 355
    Norman A. Krasnegor

Author Index   359
Subject Index 379

Preface

Scientists, physicians, and legislators have come to appreciate the fact that delivery of health care is in part dependent upon the willingness and motivation of patients to participate in the medication regimen(s) being proffered. Therefore, for effective therapy to be either given or tested, individuals who are ill must adhere to the instructions given by the dispensers of advice and/or medication. From the public health perspective, the establishment of compliance in the aggregate is also necessary for healthy people. Such individuals have to learn behaviors that help them maintain a healthy life style (e.g., proper nutrition, exercise, etc.) and avoid the initiation of risky behaviors (e.g., cigarette smoking, excessive drinking, illicit drug use, unprotected sexual intercourse, etc.), that could lead to the onset of pathology such as neoplastic, cardiovascular, and sexually transmitted diseases. In the 1970s, research on health related compliance behavior was conducted in large part on adult populations (particularly in relation to cardiovascular disease) to help gain an understanding of how such behaviors could be taught and maintained in specific target populations.

In the 1980s compliance research changed its focus to an investigation of acute diseases in pediatric populations. As the decade wore on, the emphasis continued to be on children, but researchers became interested in the relationships between compliance behaviors and chronic conditions (e.g., diabetes, asthma, obesity, hemophilia, etc.). As these studies continued, researchers became aware that the mechanisms that underpin compliance behavior(s) in children are qualitatively different from those observed in adults. Investigators have come to realize that in order to fully understand compliance behavior of pediatric populations, developmental factors have to be factored in.

This volume arose out of a conference sponsored by the Human Learning and

Behavior Branch of the National Institute of Child Health and Human Development, held in Bethesda, Maryland, in July of 1989. Although the volume is based in part on the conference proceedings, the contributions are in the form of individual chapters that provide overviews of topics on which they focus. As such, they give the reader a scholarly and, in most instances, an in-depth coverage of the subject discussed.

Norman A. Krasnegor

Developmental Aspects of Health Compliance Behavior

Introduction

Norman A. Krasnegor
National Institutes of Health

Health compliance research has been a field of interest for the past two decades. A major focus of the investigations carried out was on adults in connection with treatment received for heart disease (Haynes, Taylor, & Sackett, 1979). The classic definition of compliance was composed by Haynes (1979). He said that compliance reflects "the extent to which a person's behavior coincides with medical or health advice" (pp. 1–2). Ewart (this volume) points out, however, that compliance has at least three meanings. These are (a) the behavior(s) that is the goal of intervention, (b) a process through which behavior is changed, and (c) a behavioral product of the context in which behavioral change processes operate. This view provides a more complex picture of compliance in comparison with the definition articulated earlier by Haynes. A most recent conceptualization of compliance indicates that it is a multidimensional construct (see Johnson, this volume). This recognition has important implications for the measurement of compliance.

Whereas in the late 1970s and early 1980s health compliance research on adults represented a vigorous field of study, a marked decline of interest on the topic set in during the last part of the 1980s. By contrast, research on health compliance involving pediatric populations was less popular during the same period; however, interest on this topic is on the increase as evidenced by the contributions to this volume (for an historical perspective, see the chapter by Dunbar et al.).

Four main themes emerge from the chapters contained in this volume and are interwoven among them. They relate to theory, measurement, prevention, and intervention. These themes help to bind and unify the book into a conceptual whole. Although the sections are divided along these thematic lines, the reader should be aware that the chapters within sections are not limited to just that particular theme. Thus, contributors often include elements of some or all the themes within their work. This state of affairs reflects the interdependence of these thematic issues and suggests how important they are for the state of the art.

THEORY

Theoretical approaches for analyzing and studying compliance have been available for some time; however, what has been missing are conceptualizations that address developmental issues; that is to say, much of what has been written in the past has focused almost exclusively on adults. This work cannot be expected to generalize to children due to the special nature of pediatric populations. Inherent in the developmental trajectory are many constructs, presumably essential for certain aspects of health compliance, that become available only with the passage of time and the attainment of capacity to express the function. For example, normal cognitive development is considered essential to insure that compliance can occur. One aspect of cognitive development relates to the capacity to remember instructions (what to do) and to remember whether what needs to be done has been consummated. If the appropriate developmental stage of memory is not in place, then certain kinds of tasks cannot be made the responsibility of a child. This observation is connected to the larger point, namely, that theories of compliance for pediatric populations must take into account theories of development. The contributors to this volume are aware of this issue and provide insight into how such a marriage can take place (see Iannotti & Bush, and Johnson). Just as important as constructing theories that apply to children is the imperative that they be used to guide the drafting of hypotheses that can help to inform about mechanisms that underpin compliance behaviors.

MEASUREMENT

Assessment of compliance is a complex process. Because the construct is multidimensional, creative approaches must be used to measure the degree to which health compliance is occurring. Whereas pill count techniques and sophisticated measurement devices are becoming available (see Rudd, this volume), they are not by themselves sufficient to determine whether children are compliant to their medication regimes. Information is necessary concerning the interactions of the child patient and his or her family who may be providing help in following medical advice. As well, one needs to know what physicians know and expect about compliance for their patients. Another important point is that health status and compliance are not necessarily synonymous. On the one hand a noncompliant patient can contribute to poor health status; however, a patient can comply perfectly and still have a poor health status. Therefore health status should not be used as the gold standard for determining compliance. Reliable and valid measures of a phenomenon are the sine qua non of good science and effective clinical care. Measurement issues are therefore a topic represented, in one form or another, in almost all the contributions to this volume. The topic of measurement deserves increased attention in the years to come to insure that different investigators who are studying compliance can, with confidence, compare their results.

The development of health compliance behavior is also of relevance to the field of clinical trials research associated with the measurement of the efficacy of new drugs. Studies of this aspect of biomedicine inform manufacturers, pharmacologists, physicians, and consumers about how well new medications work. Each of these groups has a vital interest in gaining an understanding of the measurement of compliance behavior and how it develops. This is the case because an evaluation of efficacy is dependent, in part, on whether and how a patient takes the medication being tested. Whereas one strategy is to eliminate noncompliers prior to initiating a clinical trial, this approach can sometimes be counterproductive. For example, side effects to a medication can alter compliance in even the most motivated of patients. Getting an estimate of noncompliance can therefore provide an additional measure of drug efficacy.

Regarding medications designed for pediatric populations, there are many reasons why regimens are followed, or not, that may have nothing to do with a drug's effects. Therefore, it is important to elucidate why some children comply with the regimen under study and others don't. Such information can contribute to more accurate conclusions of how efficacious the regimen will be in actual usage by the pediatric populations for which it is being developed. Also, basic knowledge of health compliance behavior can help promote better research by incorporating features into the design of such studies that maximize compliance. Results from this type of study can, in turn, inform how to maximize the chances that the overall regimen will be carried out once the medication regime is approved for marketing.

PREVENTION

As we approach the year 2000, the agenda for the public health is moving increasingly toward a strategy of health promotion and disease prevention. Epidemiological research has identified certain behaviors practiced by adults and increasingly by adolescents as being linked to the onset of chronic disease. Moreover, studies have revealed that such behaviors, particularly those associated with substance use (e.g., cigarette smoking, alcohol drinking), risky sexual behavior (e.g., unprotected intercourse), diet, (e.g., unhealthy food choices), and sedentary lifestyle (e.g., lack of regular exercise) can be modified. Changes in such behaviors may reduce the risk for the morbidity and risk associated with major classes of chronic illness (e.g., cardiovascular, pulmonary, and neoplastic). Based on this understanding, a useful strategy might be to promote health compliance behaviors in pediatric populations. Exposure to educational and motivational techniques early in childhood could have life-long benefits for the individual and in the aggregate for the population as a whole. For example, school-based programs, started in Grades K–6 that promote vigorous exercise, appropriate dietary choices, and avoidance of licit substances that can become dependence producing should be high on the public health prevention agenda. Strategies should also be developed to reinforce these health compliance behaviors in the home and community environments. Theoretical and empirical research should be designed and conducted to determine how to best accomplish these goals.

INTERVENTION

Health compliance behaviors are judged to be as relevant for pediatric populations as for adults vis-à-vis the general goals of health promotion and disease prevention. Such behaviors are also of equal importance for individual patients, their families, and physicians regarding interventions for acute and chronic medical regimes. In the clinical arena, to cite just a few examples, pediatricians are acutely aware of the need of patient compliance regarding keeping of health care appointments, prevention of injuries that occur in the home, child passenger safety (e.g., seat belt usage), and medication taking associated with short-term infections (Christophersen, Finney, & Friman, 1986).

Varni (1983) has also pointed to a new trend emerging in the treatment of pediatric populations. He indicated that medical practice is gradually changing from a focus on acute, infectious diseases, to supervision of chronic health problems and disorders in which somatic factors represent but a single part of comprehensive care (see also Dunbar et al., this volume). Varni (1986) further observed that, when the goal is management of chronic symptoms rather than care, the major domains associated with intervention are health care behaviors, coping, quality of life, and promotion of independent living. If this premise is valid, then one should observe an interdependence between health-related compliance behaviors and chronic disease management. Within such a conceptual framework, the relationships of interest will be those of parent–offspring, child–peer–sibling, and child–parent–physician (Varni, 1986). Further, the establishment and maintenance of health compliance behaviors, associated with the medical regimens of chronically ill children, implies an interdisciplinary strategy. Such an approach requires a coordinated team effort among many professionals, including physicians, nurses, psychologists, and other health care providers in concert with the parent–child dyad to help intervene in the management of chronic illness.

ORGANIZATION OF THE BOOK

The book deals with a topic that is of central importance to the field of behavioral medicine and its subdiscipline, behavioral pediatrics. The various chapters contained herein help to elucidate from theoretical and empirical perspectives how developmental factors influence health compliance behavior in children.

The book is organized into six sections. These are respectively, Definition of Compliance and Overview of Health Compliance Research, Theories of Health Compliance Behavior, Measurement, Prevention, Intervention, and Future Research Directions.

DEFINITION OF COMPLIANCE AND OVERVIEW OF HEALTH COMPLIANCE RESEARCH

Norman A. Krasnegor

This section of the book contains two chapters that, respectively, address issues related to defining compliance and providing a perspective on health compliance research carried out in the 1970s and 1980s.

Chapter 1 by Paul Karoly, "Enlarging the Scope of the Compliance Construct: Toward Developmental and Motivational Relevance," has as its focus the analysis of health compliance as a construct. Karoly suggests that compliance is usually defined as a *technical problem* that is atheoretical in nature; that is to say, compliance is a problem associated with getting the patient to behave in accord with medical advice. He finds this definition to be somewhat sterile and urges that compliance should be thought of as a construct not unlike intelligence.

Karoly argues that control theory offers a useful meta-analytic framework for conceptualizing the construct. The power of this approach is that it offers the possibility of combining cause–effect models and those that attempt to analyze "properties of people and/or systems (e.g., families) that are capable of yielding consistencies in health maintaining behavior." Karoly offers a triarchic model of compliance that is analogous to Sternberg's model of the construct of intelligence. The three levels of explanation are, respectively, the componential, the contextual, and the experiential.

The *componential* model addresses the mechanisms by which an individual can manage the medical regimen required in relation to the illness. The *contextual* model addresses a child's cognitive functions as these are influenced by "situational enabling/disabling conditions." The *experiential* model focuses on the content of the processes involved in compliance behavior. These processes relate to motivational aspects (feedback, feedforward, etc.) and evaluative criteria involved in adhering to regimens.

This highly original definitional characterization provides a useful way to abstract compliance behavior as a construct. The framework preferred provides a rich source of ideas about how to isolate and conduct in-depth studies of critical aspects of health compliance behavior. The definition is important also because it can take into consideration the issue of period of development. The chapter by Karoly foreshadows the theoretical analyses of Ianotti and Bush, Anderson and Coyne, and Leventhal, presented in Part II of this volume.

The second chapter in this section by Jacqueline Dunbar, E. Jean Dunning, and Kathleen Dwyer, "Compliance Research in Pediatric and Adolescent Populations," examines research on health compliance behavior in pediatric populations. The studies discussed were carried out in the 20-year period between 1970 and 1989. The results of the survey of research undertaken revealed that just over 90 studies were published during the time-span analyzed. The authors indicate that, in the decade of the 1970s when children of all ages were studied, only one investigation on teenagers was undertaken. By contrast, in the next 10 years the vast majority of work involved health compliance behavior of school-aged children and adolescents.

The review of health compliance behavior also reveals that almost 70% of the studies investigated acute illness during the 1970s. During the decade of the 1980s, the trend was totally reversed. Almost 70% of the studies conducted has as their focus health compliance associated with chronic illness.

The health compliance behaviors studied in connection with acute illness focused principally on adherence to antibiotic regimes associated with otitis media. The chronic illnesses of greatest interest to health compliance researchers included diabetes, asthma, epilepsy, and juvenile arthritis. In the case of these diseases, the interest was in how regularly children afflicted with the illnesses took their medication and, where appropriate, whether bodily fluid specimens were tested according to prescribed regimes.

Dunbar and her co-authors report that the researchers employed biological assays (e.g., blood, saliva), pill counting, and self-reports to determine that rate of compliance to the regimes prescribed. The most frequently employed research design employed intervention approaches to examine the efficacy of behavioral or educational techniques to influence the rate of compliance. Other designs of interest included purely descriptive studies and case control procedures.

The chapter contains four useful tables. Each of these describes the studies conducted on health compliance behavior in epochs of 5 years. Researchers will

I. DEFINITION OF COMPLIANCE AND OVERVIEW OF HEALTH COMPLIANCE

find the tabular material of great value because the authors have enumerated subject age, theoretical approach used, level of disease, type of behavior, dependent measures, rates of compliance, type of design, level of intervention, and outcome in terms of improvement. There is a complete bibliography that complements the thoroughly compiled tabular material. Although the authors do not provide an in-depth critique of the studies included, the reader will find the assembled material useful for getting the big picture on trends in pediatric health compliance research during the past 20 years.

1 Enlarging the Scope of the Compliance Construct: Toward Developmental and Motivational Relevance

Paul Karoly
Arizona State University

SETTING THE STAGE

One of the oldest and least productive recurrent dichotomies is that which distinguishes *determinism* (as a concept and/or a set of causal mechanisms) from *free will* (as a concept and/or a set of causal mechanisms). Among the problems generated by a belief in the validity of this categorical distinction is the assumption that science and "scientific method" are predicated upon the former, and require a renunciation of free will in any of its manifestations. As noted by Howard and Myers (1989), free will is not synonymous with the doctrine of *nondeterminism,* which is, in fact, the true opposite of deterministic models in science. The belief that events (including human actions, thoughts, and feelings) result from some cause(s)—the essence of a deterministic philosophy—is not innately incompatible with a belief in internal (personal, under-the-skin) sources of causation (the philosophy of *agency, self-determination, internal control,* or, more commonly, *free will*). Clearly, then, one can maintain a belief in the doctrine of determinism while simultaneously believing that some event antecedents (some of the time) are person centered.

Hence, the converse of determinism is nondeterminism, or the view that events "just happen" in an unknowable manner (a truly nonscientific stance), whereas the opposite of free will is *nonagentic mechanism,* or, according to Howard and Myers (1989), the position that: "our actions are the result of mechanisms (e.g., environmental, physiological, genetic, cultural) which are completely coercive" (p. 337). A serious, subtle, and pervasive problem in contemporary social science is the dual tendency to remain suspicious of concepts that smack of self-determination while conflating valid causal analysis with the notion of nonagentic mechanism. Nowhere is this problem more palpable than in the study of patient nonadherence/noncompliance. I argue in this chapter that the widespread tendency of patients (both young and old, informed and uninformed, with either serious or mild medical problems) to appear "noncompliant" results from the conceptual and technical failures of a *coercive (social power-based) model*—that is, a model built upon the necessity of nonagentic mechanism. I offer, as an alternative, a *control systems model*, wherein *both* external and internal sources of influence are seen as necessary, and wherein the nature of the relation between diverse elements in the causal stream becomes a central analytic target.

DEFINITIONS

As a technical concept, adherence or compliance has meant different things to different investigators. For example, it has been defined alternatively as appointment keeping, medication taking, diet or exercise management, and the like. As a broad descriptive concept, however, the received view is that, in all its manifestations, compliance refers to the *goodness of fit between a program of health/illness management designed primarily by a health professional and the program-specific behaviors enacted by a patient (or patients) and/or those individuals in a caretaking role.* This is but a slightly elaborated version of Haynes' (1979) often cited definition that compliance reflects "the extent to which a person's behavior (in terms of taking medications, following diets, or executing lifestyle changes) coincides with medical or health advice" (pp. 1–2).

As pragmatically useful as such working definitions have been (cf. Haynes, Taylor, & Sackett, 1979), they are not without limitations. Although frequently criticized on semantic grounds for their connotation of authoritarian control (e.g., DiMatteo & DiNicola, 1982) along with an associated "blaming the victim" or "patient irresponsibility" mindset, the goodness-of-fit definitions have produced operationalizations that have, at once, given tangible meaning to the alliance of doctor and patient while perhaps prematurely setting the focus for the empirical examination of that alliance. Specifically, compliance has come to be seen as a *technical problem*, one that is pursued largely in a *theoretical vacuum*. It is a concept defined (its foci and boundaries delineated) by the specific management parameters associated with the illnesses or health objectives toward which it is directed.

When a construct takes its identity from its surrounds, it is apt to depend for heuristic support on implicit, sometimes lightweight, methatheoretic structures that, like savings and loans (S & L's), may occasionally find themselves in need of a bailout from a more credit-worthy source. The S & L's from which compliance research has drawn its capital have been (from a philosophy-of-science perspective) mainly materialist in nature, built on the assumption of linear causality and directed toward the establishment of universal (context-independent) laws. Although certainly not implying an imminent congressional investigation, this chapter is predicated on the position, stated succinctly by Leventhal, Zimmerman, and Gutmann (1984) in their review of compliance, that "slight changes in perspective can lead to major changes in theory and research" (p. 371).

Five related areas of concern associated with compliance metatheory are briefly reviewed. It is asserted that theory building, assessment, research, and clinical application have been needlessly constrained as a result of the tendency of compliance investigations to be: (a) unidimensional, (b) practitioner centered, (c) reductionistic, (d) stability (consistency) oriented, and (e) amotivational. The problem listing is then followed by a discussion of potential conceptual alternatives, and by the presentation of a tentative family of terms to replace the current overextended usage of the compliance label.

SOME CONCEPTUAL PROBLEMS

The Problem of Unidimensionality. Despite the existence of multiple forms or modalities of noncompliance—from appointment breaking to nonparticipation in preventive programs—the tendency exists, within any single camp, to approach the subject one-dimensionally. Diverse patterns of activity extended in time and space are described or indexed in the form of a *summary* score. What is essentially a dynamic, transactional, multitiered system of unfolding events becomes a singular product or outcome taken out of context largely for purposes of bookkeeping. Even when investigators employ several distinct measures, the associated scores are typically viewed as converging upon the uniform construct of "doing or not doing as instructed."

To further the cause of homogenization, some investigators render the continuity of the single score into a dichotomous judgment, classifying patients as either *compliers* or *noncompliers*. This practice was once considered "essential" (Gordis, 1979). As Gordis explains: "One approach to classifying a patient is to carry out a series of tests and calculate the percentage of tests which are positive. The population may then dichotomized into compliers and noncompliers. Ideally, this should be done on the basis of a biologic rationale such as the level of compliance required to achieve a therapeutic response" (p. 40). However, Gordis acknowledges that the "biologic rationale" is often lacking and goes on to state that the more common practice has been to select arbitrary cutoffs. To his credit, Gordis notes the intractable conceptual problems inherent in the use of discretionary nominal judgments by illustrating how several diverse behavioral patterns could yield the identical label of "50% compliance."

A contemporary manifestation of the construction of homogeneous patient groups (but one that appears less arbitrary) is the comparative analysis of illness survivors and nonsurvivors via archival records. Indeed, one reason for the continued interest in compliance is its presumed association with survivorship. However, this relation may be neither causal nor easily interpreted (cf. Epstein & Cluss, 1982; Meichenbaum & Turk, 1987).

Whether a box score quantitative model is used or a categorical qualitative approach is taken, the concept of compliance resembles the concept of "intelligence" in the early stage of its evolution—when it was viewed as a monistic capacity or higher order analytic entity whose many surface manifestations were believed to merely reflect the underlying *core* construct (cf. Sternberg, 1985). And like the early intelligence research, efforts in the compliance area have often been directed at discovering the best "indicators" of the construct, with "objective" (bioassay) and "subjective" (clinical rating) types vying for their share of attention.

The Practitioner-Centeredness Problem. Although it is the patient who must comply, it is the physician or allied health professional who establishes the conditions whereby the correctness of patient behavior can be determined. The doctor asks "Is this patient doing as I instructed?", and the patient is likewise concerned "Am I doing as my doctor advised?" It is tacitly assumed that patients, both children and adults, recognize the validity of physician-based rule systems and *internalize* these rules for use outside the immediate press of the doctor–patient encounter. And by *internalization* is meant more than memorization; rather, the term denotes the establishment of health-maintenance or illness-containment objectives consistent with sound medical practice as well as the recruitment of behavioral skills capable of overcoming (a) motivational inertia, (b) the absence of tangible and immediate feedback concerning the effects of noncompliance, and (c) everyday obstacles to the performance of complex self-care regimens.

The proactive and self-referential processes of health-relevant goal selection, goal monitoring, and goal modulation on the part of the patient have been relatively neglected. This follows from the practitioner centeredness of the compliance construct. Even the widespread attempts to *train* patients in the mechanics of self-care fail to directly address the problem of internalization/noninternalization because both the rules and the means for adhering to them derive almost exclusively from the practitioner's representational model of illness.

Compliance as a construct bears a striking resemblance to the concept of "self-regulation" as used in the clinical/developmental literature; that is, both are designed to describe the process of goal directedness in the absence of immediate external supports or directives. Not surprisingly, the present critique of compliance is reminiscent of an earlier critical analysis of research on children's self-regulation. As I noted over a decade ago (Karoly, 1980): "What is known about children's rule following has come from experimentation in which adults have engaged in direct and explicit rule giving. The focus on experimenter-imposition of rules severely limits our knowledge of how and when children learn to recognize (or detect) situational requirements for self-regulation in their natural environments" (p. 89).

Because compliance with medical regimes clearly requires that the practitioner's "script" becomes the patient's, investigators must address children's mediational networks when defining the boundaries of expectable progress. Again, as I pointed out with reference to socialization research (Karoly, 1980): "Because youngsters can be rule users when the task requirements and motivational options are clearly laid out . . . it cannot be assumed that children have *accepted* the rule, that they will *preserve* it for future use, that they will *recognize its applicability* in other (noncontrived) contexts, or that they would *modify or revise* it when circumstances so warranted" (p. 89, italics added).

The Problem of Reductionism. Given what has just been said, it would be quite natural to assume that a *child-centered* (or patient-centered) definition of compliance is being advocated. However, no such resolution of the problem of practitioner centeredness is proposed. To do so would only compound or abet the third type of conceptual obstruction to which the field of compliance is heir—and that is *reductionism*.

As an empirical index, compliance is often "reduced down" to a set of instrumental actions whose topography is judged to be in accord with predetermined standards. Alternatively, to define compliance as a cognitive construction—either of the practitioner or of the child patient (or of the child's parents)—would amount to upward reductionism. In the first instance (downward reduction), we must contend with the possibility of *compliance without awareness* (or "inadvertent compliance"—a conceptual cousin to what Suzanne Johnson calls *inadvertent noncompliance*). Whatever it is called, the idea that one can follow rules (or not follow them) without intending to do so places the concept of compliance outside the practitioner's or the patient's stream of consciousness. On the other hand, viewing compliance as a pure mental representation places it outside the stream of behavior. In either case, the concept becomes decontextualized, thereby reducing much of its value as a pragmatic tool. The "solution" to the problem of reductionism (as I elaborate later) is to consider compliance within a transactional framework (e.g., Bugenthal & Shennum, 1984; Fiese & Sameroff, 1989; Karoly, 1989), wherein the smallest unit of analysis can neither be the clinician's prescription nor the patient's intentions, but rather the dynamic interconnection of the two.

The difficulties associated with reductionism can manifest themselves in several additional forms. For example, when adherence is defined in purely behavioral terms, there is a tendency to concentrate solely on the diverse activities the child must pursue over the course of managing his or her health regimen, with particular emphasis on the complex relations between specific actions. From an engineering or human factors perspective, a *workload* problem is being addressed. However, a materialist emphasis serves to obscure the fact that a child, who has many things *to do* in the purchase of say diabetes or asthma self-regulation, also has many things *to think about,* monitor, and/or process. Defining compliance relationally (in terms of the fit between internalized goals and situation-specific task requirements) might help to highlight the possibility that acting in accord with medical advice can constitute a case of *mental overload.* It is well to think of medical compliance as a complex, multilevel skill akin to such things as flying an aircraft or operating an intricate piece of machinery (tasks that are often simulated in applied psychology research). By so doing, many of the factors found to influence performance in such settings can be justifiably promoted from the ignoble status of error variance to the honorable status of measured variable (cf. Barber, 1988; Wickens, 1984). Apropos of the earlier discussion of unidimensionality, it is noteworthy that human factors researchers have, for the most part, abandoned the search for a universal index of mental workload—preferring instead to examine the relations among self-report, physiological, and various primary and secondary task performance measures.

The Problem of Stability-Centeredness. A fourth concern that arises vis-à-vis the traditional definition of compliance is its misplaced emphasis on performance stability and the discrepancy-reducing capacity of the organism, in contrast to the possibility of destabilization, growth, and flexibility. The compliance or adherence construct has given rise to a *matching-to-sample,* negative feedback, or deviation reduction paradigm that is, in essence, conservative. Although medical prescriptions are periodically altered and updated, the task of most compliance training has been to establish behavioral allegiance to a *fixed set of rules* by means of a *well-learned* (stable) *set of responses.* Thus, compliance takes on a static, immutable quality, reflecting a lifestyle alteration that, once achieved, is expected to continue in much the same form for an indeterminate period. Such an arrangement makes sense only in a highly predictable or invariant environment (Ford, 1987).

Compliance is also largely ahistorical (or nontemporal) by virtue of a unitary outcome orientation that fails to call attention to the action sequences or fluctuating pattern of events that ultimately come to influence health status. From an interventionist point of view, compliance is a *nondevelopmental construct,* more clearly representing action repetition across similar circumstances than creative problem solving under changing circumstances. Being nondevelopmental, the traditional view of compliance has stimulated little interest in the effects on learning or performance of maturation, social experience, or cognitive readiness *except as they represent covariates to be controlled.*

A potential solution to the stability problem is to seek a balance between a programmed approach to compliance and a flexibility-centered perspective based on inductive reasoning and dynamic problem solving (cf. Holland, Holyoak, Nisbett, & Thagard, 1986; Kanfer & Busemeyer, 1982; Karoly, 1991a).

The Motivation Problem. Precisely where are the incentives for the lifestyle changes mandated under the banner of compliance? The conventional wisdom (e.g., DiMatteo & DiNicola, 1982; Haynes, 1982; Meichenbaum & Turk, 1987) seems to be characterized by diversity of opinions—from internal (self-generated) sources to interpersonal (especially doctor–patient and familial) and societal (normative) pressures, each of which is readily associated with a distinct (although not incompatible) mode of clinical intervention. However, these views on the nature of reinforcement for medical compliance may not be quite as divergent as they first appear. As a discrepancy-reducing, homeostatic kind of concept, compliance is associated, on an interventive level, almost exclusively with *feedback-driven performance*. Regardless of whether the evaluative source is the patient or an external agent, the field nonetheless construes the *processes* underlying compliance mainly in terms of *task accomplishment*, and the mechanisms attendant to the voluntary translation of intentions into persistent, effortful actions.

This emphasis is hardly surprising, given the prescriptive, bottom line, service–delivery orientation of medicine and applied psychology. However, the metatheoretical problem, as herein conceived, is that compliance becomes, in the parlance of the German action theorists (Heckhausen, 1986; Kuhl & Beckmann, 1985), a purely *volitional* construct. What tends to be omitted is the *motivational* side of the equation, or a concern for predecisional, preperformance goal cognition. Despite the reasonableness of the "getting the job done" mentality that pervades research and conceptualization in health compliance, putting all or most of our eggs in the "doing" side of the *wanting–doing continuum* has meant a relative neglect of motivational initiators or so-called "anticipatory cognitive regulators" that precede and provide the energy for the skilled, feedback-sensitive performance of self-care or preventive health behaviors. Such concepts as expectancy, goal, need, value, preference, and the like, which relate to the *activation of action*, need to be brought more fully in the empirical fold (cf. Bandura, 1989; Heckhausen, 1986; Karoly, 1989, 1991b).

The five correlated problems that have just been proposed to be implicit in contemporary uses of the compliance construct need not continue to constrain research and theory building. Next, some ideas are offered for ways of reconfiguring our analytic focus and hopefully reducing the compartmentalization that presently characterizes the field.

AN ALTERNATIVE FRAMEWORK

Underlying the present set of critical appraisals of the compliance construct is a sense of disappointment—disappointment both with the atheoretical nature of the field and with the resultant tendency to rely upon a relatively physicalistic, action-oriented metatheory (cf. Mandler & Kessen, 1959) to guide our empirical efforts. Compliance is a thing. It is a thing that happens. It is a thing that happens that is composed of tangible characteristics. It is a thing that happens whose characteristics can be identified (decomposed), and subsequently taught and reinforced. Because we can often get along quite well with only metatheory (or no theory at all), the compliance notion that emerges is not so much viewed as *in crisis* as it is *in a rut*.

Is there a coherent framework upon which to erect our theoretical models that can cleanly address the five "structural" problems noted previously? It is here asserted that we might escape the aforementioned rut if we can manage to think in terms of: (a) children's representations of future outcomes and their incentive anticipation as well as the more familiar process of task-specific reward or punishment under the control of self or others; (b) flexible, hierarchically organized rule systems that admit exceptions and default options rather than in terms of fixed habit patterns and all-or-none rules designed to operate in what the ego psychologists used to call an "average expectable environment"; (c) transactional networks, reflecting not the imperative power of controlling versus countercontrolling forces (or loci), but the relational interplay of patient (person) variables (e.g., Mischel, 1973) and social setting variables operating in real time. In this sense, compliance is (or can be) an emergent characteristic of a dynamic system—neither an attribute of the actor nor of the environment, nor a quality frozen outside of time; (d) the need to coordinate the practitioner's conception of the requisite prohealth behaviors with the representational models of the pediatric patient and of his/her caretakers; and, finally, (e) the fact that, although compliance most often seems to be a noun (a state), it has also been rendered as a verb (a process) and as an adjective (an individual difference factor), depending on the investigator's aims and methodological commitments. Consequently, a view that enables a researcher to select the level of analysis appropriate to the question being addressed is preferable to an approach that defines reality monolithically.

Control Theory as a Framework. In recent years, control theory has been put forward as a guiding framework for health psychology in general (Schwartz, 1984), for addictive disorders and self-destructive lifestyles (Marlatt & Parks, 1982), as well as for the domain of medical compliance (Leventhal, Zimmerman, & Gutmann, 1984). By now, its basic tenets are well known, as are the practical interventive implications of self-monitoring, the standard-setting process, self-generated incentives, and the like (cf. Holroyd & Creer, 1986; Karoly & Kanfer, 1982). However, as a metatheoretical scaffold for a "living systems" conception of human adaptation, a framework capable of relaxing the grip of formistic and mechanistic thinking on the field of compliance, the control systems model may also provide the analytic justification for integrating our research efforts and putting an end to the isolation and compartmentalization that currently exists (cf. Pepper, 1942; Schwartz, 1984).

Several fundamental control systems concepts can assist in setting the stage for a definitional reformulation of compliance. First, the idea of an *open system* denotes a human or mechanical entity that exchanges material, energy, or information with its surrounds. Humans are open systems as long as they are alive, implying that they do not move toward states of balance, equilibrium, or equal energy distribution but rather toward states of increasingly complex organization. As Ford (1987) notes: "Living systems are never in simple equilibrium, like a clock that has run down. They are more like a clock that is wound up . . . In fact, a unique thing about living systems is that *they* keep *themselves* wound up" (p. 42). Thus, whereas a stable structural and functional organization (defined as a relatedness among parts) is basic to control theory, so too is the idea that the processes that maintain this organized stability also act to disrupt the system's state—thereby producing a *dynamic equilibrium.* Not only does the organism import and export energy and information, thereby keeping the system variable, but the environment itself changes, forcing further movement away from perfect balance or entropy. Thus, consistency and variability are working partners, not opposites. Most psychological models, including trait conceptions of personality and behavioral formulations, deal in *finished products, fixed criteria, end states, outcomes, completed tasks, asymptotes, threshold levels,* or other presumed continuities in the content and style of performance or in the status of knowledge and value. The control theory alternative is to seek consistency in patterns of changing states, and to focus on the organismic processes through which individuals establish and maintain specified conditions while living amidst a variable internal and external environment (cf. Ford, 1987).

Perhaps the most well-known control process is that associated with the operation of the *negative feedback loop.* Although the most visible element of control theory, it is also the most overworked. A feedback loop is a closed causal chain relating information about action-on-the-environment back to the actor. Often, a system is set to detect discrepancies between current environmental events (perceptual input signals) and desired states (goals, standards, or reference signals) by means of a comparator that generates an error signal. When the detected error leads to actions that *reduce the discrepancy,* the process is labeled *negative feedback* (Powers, 1973).

The discrepancy-reducing function of control systems has been both oversimplified and overcelebrated. It has been oversimplified to the extent that investigators have neglected the fact that a reference signal (or standard) can come in many forms. For example, it can stand for a desired end state, the manner by which the state is to be achieved, the rate of progress toward the goal, or a way of feeling or of perceiving oneself over the course of goal-directed activity (Hyland, 1988; Karoly, 1985). Thus, the process of comparing input to standards requires particular attention to the content or nature of those standards. Secondly, attention to the negative feedback (discrepancy reduction) process has obscured the important role of the *feedforward* process. Feedforward represents the *directive* power of the goal, standard, or reference signal in the sense that this signal tells the system where to go—in contrast to a feedback signal that can only tell the system where it has been (Ford, 1987). It is only the *combination* of feedback and feedforward that permits *flexible adaptation*. As Ford (1987) noted: "When feedback and feedforward are combined, a dynamic control system potential emerges that can combine information about past, present, and projected future events to guide the flow of its current activity in a variable environment to either maintain or alter its current steady states" (p. 69).

Thus, armed with the concepts of open system, dynamic equilibria (steady states), reference standards, feedforward, and feedback, we are poised to reconsider what it means for an asthmatic or diabetic youngster to be charged with the responsibility of managing medications, activity level, or exposure to stressful events and stimuli in accordance with the multiple objectives of satisfying family, physician, teachers, peers, and ultimately her or himself. However, to complete our control theory reframing we need to consider in more detail the specific functional capacities that make the system work—some of which we have explicitly noted (like the feedforward function) and others of which have only been implied.

Describing the interrelated system functions that enable the individual to manage steady state transitions is aided by the integrative account of human adaptation offered by Donald H. Ford (1987).

Essentially, Ford (1987) proposes six interrelated "functions" including:

1. *the directive* (command, set point, or feedforward) *function,* which refers to those cognitive or imaginal operations that specify a desired or intended future state or set of consequences. It is assumed that individuals construct mental representations of future states of self, world, or self–world relations and that these representations come to direct their environmental transactions.

2. *the information collection function,* reflecting the organism's ability to monitor the status of the condition to be controlled. This is the knowledge-of-results sensor.

3. *the regulatory function,* which acts as the comparator, taking the information from the data collection function and comparing it against the standard set by the directive or command function. If there is a sensed discrepancy, the regulating function sends a signal forward to the next functional component.

4. *the control function,* which receives the feedforward signal from the regulatory (or comparator) function and selects a course of action that will reduce the sensed discrepancy.

5. *the action function,* which triggers the appropriate course of action in the environment that will explicitly influence the goal state.

6. *the energizing function,* which provides the energy for the continuous operation of all the other functions. The energy for human control systems derives from CNS activation and emotional modulation.

The model that emerges as a result of these six processes operating in a variable (changing) environment cannot, by its very nature, fall victim to any of the analytic problems previously linked to the compliance construct. In a control systems framework, fixed or unidimensional outcomes are secondary to continuous transactions. Similarly, one can choose to examine the processes underlying goal directedness at any one of a number of different levels reflecting any of the six functions and/or the movement of information through the system. No single function or process represents the "essence" or "core" of compliance—only the organized pattern of events in real time truly reflects its meaning. Because the actor imports information from and exports information to the environment, he or she exists in a reciprocal relationship with significant others. No source—person or other—is primary, even when the other is a powerful, authoritative physician and the actor is a 10-year-old diabetic child. The model of control systems likewise so clearly reflects the person as an organized set of interdependent components that downward or upward reductionism is also precluded. Because of the negative feedback and regulating components, the approach recognizes the stabilizing or discrepancy-reducing aspects of adaptation, yet is not centered upon them inasmuch as it depends equally on the destabilizing influence of feedforward. If compliance is an adaptive process, it will not be captured in a fixed set of skills, attitudes, rules, or behavior–outcome expectancies. And, finally, because control theory recognizes the directive capacity of goals as feedforward signals, it is in tune with motivational, "wanting," or anticipatory aspects of human self-regulation.

The control perspective not only sharpens the metatheoretic foundations of compliance; it can also provide a more precise terminology for describing this self-motivational process. A brief account of such an analytic scheme is presented next.

TOWARD A TRIARCHIC ANALYSIS OF COMPLIANCE

Compliance has been approached both from the *outside in,* in terms of coercive, linear, cause–effect models, and from the *inside out,* by virtue of attempts to analyze the properties of people and/or systems (e.g., families) that are capable of yielding consistencies in health-maintaining behavior under variable circumstances. Social influence theories represent the former (outside in) type, whereas single-case experiments, information processing, and personality theories represent the latter (cf. Cummins, 1983). The former framework benefits from being specific, operational, quantitative, and practical. The latter yields more idiographic, ecologically valid, and contextually relevant insights. In a sense, each approach addresses the limitations of the other.

What has been presented under the rubric of control systems theory has the potential to combine the two viewpoints. Control theory concerns itself *both* with explaining state transitions as a function of manipulable events as well as with exploring the properties of self-regulating systems that underlie successful and dysfunctional adaptation (cf. Ford, 1987).

It is important that we seek to integrate inside-out and outside-in models because they, at base, represent the proverbial blind men examining the elephant. The deductive, functionalist models of the "outside-in" variety tell us that X increases compliance and that Y decreases it. The mediational, constructivist, time intensive perspective, on the other hand, informs us what it's like to be a patient with a chronic illness, thinking, planning, coping, encountering obstacles, and feeling demoralized, embarrassed, and misunderstood. It should be clear that an analytic or diagnostic approach based solely on one *or* the other perspective is painfully deficient. When the X that enhanced compliance in a published experiment fails to do so for your patient, or when a patient's multidimensionally scaled map of illness fails to jibe with that of his or her family, we begin to appreciate the limitations of our methodological commitments.

Earlier, a comparison between compliance and intelligence was offered. This was not a passing reflection. What Sternberg (1985) did for intelligence may be just the shot-in-the-arm that is needed to move the compliance construct ahead. Specifically, the control systems formulation when plugged into a framework modeled after Sternberg's triarchic theory of intelligence may provide a richer descriptive (diagnostic) and analytic scaffold than the diverse and nonoverlapping conceptions now being applied to compliance. The descriptive richness comes from the built-in respect for both the cause–effect and analytical strategies and from the explicit identification of the level at which one is working. The explanatory richness derives from the immunity of control theory to the logical dilemmas outlined in the first part of this chapter and its explicit putting together of heretofore separate structures and functions.

Consequently, rather equating compliance with a goodness-of-fit index and then seeking to approach it from orthogonal (inside vs. outside) strategies, it is proposed that three compatible *submodels* be brought to bear. Analogous to Sternberg's (1985) program, the three levels of explanation can be labeled the Componential, the Contextual, and the Experiential models. Although the term *compliance* can usefully be employed to denote a field of study, it need no longer be used to denote the *how, what, or why* of research in that field.

The Componential Model. This approach to compliance specifies the mechanisms (the processes and structures) that enable an individual to manage his or her medication or preventive response regimen. As in Sternberg's model, the basic unit of analysis is *information,* and the fundamental components operating upon this unit are the six (previously described) functions along with the feedback and feedforward signals that tie them together in an organized, interdependent system.

Most prior conceptual approaches will find a base of operation in one or more of the six functions. For example, many investigators have emphasized knowledge gathering as vital to compliance. The information collection function represents their concerns. Other research has been directed at skills building (the action function), decision making (the control function), motivation (the energizing function), value-expectancy parameters (the directive function), or self-evaluational processes (the regulatory function). The varied concerns of contemporary researchers/clinicians are not seen as *incorrect,* but rather as incomplete. Should investigators continue to "specialize" in one of the systems functions, they will nevertheless be better able to identify the boundaries of its effectiveness. An integrative componential approach could, however, stimulate task analytic or error analytic studies designed to examine the conditions under which the hypothesized linkages between functions are strengthened and/or weakened.

Further, from a developmental perspective, the componential model provides a blueprint for the study of age-related changes in the content and structural organization of each of Ford's (1987) six functions as well as changes in the relations between the components (Miller, 1989). Such a research program could be genuinely developmental, in contrast to the many investigations in the compliance realm that incorporate data on age or experience primarily to reduce error variance.

In short, the componential model organizes the content, structure, and function of self-regulating systems in a manner designed to enhance the diagnostic, predictive, and interventive powers of compliance investigators.

The Contextual Model. Just as Sternberg (1985) views intelligence as involving active adaptation to, selection of, and shaping of the environment so as to attain a better "contextual fit," so too a control theory-inspired account of compliance emphasizes the need to examine real-world constraints upon adaptation. Included among the noncognitive constraints would be not only ecological parameters but biological (genetic, temperamental) factors as well.

Understanding compliance means gauging general social norms and expectations and familial (local) competence criteria prior to deciding what a child or adolescent can be expected to do, with and without assistance (Karoly, 1982). In addition, as people are the most significant constituents of a child's environment, particularly family members and peers, the intersection of a self-regulating child and a set of significant others who are seeking to self-regulate different and even incompatible inputs needs to be more fully explored. It is not necessarily true, for example, that a chronically ill child, managing his or her medications, and that child's family—all of whom are also interested in seeing that the medical regimen is being followed—are working to control the same inputs or reacting to the same environmental disturbances.

What would developmentally informed contextual research look like? First, it would seek to examine children's cognitive component capacities (e.g., the six control functions) as they are influenced by situational enabling/disabling conditions. Compliance is known to be disrupted by large-scale, predictable developmental crises and transitions (e.g., puberty, the move from one school to another), but the microstructure of daily behavior-environment patterns remains largely unexplored. The manner by which children's significant others provide what systems theorists call *transition protection* during times of crisis is likewise unexplored. Control theory also postulates that environmentally wrought disorganization of well-learned patterns (e.g., medical compliance behaviors in young, rule-oriented patients) also leads to behavioral exploration and to the development of alternative patterns. Charting this process is yet another agenda item for the contextual compliance researcher (cf. Ford, 1987, Chap. 4 & 5; Larsen, 1989).

The Experiential Model. The final model focuses on *content* in contrast to transactional processes. Not only does compliance differ as a function of the particular illness or health management task at hand (which must be formally studied), but also as a function of the precise nature of the feedback and feedforward reference signals employed, and as a consequence of the activation of differing regulatory criteria (Ford, 1987). Further, with the passage of time and practice, stylistic differences emerge in the topography of the child's or adolescent's compliance routines.

Analyses of the content of feedforward, directive reference signals is rapidly developing in the field of motivational psychology (e.g., Bandura, 1989; Karoly, 1991b; Pervin, 1989). Systems for coding not only what goals people have but how they construe various goal dimensions (such as perceived difficulty, importance, self-relevance, likelihood of support from others, etc.) are now available. Research in our laboratory is underway to address the contents not only of the directive reference signals, but of the regulatory, control, and arousal (energizing) signals as well. Studies of age-related changes in the content of such representations are, as yet, nonexistent.

The self-regulatory system is significantly affected also by the evaluative criteria used to appraise postperformance feedback. The experiential compliance researcher would need to know, for example, both the level of stringency/leniency of standards as well as their source (i.e., Are they self-selected or do they represent parent, physician, or peer influences?).

A number of writers have emphasized the hierarchial organization of reference values (e.g., Powers, 1973). Leventhal and his colleagues (Leventhal, Zimmerman, & Gutmann, 1984), for example, highlight the nature of higher order illness schemata or representational models that provide the reference signals for the control of lower order health-relevant action. Assessing the content of such mental models across ages and contexts is critical, as such structures probably determine the level of flexibility with which children pursue their own (or their caretaker's) health lifestyle objectives.

SUMMARY

This chapter provided a methatheoretic analysis of the contemporary research in compliance/adherence. Five conceptual/logical deficiencies in the conduct of compliance investigations were noted; and, in the process of explicating their nature, origins, and alternatives, an overreliance upon rigidly deterministic models was identified as a significant etiologic factor (Cummins, 1983). Subsequently, modern control theory (e.g., Ford, 1987) was touted as a potential epistemic antidote. Several key control systems concepts were described (e.g., open systems, feedback, feedforward, dynamic equilibrium, and the directive, regulatory, control, action, energizing, and information-collection functions) and their value for clarifying the compliance construct considered. Finally, a triarchic analysis of compliance was presented modeled on Sternberg's (1985) triarchic conception of intelligence, but utilizing the control systems rationale previously described. The triarchic analysis offers not a new set of compliance terms, but rather (a) a new way of categorizing what compliance researchers do and (b) some suggestions for doing it more systematically.

REFERENCES

Bandura, A. (1989). Self-regulation of motivation and action through internal standards and goal systems. In L. A. Pervin (Ed.), *Goal concepts in personality and social psychology* (pp. 19–85). Hillsdale, NJ: Lawrence Erlbaum Associates.

Barber, P. (1988). *Applied cognitive psychology: An information-processing framework.* London: Methuen.

Bugenthal, D. B., & Shennum, W. A. (1984). "Difficult" children as elicitors and targets of adult communication patterns: An attributional-behavioral transactional analysis. *Monographs of the Society for Research in Child Development, 49,* Serial No. 205.

Cummins, R. (1983). *The nature of psychological explanation.* Cambridge, MA: MIT Press.

DiMatteo, M. R., & DiNicola, D. D. (1982). *Achieving patient compliance.* New York: Pergamon Press.

Epstein, L. H., & Cluss, P. A. (1982). A behavioral medicine perspective on adherence to long term medical regimens. *Journal of Consulting and Clinical Psychology, 50,* 960–971.

Fiese, B. H., & Sameroff, A. J. (1989). Family context in pediatric psychology: A transactional perspective. *Journal of Pediatric Psychology, 14,* 293–314.

Ford, D. H. (1987). *Humans as self-constructing living systems: A developmental perspective on behavior and personality.* Hillsdale, NJ: Lawrence Erlbaum Associates.

Gordis, L. (1979). Conceptual and methodologic problems in measuring patient compliance. In R. B. Haynes, D. S. Taylor, & D. L. Sackett (Eds.), *Compliance in health care* (pp. 23–45). Baltimore: Johns Hopkins University Press.

Haynes, R. B. (1979). Introduction. In R. B. Haynes, D. W. Taylor, & D. L. Sackett (Eds.), *Compliance in health care* (pp. 1–7). Baltimore: Johns Hopkins University Press.

Haynes, R. B. (1982). Improving patient compliance: An empirical view. In R. B. Stuart (Ed.), *Adherence, compliance, and generalization in behavioral medicine* (pp. 56–78). New York: Brunner/Mazel.

Haynes, R. B., Taylor, D. W., & Sackett, D. L. (Eds.). (1979). *Compliance in health care.* Baltimore: Johns Hopkins University Press.

Heckhausen, H. (1986). Why some time out might benefit achievement motivation research. In J. H. L. van den Bercken, E. E. J. DeBruyn, & Th. C. M. Bergen (Eds.), *Achievement and task motivation* (pp. 7–39). Berwyn: Swets North America.

Holland, J. H., Holyoak, K. J., Nisbett, R. E., & Thagard, P. R. (1986). *Induction: Processes of inference, learning, and discovery.* Cambridge, MA: MIT Press.
Holroyd, K. A., & Creer, T. L. (Eds.). (1986). *Self-management of chronic disease: Handbook of clinical interventions and research.* Orlando, FL: Academic Press.
Howard, G. S., & Myers, P. R. (1989). Some experimental investigations of volition. In W. A. Hershberger (Ed.), *Volitional action: Conation and control* (pp. 335–352). Amsterdam: Elsevier/North Holland.
Hyland, M. E. (1988). Motivational control theory: An integrated framework. *Journal of Personality and Social Psychology, 55,* 642–651.
Kanfer, F. H., & Busemeyer, J. R. (1982). The use of problem solving and decision making in behavior therapy. *Clinical Psychology Review, 2,* 239–266.
Karoly, P. (1980). Self-management problems in children. In E. J. Mash & L. G. Terdal (Eds.), *Behavioral assessment of childhood disorders* (pp. 79–126). New York: Guilford Press.
Karoly, P. (1982). Developmental pediatrics: A process-oriented approach to the analysis of health competence. In P. Karoly, J. J. Steffen, & D. J. O'Grady (Eds.), *Child health psychology: Concepts and issues* (pp. 29–57). New York: Pergamon Press.
Karoly, P. (1985). The logic and character of assessment in health psychology: Perspectives and possibilities. In P. Karoly (Ed.), *Measurement strategies in health psychology* (pp. 3–45). New York: Wiley.
Karoly, P. (1989, April). *Compliance/persistence in health care: A goal systems perspective.* Paper presented at the 5th Annual Conference of the Society for the Exploration of Psychotherapy Integration, Berkeley, CA.
Karoly, P. (1991a). On the robustness and flexibility of clinical health interventions. In C. R. Snyder & D. R. Forsyth (Eds.), *Handbook of social and clinical psychology: The health perspective* (pp. 717–736). New York: Pergamon Press.
Karoly, P. (1991b). Goal systems and health outcomes across the life-span: A proposal. In H. E. Schroeder (Ed.), *New directions in health psychology: Assessment* (pp. 65–93). New York: Hemisphere.
Karoly, P., & Kanfer, F. H. (Eds.). (1982). *Self-management and behavior change: From theory to practice.* New York: Pergamon Press.
Kuhl, J., & Beckmann, J. (1985). *Action control: From cognition to behavior.* Berlin: Springer Verlag.
Larsen, R. J. (1989). A process approach to personality psychology: Utilizing time as a facet of data. In D. M. Buss & N. Cantor (Eds.), *Personality psychology: Recent trends and emerging directions* (pp. 177–193). New York: Springer Verlag.
Leventhal, H., Zimmerman, R., & Gutmann, M. (1984). Compliance: A self-regulatory perspective. In W. D. Gentry (Ed.), *Handbook of behavioral medicine* (pp. 369–436). New York: Guilford Press.
Mandler, G., & Kessen, W. (1959). *The language of psychology.* New York: Wiley.
Marlatt, G. A., & Parks, G. A. (1982). Self-management of additive behaviors. In P. Karoly & F. H. Kanfer (Eds.), *Self-management and behavior change: From theory to practice* (pp. 443–488). New York: Pergamon Press.
Meichenbaum, D., & Turk, D. C. (1987). *Facilitating treatment adherence: A practitioner's guidebook.* New York: Plenum Press.
Miller, P. H. (1989). *Theories of developmental psychology.* New York: W. H. Freeman.
Mischel, W. (1973). Toward a cognitive social learning reconceptualization of personality. *Psychological Review, 80,* 252–283.
Pepper, S. C. (1942). *World hypotheses.* Berkeley, CA: University of California Press.
Pervin, L. A. (Ed.). (1989). *Goal concepts in personality and social psychology.* Hillsdale, NJ: Lawrence Erlbaum Associates.
Powers, W. T. (1973). *Behavior: The control of perception.* Chicago: Aldine.

Schwartz, G. E. (1984). Psychobiology of health: A new synthesis. In B. L. Hammonds & C. J. Scheirer (Eds.), *Psychology and health: The master lecture series* (Vol. 3, pp. 149–193). Washington, DC: American Psychological Association.

Sternberg, R. J. (1985). *Beyond I.Q.: A triarchic theory of human intelligence*. Cambridge: Cambridge University Press.

Wickens, C. D. (1984). *Engineering psychology and human performance*. Columbus, OH: Charles E. Merrill.

2 Compliance Research in Pediatric and Adolescent Populations: Two Decades of Research

Jacqueline Dunbar-Jacob
E. Jean Dunning
Kathleen Dwyer
University of Pittsburgh

The systematic study of adherence in pediatric populations has gained in popularity over the past two decades. Increasingly, researchers have become aware of the positive effects that interventions, aimed at increasing treatment compliance, can have on child health outcomes. A review of the state of the art in pediatric adherence, however, reveals existing gaps in knowledge. Pediatric adherence research has primarily focused on the older age groups and on the chronically ill population. The changing trends in pediatric patient populations and in health care delivery may suggest that a review of current knowledge is warranted.

This chapter addresses the evolution of published pediatric compliance research during the past two decades. Attention was directed toward identifying the theoretical underpinnings of the research, the research designs commonly used, the types of behaviors studied, the ages and pathology of the populations, and the measurement of compliance. The trends over time in each of the categories and the current state of adherence research in pediatric populations are identified.

REVIEW PROCESS

A Medline search was conducted to identify studies related to adherence in pediatric populations published from 1970 to 1989. Given an emphasis on compliance to treatment or preventive regimen for medical conditions, studies on compliance with abstinence from substance abuse, alcohol, illicit drugs, or tobacco were not addressed. Review papers, thought pieces, and advice types of articles also were excluded. Research papers that included adults with children or adolescents in the analyses were omitted. Ninety-one research articles were identified.

The articles were summarized by 5-year intervals to facilitate observing trends over time. Information from the studies was entered into a database management system. This information consisted of the illness and behavior that was studied, the age of the sample, the design of the study, the target of intervention if any, the nature of the intervention if any, the theoretical nature of the study, measurement strategies, and adherence rates. This information was subsequently categorized and frequencies for each category were tabulated. Trends were identified and related to current data from the National Health Interview regarding child health and illness care.

EVOLUTION OF PEDIATRIC COMPLIANCE RESEARCH

During the two decades spanned by this review, 91 research papers on compliance were published. These papers represent the results of 81 separate investigations. The numbers of papers published increased progressively over the 15-year interval, 1970 through 1984. There were 9 research papers published between 1970–1974, representing 7 investigations (see Table 2.1). This number doubled in the latter half of the decade with 16 papers published, representing 15 studies (see Table 2.2). The early 1980s saw another doubling of work with 37 papers, 35 studies, published between 1980 and 1984 (see Table 2.3). Since that time there appears to have been a leveling off in the numbers of publications. The period from 1985 through 1988 saw 29 papers, representing 27 studies, appear in the literature (see Table 2.4).

Age Levels Addressed Over Time

Over time the ages addressed in the research on pediatric compliance have become increasingly older. In the 1970s, children of all ages were represented, but only one study related to adolescents. By the 1980s the proportion of research focused on the adolescent and school-age child far exceeded that being carried out on the infant and preschooler. Indeed, over half the research in the 1980s focused on the adolescent with just 20% of the research directed to the preschool child and infants. As is noted later, this shift to research on the older child appeared to have significant implications for a shift in focus of the research itself during this time period.

The Use of Theory Over Time

The majority of the research has been atheoretical. This has not changed over time. In fact, as the absolute number of studies has increased, the proportion of

TABLE 2.1
Compliance Articles 1970-1974

Author/Year	Age	Theory	Level of Illness	Disease	Behavior	Measure	Rates Reported	Design Type	Exp	Level of Intervention	Improvement
Arnhold et al. (1970)	<2-10+yrs	none	other		Meds	Pill ct.	Yes	D	No		—
Barnes et al. (1971)	6-13	none	Prev		Dental	Other	No	I	Yes	Parents	+DO,42 checkups
Becker et al. (1972a)	6 wks-10 yrs	HBM	Acute	Otitis	Meds Appt	Bio/Chart	Yes	C	No		—
Becker et al. (1972b)	6 wks-10 yrs	HBM	Acute	Otitis	Meds Appt	Bio/Chart	Yes	C	No		—
Becker et al. (1974)	6 wks-10 yrs	HBM	Acute	Otitis	Meds	Bio/Chart	Yes	C	No		—
Colcher & Bass (1972)	1-15 yrs	none	Acute	Pharyngitis	Meds	Bio	Yes	I	Yes	Parents	+22% compliance
Dawson & Jamison (1971)	6 mos-12 yrs	none	Chronic	Epilepsy	Meds	Bio	Yes	D	No		—
Korsch & Negrete (1972)	Unsp.	none	Acute		Other	Self	Yes	D	No		—
Shmarak (1971)	0-19 yrs	none	Acute	Dental	Appt	Other	Yes	I	No	Parents	+21% appt keeping

LEGEND Age: Unsp. = Unspecified

Measure: Pill ct = Pill Count
Chart = Chart Review
Bio = Biologic Assay
Self = Self-Report
Unsp. = Unspecified

Design: C = Correlational
D = Descriptive
I = Intervention
CS = Case Study

Theory: HBM = Health Belief Model
SL = Social Learning Theory
RA = Theory of Reasoned Action
PSY = Psychoeducational Theory

Exp: Yes = Experimental Design
No = Nonexperimental Design

Behavior: Meds = Medication Taking
Appt = Appointment Keeping
Imm = Immunization
CR = Complex Treatment Regimen

Disease: IDDM = insulin dependent Diabetes Mellitus
CF = Cystic Fibrosis
JRA = Juvenile Rheumatoid Arthritis

TABLE 2.2
Compliance Articles 1975-1979

Author/Year	Age	Theory	Level of Illness	Disease	Behavior	Measure	Rates Reported	Design Type	Exp	Level of Intervention	Improvement
Barkin et al. (1977)	birth-9 mos	none	Prev		Imm	Chart	Yes	D	No		—
Becker, Nathenson et al (1977)	Unsp.	HBM	Prev		Appt other	Unsp	No	C	No		—
Becker, Maiman et al. (1977)	19 mos-17 yrs	HBM	Chronic	Obesity	Meds	Unsp	Yes	I	Yes	Parent	NR
Becker et al. (1978)	9 mos-17 yrs	HBM	Chronic	Asthma	Meds	Bio	No	C	No		—
Buchanan & Mashigo (1977)	Unsp.	none	Prev		Meds	Pill Ct	Yes	D	No		—
Dickey et al. (1975)	1-12 yrs	none	Acute	Otitis	Meds	Pill Ct	Yes	I	No	Parent	+45% compliance
Eney & Goldstein (1975)	Unsp	none	Chronic	Asthma	Meds	Bio	Yes	I	No	Parent	+31% compliance
Freiman & Buchanan (1978)	8 mos-13 yrs	none	Chronic	Epilepsy	Meds	Bio	Yes	D	No		—
Korsch et al. (1978)	>12 yrs	none	Chronic	Renal	Meds	Other	Yes	C	No		—
Magrab & Papadopoulous (1977)	11-18 yrs	none	Chronic	Renal	Diet	Bio/Other	Yes	I	No	Child	-45% wt gain
Mattar et al. (1975)	1-12 yrs	none	Acute	Otitis	Meds	Pill Ct	Yes	I	No	Parents	+42.5% compliance
Meyers et al. (1975)	4-20 yrs	none	Chronic	C.F.	Meds	Bio	Yes	D	No		—
Radius (1978)	9 mos-17 yrs	HBM	Chronic	Asthma	Meds	Bio/Self	Yes	C	No		—
Smith et al. (1979)	8 mos-17 yrs	none	Chronic	Cancer	Meds	Bio	Yes	D	No		—
Sublett et al. (1979)	8 mos-14 yrs	none	Chronic	Asthma	Meds	Bio	Yes	D	No		—
Summey (1978)	5-14 yrs	HBM	Other		Other	Other	Yes	I	No	Par/Child	-16% get glasses

TABLE 2.3
Compliance Articles 1980-1984

Author/ Year	Age	Theory	Level of Illness	Disease	Behavior	Measure	Rates Reported	Design Type	Exp	Level of Intervention	Improvement
Barglow et al. (1983)	13.4 ± 3.3 yrs	none	Chronic	IDDM	CR	Bio	No	I	No	Child	NR
Belmonte et al. (1981)	8-16 yrs	none	Chronic	IDDM	CR	Bio	No	D	No	–	–
Blount et al. (1984)	6-14 yrs	none	Prev		Meds	Other	No	CS	No	–	NR
Carney et al. (1983)	10-14 yrs	none	Chronic	IDDM	CR	Bio	Yes	I	No	Par/Child	+ 82-88% SBGM
Carstenson & O'Grady (1980)	15-18 yrs	none	Prev		Other	Self	Yes	I	No	Child	+ 32% BSE
Cluss & Epstein (1984)	7-12 yrs	none	Other		Meds	Bio	Yes	CS	No	–	NR
Cluss et al. ((1984)	7-12 yrs	none	Chronic	Asthma	Meds	Bio	No	C	No	–	–
Cohen et al. (1980)	10-17 yrs	none	Chronic	Obesity	Diet	Self	No	C	No	–	–
Daneman et al. (1984)	8-12 yrs	none	Chronic	IDDM	CR	Other	Yes	I	No	Par/Child	No Δ GHb
Durant et al. (1984)	14-19 yrs	none	Prev		Meds/Appt	Self/Pillct Bio/Other	No	C	No	–	–
Epstein et al. (1981)	8-12 yrs	none	Chronic	IDDM	CR	Other	No	I	Yes	Par/Child	+ 0.8% GHb
Gross (1982)	10-12 yrs	none	Chronic	IDDM	CR	Other	No	CS	No	–	+ 65% urine testing
Gross et al. (1984)	9-12 yrs	none	Chronic	IDDM	CR	Bio/Other	No	CS	No	–	–
Hamburg & Inoff (1982)	9-12 yrs	none	Chronic	IDDM	CR	Other	No	C	No	–	–
Harris et al. (1980)	12-25 yrs	none	Chronic	Obesity	Diet	Bio/Self/Other	No	I	No	Child	- Δ 16.42... wt loss
Jones & Caldwell (1981)	Unsp	none	Other		Other	Other	Yes	C	No	–	–
Killam et al. (1983)	7-12 yrs	none	Chronic	Spina Bifida	Diet	Bio/Self Other	No	CS	No	–	- Δ 13. Wt loss
Kruger & Rawlins (1984)	Unsp	none	Other		Other	Other	No	I	No	Parent	+ Δ 28 Knowledge

(*Continued*)

TABLE 2.3 (Continued)

Author/Year	Age	Theory	Level of Illness	Disease	Behavior	Measure	Rates Reported	Design Type	Exp	Level of Intervention	Improvement
Litt & Cuskey (1981)	12.12± 2.01 yrs	none	Chronic	JRA	Meds	Bio	Yes	C	No		—
Litt & Cuskey (1983)	mean age 14.9 yrs	none	Other		Appt	Self	No	C	No		—
Litt et al. (1982)	14.2± 2.8 yrs	none	Chronic	JRA	Meds	Bio	Yes	C	Np		—
Litt et al. (1980)	12 - 21 yrs	none	Prev		Meds	Self/Other	Yes	C	No		—
Lund & Kegeles (1982)	Unsp	none	Prev		Other	Other	Yes	I	Yes	Child	+ 17% bottle count
McCaul & Glascow (1983)	12 & 14 yrs	SL	Chronic	IDDM	CR	Bio/Other	No	C	No		—
McLean & McLorie (1984)	Unsp	none	Acute	Hernia	Other	Other	Yes	I	No	Parent	+ 31% pre-op behaviors
Rapoff et al. (1984)	7 yrs	none	Chronic	JRA	CR	Other	No	I	No	Child	+ 36% compliance
Weinstein (1982)	9 - 17 yrs	none	Prev		Appt	Other	Yes	I	No	Child	+ 50% appt kept
Schafer et al. (1982)	16 - 18 yrs	SL	Chronic	IDDM	CR	Self/Bio	Yes	CS	No		+ Δ 12.0 urines neg
Schafer et al. (1983)	12 - 14 yrs	SL	Chronic	IDDM	CR	Bio/Other	No	C	No		—
Sergis-Deavenport & Varni (1983)	3.5 - 6 yrs	none	Chronic	Hemophilia	Other	Other	Yes	I	No	Parent	+ 77% skill improvement
Shope (1980)	< 16 yrs	none	Chronic	Epilepsy	Meds	Bio	Yes	I	Yes	Parent	+ 0.7 compliance
Smith et al. (1984)	1.5 - 17.3 yrs	none	Chronic	Asthma	Meds	Bio	Yes	C	No		—
Tinkleman et al. (1980)	11 - 18 yrs	none	Chronic	Asthma	Meds	Bio	Yes	I	Yes	Child	NR
Trostle et al. (1983)	16 - 42 yrs	none	Chronic	Epilepsy	Meds	Self/Other	No	CS	No		NR
Warren-Boulton et al. (1981)	17 - 23 yrs	none	Chronic	IDDM	CR	Bio	No	CS	No		- Δ 106 BG
Williams & Forehand (1984)	2.5 - 8 yrs	SL	Prev		Other	Other	Yes	C	No		—
Yokdey & Glenwick (1984)	< 5 yrs	none	Prev		Imm	Chart	No	I	No	Parent	+ 1.6-34.4% compliance

TABLE 2.4
Compliance Articles 1985-1989

Author/ Year	Age	Theory	Level of Illness	Disease	Behavior	Measure	Rates Reported	Design Type	Exp	Level of Intervention	Improvement
Baum & Creer (1986)	6-16 yrs	none	Chronic	Asthma	Meds	Bio/Other	No	I	Yes	Par/Child	No Δ
Bennett-Johnson et al. (1986)	6-19 yrs	none	Chronic	IDDM	CR	Self	No	C	No		–
Blotcky et al. (1985)	13-17 yrs	none	Chronic	Cancer	Other	Self	No	C	No		–
Brown et al. (1985)	6-12 yrs	none	Chronic	ADD	Meds	Other	Yes	D	No		–
Cipes (1985)	7- 8 yrs	HBM	Prev		Other	Pill ct	No	I	Yes	Par/Child	+ 11 - 13% compliance
Cipes & Miraglia (1985)	7 yrs	none	Prev		Other	Pill ct	Yes	I	Yes	Par/Child	+ 6.2% bottle count
Deaton (1985)	6-14 yrs	none	Chronic	Asthma	Meds	Self/Other	No	C	No		–
Dolgin et al. (1986)	3-18 yrs	none	Chronic	Cancer	CR	Chart/Other	No	D	No		–
Eisen et al. (1985)	13-17 yrs	HBM	Prev		Meds	Self	No	I	No	Child	NR
Fosarelli et al. (1985)	Unsp.	none	Other		Appt	Chart	Yes	D	No		–
Finklestein et al. (1986)	Unsp.	none	Chronic	CF	Other	Self	Yes	C	No		–
Friedman et al. (1986)	9-17yrs	none	Chronic	Epilepsy	Meds	Bio/Other	No	CX	No		–
Gross et al. (1985)	9-17 yrs	none	Chronic	IDDM	CR	Bio/Other	No	I	Yes	Par/Child	+ Δ .7 parent – 2.5 behav rating
Jamison et al. (1986)	12-18 yrs	none	Chronic	Cancer	CR	Self/Other	No	C	No		–
Kaplan et al. (1985)	13-18 yrs	SL	Chronic	IDDM	CR	Bio	No	I	Yes	Child	– Δ 2.70.GHb
Lisk & Greene (1985)	10 mos - 14 yrs	none	Chronic	Epilepsy	Meds	Self/Pill ct/Bio	Yes	D	No	–	
Litt (1985)	16.4 ± 1.3 yrs	none	Prev		Meds	Self	Yes	C	No		–

(Continued)

TABLE 2.4 (Continued)

Author/Year	Age	Theory	Level of Illness	Disease	Behavior	Measure	Rates Reported	Design Type	Exp	Level of Intervention	Improvement
Maiman et al. (1988)	6 mos - 10 yrs	none	Acute	Otitis	Meds	Self/Pill ct	No	I	Yes	MD	+ 26.4% compliance
Marteau et al. (1987)	5 - 16 yrs	HBM	Chronic	IDDM	CR	Other	No	C	No		—
Neel et al. (1985)	Ave 16.1 yrs	none	Prev		Meds	Bio/Self	No	C	No		—
Parrish et al. (1986)	Unsp.	none	Prev		Appt	Chart	No	I	Yes	Par/Child	+ 19 - 40% appt keeping
Rapoff et al. (1985)	2 - 25 yrs	none	Chronic	JRA	CR	Self	Yes	D	No		—
Rapoff et al. (1988)	3 - 13 yrs	none	Chronic	JRA	Meds	Self/Pill ct	No	CS	No		+ Δ 37.0 compliance
Shenkel et al. (1986)	12 yrs +	RA	Chronic	IDDM	Diet	Self	No	C	No		—
Smith et al. (1986)	5 mos - 16.3 yrs	HBM	Chronic	Asthma	Meds	Self	Yes	I	Yes	Parent	+ 23.5% compliance
Tebbi et al. (1986)	2.5 - 23 yrs	none	Chronic	Cancer	Meds	Self/Bio	Yes	C	No		—
Waszak (1987)	8 - 11 yrs	PSY	Chronic	IDDM	Cr	Self/Bio	No	I	No	Par/Child	No Δ compliance
Weinstein & Cuskey (1985)	1 - 18 yrs	none	Chronic	Asthma	Meds	Bio	No	I	No	Par/Child	NR
Williams et al. (1986)	2 - 24 mos	none	Acute	Otitis	Meds	Self/Pill ct/Bio	No	I	No	Parent	2 - 5% compliance

studies that have been theory driven has decreased. Overall, 79% of studies have been atheoretical. For those 19 studies that did focus on some theoretical formulation, the Health Belief Model has been and continues to predominate. The majority of these studies have centered about the health beliefs of the mother. In the 1980s Social Learning Theory made its appearance and comprises the second most utilized formulation. More recently, the Fishbein and Ajzen Theory of Reasoned Action and psychoeducational models have been introduced into the pediatric compliance research literature.

The majority of the studies (58%) that have been theory driven have been correlational in nature, regardless of the theoretical formulation. Just 23% of the intervention or single-case studies were theory driven, with the health belief model predominating. The numbers of studies are too small and the nature of the reporting of compliance outcomes too disparate to examine the efficacy of one model over another. However, of the eight studies examined, four reported positive findings (health belief and social learning models), one negative findings (health belief), one no effect (psychoeducational), and two did not report outcomes (health belief).

The field of research in pediatric compliance suffers from a lack of organizing frameworks to direct investigations. No studies were identified that compared the efficacy of different models in predicting nor in improving compliance. The use of theoretical models to guide research in this area very likely would further our understanding of this important health behavior.

Illness Areas of Interest Over Time

Over time a shift in illness focus has moved from the study of compliance in acute illness to chronic disease. In the early 1970s, two thirds of the research was directed to acute illness. Admittedly, the number of studies during that time period was small. By the late 1970s, the proportion of acute illness studies had dropped to 12.5%, although 62% of studies were now focused on chronic disease. The proportion continued to rise in the 1980s such that 64% of studies in the early half of the decade and nearly 70% of studies in the latter half of the decade concerned chronic illness.

Prevention has generated some interest among pediatric compliance researchers. However, the proportion of studies devoted to this important aspect of pediatric care has remained low. The study of compliance with prevention activities seemed to peak in the early 1980s when somewhat less than one third of published investigations focused in this direction. The majority of the prevention studies that have been conducted centered about adolescent's lifestyle and contraceptive behaviors.

Whereas illness has been spotlighted in pediatric compliance research, few specific illnesses have been studied. Among the acute illnesses, otitis media has consistently been addressed. It has been the illness of interest in 64% of the studies. Pharyngitis, dental problems, and outpatient surgery have each been addressed in single studies.

Among the chronic illnesses, diabetes has ranked first in attention. It has been addressed in one third of the studies. Interest in adherence to diabetes regimen among children and adolescents was not seen, however, before 1980. The interest in diabetes regimen appears to parallel the rise in the number of studies addressing school-age and adolescent children.

Asthma ranks second with 20% of studies examining compliance with asthma regimen. Interest in asthma appeared in the late 1970s and has persisted at a steady level. Epilepsy comprises the third most frequently studied chronic disease, 11% of studies, with studies appearing consistently over the past two decades. Epilepsy is closely followed by juvenile arthritis in frequency (9%), with studies in this area not appearing before the 1980s. Few other chronic diseases have been addressed.

Most of what we know about compliance with pediatric regimen has come from studies of compliance to antibiotic regimen for otitis media and from the studies of compliance to diabetic and asthma regimens, principally focused on medication and urine/blood testing. The acute disease studies have contributed principally to those studies with infants and toddlers, whereas the chronic disease studies have contributed principally to those studies of school-age and adolescent children. The prevention studies have further contributed to those studies focused on very young children and on adolescents. Thus, there appears to be a direct linkage between the illness studied and the age of the child. None of the studies have addressed the nature of the changes, if any, in compliance to acute or chronic disease as the child matures.

Behavioral Focus Over Time

As suggested by the diseases studied over time, the major regimen behavior of interest has been medication taking (46% of studies). Medication taking has been studied in both acute and chronic disease. This is followed by studies of compliance to complex or multicomponent regimen (23% of studies). These studies have addressed primarily diabetes regimen. Of lesser importance and in declining order have been studies examining appointment keeping, compliance to therapeutic or weight loss diets, and immunizations. On a more limited basis, studies have addressed dental regimens, administration of factor VIII, breast self-examination, and preoperative behaviors.

One might predict that these regimen behaviors of interest would have changed over time as the shift from studying acute to studying chronic disease was made. However, this does not appear to be the case. Medication taking has formed a major, if not the major, behavior of interest over time. Appointment keeping has appeared at a steady, albeit low, rate over the past two decades. Dietary studies appeared in the mid-1970s and have persisted, although they remain few in number. As might be expected, however, the interest in compliance with complex regimen appeared in the 1980s, paralleling the rise in interest in diabetes. During the 1980s it is reasonable to state that medication taking and complex regimen formed the major focus of study. Collectively, they have been addressed by over two thirds of studies published in the last decade. Thus, our knowledge of compliance behaviors has been formed by the examination of a few behaviors in a very few illnesses at relatively discrete stages of development.

Measurement of Compliance Over Time

Over time, the predominant compliance assessment strategy has been the use of biological assays. These have consisted of the detection of drugs in serum, urine or saliva, or the level of diabetes control assessed through blood glucose or hemoglobin A_1c. The problems of biological assays as measures of compliance behavior are well known. Multiple factors can moderate the behavior–outcome relationship, including such things as individual variation in drug absorption and/or metabolism or inadequate prescription and, for diabetes variations in activity and stress levels, the presence of illness or a host of other factors.

Over time, self-report has played an increasing role in the assessment of pediatric compliance, particularly in the past 5 years and with the adolescent age group. Problems also exist in the reliance on self-report. These problems include, among others, faulty memory, inaccurate self-assessment, and unwillingness to report regimen errors. In addition, little is known about how the accuracy of self-report measures of adolescents compares with those of adult populations. During the past 5 years, however, self-report has become the major assessment strategy, having been used in one-third of studies conducted during that time period. Most often, self-report was used in combination with biologic measures.

To a lesser extent pill counts have been used (10.3%) to evaluate medication adherence, and chart reviews have been used (6.8%) to evaluate appointment keeping. Other measures have been used to a very small degree. These include such things as dental scores, direct observation, and various outcome measures such as pregnancy, throat culture results, weight, and physical status indices.

Unfortunately, a substantial number of research reports do not report compliance rates. The trend is problematic. In the early 1970s two thirds of studies reported compliance rates. In the latter half of the decade 91% of studies reported compliance rates. In the first half of the 1980s just 55% of studies were reporting adherence rates. Most recently in the latter half of the 1980s, just 29% of studies reported adherence rates. Clearly, the ability to examine differences or similarities across studies in terms of predictors of compliance or intervention efficacy is imperiled by the failure to report adherence rates. Systematic and consistent reporting of outcomes is necessary if knowledge is to advance.

Upon examination of the medication compliance rates that are reported, either as the compliance level in a descriptive study or the baseline or control condition rates for intervention studies, it does not appear that what we have learned has had a substantial impact on health practices among the pediatric group. The studies of the early 1970s reported compliance ranges from 25% to 58%, with a median of approximately 50%. A slight drop was seen in the latter half of the decade although the range was much broader. During this time interval, studies reported a range of 5% to 82.5% with a median somewhat over 40%. In the early 1980s the reported compliance rates ranged from 50% to 83% with a median between 55% and 65%. Similar rates were reported for the latter part of this decade. The ranges were 25% to 81.2% with a median between 54% and 62%. Thus, over time, for those studies that reported adherence rates, the averages as reflected by the median of the reported rates has not changed to any degree. The average adherence persists near 50%.

Designs for Pediatric Compliance Research Over Time

Of the 91 compliance studies reviewed the majority were intervention in nature. Thirty-six group studies evaluated interventions, while an additional 8 single-case studies brings this total to 44 or 48% of the studies. Just 15 of these studies used experimental designs however; that is, just 15 used a randomized, control group design. Attention was not directed to the maintenance of compliance following intervention in any of the studies. Slightly over one third (35%) or 32 of the studies were correlational in nature, primarily examining health beliefs or other factors associated with compliance behavior. An additional 16% (15) were simple descriptive studies.

The majority of the intervention studies reported improvement in outcome, although the outcome was as likely to be physical status as it was to be adherence. Where adherence was directly examined, improvement averaged about 33%. Improvement was also reported in weight change, glycoselated hemoglobin, blood glucose, knowledge, and skill as compliance surrogates. One needs to consider, of course, the publication bias in examining intervention effectiveness, as negative findings are less likely to appear in the literature. Further, as noted, the studies did not evaluate the maintenance of compliance behavior.

The nature of the research designs has shown some change over time. Intervention studies have grown in popularity in the 1980s. They currently comprise the most commonly used designs. Following very closely, however, is the additional increased interest in correlational studies. These also have grown in the 1980s. Interestingly, single-case studies did not appear in the literature until the 1980s. Thus, in the most recent time interval the most variety is seen in research designs, with intervention studies and correlational studies nearly equal in popularity. It appears that we still have much to learn about the determinants of health behavior compliance among the pediatric set, and that we still need to learn how best to improve compliance behavior.

Interventions in Pediatric Compliance Over Time

The target for intervention in the compliance intervention studies has shown some shift over time. During the decade of the 1970s the primary focus of attention was the parent. Just two studies addressed the child or parent–child dyad. However, in the 1980s this focus tended to shift from the child and parent–child dyad as the target of intervention during the early half of the decade to predominantly the parent–child dyad during the latter half of the decade. In part, this shift can be explained by the shift from studies of the infant and preschooler to studies of the school-age child and adolescent. The study of compliance with diabetes regimen particularly influenced the focus on the parent–child dyad seen in the 1980s. Interventions targeted simply to the parent declined in interest most recently. Interestingly, the late 1980s saw the first, and to date the only, study that directed intervention to the health care provider, in this case the physician (Maiman, Becker, Liptak, Nazarian, & Rounds, 1988).

The type of interventions have also changed over time. Both educational and behavioral interventions have grown in favor, with behavioral interventions somewhat more studied. Multicomponent interventions came into use in the 1980s, often combining educational and behavioral strategies. Fear arousal was tested in the 1970s, when mothers were the major intervention targets, but dropped out of favor. Other strategies such as triage systems or the use of short- versus long-acting drugs have been tried in a limited number of studies. As noted, the intervention studies nearly all reported improvement in compliance or its surrogate. Comparison studies examining the relative contribution of various strategies to compliance improvement have not been carried out with the pediatric population.

Summary

The nature of the research in compliance has changed over the past two decades. The absolute number of studies has grown substantially. The early attention to acute illness has shifted to a study of chronic illness and to a lesser extent to preventive regimen. Paralleling this is a shift from the study of young children to the study of school-age and adolescent children, as well as a shift from the parent as the target of intervention to the child or the parent–child dyad. More recently, a study has been reported that targeted the health care provider for intervention. Behavioral and educational intervention strategies have dominated. Medication taking has been the major behavior of interest, followed by the study of compliance with complex regimens. The study designs have been primarily intervention in nature, although less than half of these have been randomized, controlled studies. More recently, single-case studies have been used to study compliance interventions. Correlational studies have continued to be of interest. Within these studies, adherence has been assessed by a variety of strategies with biological and more recently self-report measures playing a dominant role. There has, however, been a decline during the 1980s in the proportion of studies that actually report adherence rates. Where those have been reported it appears that there have not been any significant changes over time in compliance behaviors.

Efforts to move the field forward will need to address some of the omissions of the previous work. For example, it is very important that studies address the measurement of compliance and report those data. If surrogate biological measures are used, they should be used in addition to rather than instead of measures of compliance behaviors. The field will also benefit from the evaluation of various models, both theoretical and illness models, in predicting compliance as well as in improving compliance rates. Similarly, the field needs to move to the use of more rigorous experimental designs in evaluating models and intervention strategies. And, lastly, the field of pediatric compliance in particular would benefit from a developmental approach to the study of compliance. We know very little about how compliance behaviors or the factors impinging upon them vary as a function of the development of the child.

PEDIATRIC PROBLEMS AND MEDICAL VISITS

Current Status

Compliance behaviors need to be viewed in the context of what happens among children with regard to their health and to the health care system that manages their care. They also need to be viewed in the context of the health care goals for this population. This section reviews the health status of children and their health care using data from the 1980–1981 National Health Survey and reviews the goals for health using the 1979 Surgeon General's goals for a healthy nation.

Health Problems Among the Pediatric/Adolescent Population

Reasons for Medical Visits. According to the 1980–1981 National Health Survey, the major reason for medical visits among children is acute illness (53.7%). The next highest category is for nonillness care (31.2%). Only 13.5% of visits are for chronic disease management. The remaining 1.7% of visits are for postsurgical care or for injuries.

Acute Illness. As noted previously, the majority of the studies dealing with acute illness have investigated otitis media. This illness can be a serious condition for young children, particularly if there are repeated infections. Recurrent infections can result in hearing loss and difficulty in school performance. According to the National Center for Health Statics (1986), acute ear infections rank as the third most common acute illness for children under 5 years of age (51.2 of 100 children) but occur in a relatively small proportion of older children (11.7 of 100 children). The major problems for younger and older children are respiratory conditions. Such illnesses account for 125,000,000 pupil days lost to school each year. The next most common categories are infective and parasitic conditions. Digestive conditions rank fifth in importance among acute illness for children. Injuries play a substantial role for both young and older children. Although they do not account for a large portion of medical visits, accidents are the leading cause of death for the pediatric age group. There is a paucity of studies of compliance with treatment or preventive regimens in these areas.

Chronic Illness. In the chronic disease arena, most of the compliance research is directed at diabetes and asthma. The most prevalent chronic illnesses among the pediatric set are the respiratory conditions according to the National Center for Health Statistics (1986). These include chronic sinusitis (occurring in 59.6 of 1000 children), chronic bronchitis (55.5 of 1000 children), and hay fever/bronchitis without asthma (50.3 of 1000 children). Asthma follows these conditions in prevalence. Diabetes occurs in 1.9 of 1000 children under 18 years of age, whereas arthritis occurs in 2.2 of 1000 and epilepsy in 4.5 of 1000. Other chronic diseases of significance for pediatric populations include dermatitis, acne, chronic tonsillitis or adenoiditis, heart disease, migraine headache, anemia, frequent constipation, enteritis/colitis, and high blood pressure. The field of pediatric compliance would benefit from the study of compliance in the broad range of chronic illness in children as well as the study of compliance changes over time as the children with chronic illness develop.

Prevention. As noted, little of the research on compliance with preventive regimen has centered on immunization and much has focused on contraceptive use. Data for 1985 from the Center for Disease Control show inadequate immunization status persists for children in all age groups for measles, mumps, rubella, polio, as well as DPT. Inadequate immunization was most likely to be found in the group from 1 to 4 years of age, and secondly in the older adolescent group (Miller, Fine, & Adams-Taylor, 1989). Similarly, adolescent pregnancies remain a major concern. In 1978 the adolescent birth rate ranged from approximately 15 births per 1000 for 15-year-olds to over 51 per 1000 for 17-year-olds. (Surgeon General's Report, 1979).

In addition to improved immunization status and the prevention of adolescent pregnancy, the surgeon general has identified a number of other categories of disease in need of prevention. These include control of pediatric essential hypertension, including dietary prevention, accident prevention, dental diseases, prevention of acute upper respiratory disease, the prevention of sexually transmitted diseases, and gastrointestinal infections. Categories for health promotion include: breastfeeding, adolescent physical fitness, healthy dietary practices, prenatal care, and nutrition. All the listings just mentioned are priorities for the promotion of the health of children and/or adolescents (Public Health Service, 1988; Surgeon General's Report, 1979). These areas have not been well studied vis-à-vis compliance behavior.

Differences by Age. In examining compliance behaviors in children, differences can be found by age groups. The National Health Survey data on reasons for medical visits demonstrates that the acute illnesses persist throughout childhood and adolescence. However, chronic disease visits, particularly routine chronic disease visits, increase with increasing age. In contrast, prevention visits seem to decline with age (National Center for Health Statistics, 1983). Thus, the study of compliance and acute illness can be examined across the span of childhood and adolescence, whereas the study of chronic illness is more likely to be addressed in the older child or adolescent. The study of compliance for preventive regimens varies by age. However, a potential problem with older aged children is that, unless they are ill, they are less likely to be seen by health care professionals for routine preventive care.

Physician Visits for the Pediatric Population

Young children are for the most part seen by physicians. According to the National Health Interview Survey (1983), children under 5 years of age have 6.7 physician contacts per year on average. Older children see a doctor less often. Those children 5 to 17 years have 3.3 contacts per year. Income does not appear to influence contact with the physician; however, race does. Black children are likely to have fewer physician contacts per year than White children (3.0 vs. 4.5; National Center for Health Statistics, 1986).

For those children visiting pediatrician's offices, the majority are making return visits. Indeed, 92% of visits are made by returning patients. This figure suggests that patients are not only in the health care system but they remain there. For 54% of patients, the visit concerns a previously treated health problem, whereas 38% return with new health problems (National Center for Health Statistics, 1983). These data also suggest that the health care provider likely has an established relationship with the child. This notion is further reinforced by the finding of the National Health Survey that for over half the visits (53.6%) the physician makes a specific follow-up recommendation either by visit or telephone. Another 30.6% are advised to return as needed. In only 15.8% of cases is no follow-up advice given at all (National Center for Health Statistics, 1983).

At these visits the children are most likely (71.9%) to be prescribed medication. This finding is consistent with the major emphasis of compliance research being on medication taking. The second most common (11.5%) prescription for the children is some form of dietary intervention. As noted before, considerably less attention has been given to dietary compliance research. Numerous other therapies may be prescribed for various problems, but the rates for each fall well below the 11.5% for dietary advice (National Center for Health Statistics, 1983).

Although the child is likely to be returning multiple times during the course of the year, the advice offered to the child or parent is most likely to occur in a less than 10-minute visit with the physician. In over half (56.4%) of all pediatric physician visits, the amount spent with the child is less than 10 minutes (National Center for Health Statistics, 1983). This finding suggests that interventions that are developed need to be those that fit into a brief office visit, unless other health care providers assume the responsibility of maximizing compliance among the pediatric and adolescent group. Studies examining the efficacy of brief interventions or the delivery of interventions by different health providers are generally absent in the literature.

SUMMARY

Research related to pediatric compliance began in earnest in the 1970s. The research has continued and grown over the last two decades. A review of this literature revealed a number of trends in the direction this research has taken.

The majority of the studies found in the literature were conducted in the last decade. Most of the studies focused on treatment compliance in chronic illness in the school-age or adolescent population. Little attention has been directed toward the acute illnesses. The behavior most often studied in both the acute and chronically ill populations has been compliance with taking prescribed medications. Researchers have most often measured compliance by biological assay alone or in combination with self-report methods.

Many of the studies examined the efficacy of a variety of behavioral or educational interventions on the child or parent–child dyad. Correlational study designs were the second most common type of study found in the literature. Attempts were made to identify psychological factors that may relate to high- or low-compliance rates. Very few of the published studies used a theory to guide the research process. To date, the Health Belief Model is the theory that has been used most often. Little data are available to provide a comparison of the utility of various models in explaining or remediating compliance among the pediatric population.

Current national health data reveal that children are frequent consumers of health care for the treatment of predominately acute upper respiratory or gastrointestinal infections. Most of the visits to physician's offices are for repeat visits; however, generally the visits do not last longer than 10 minutes. Most of the visits result in prescriptions for medication or a diet regimen. There have been a paucity of studies that examine compliance with health-promoting or disease-prevention activities, and yet multiple areas have been targeted for disease prevention by the Surgeon General. The dissonance between the current trends in pediatric compliance research and the trends in the utilization of health delivery systems by the pediatric population suggest an examination of the direction of research efforts is warranted.

The research to date leaves many areas that need to be addressed. There are numerous common acute and chronic illness about which we know very little in terms of compliance. Similarly, we know very little about changing compliance or factors associated with compliance as children age. The problem of omissions of reports of compliance data in intervention studies combined with the limited use of experimental designs and theoretical models leaves us with little knowledge about how best to improve compliance. In addition, the lack of attention to the evaluation of interventions that would be useful in the current care delivery system raises questions about the ability to generalize successful studies into the practice setting. The past decade has continued to develop the field, but the omissions of the past point out the need for a focused and systematic examination of compliance in pediatrics in the future.

REFERENCES

Arnhold, R. G., Adebonojo, F. O., Callas, E. R., Callas, J., & Carte, E. (1970). Patients and prescriptions: Comprehension and compliance with medical instructions in a suburban pediatric practice. *Clinical Pediatrics, 9*(11), 648–651.

Barglow, P., Edidin, D. V., Budlong-Springer, A. S., Berndt, D., Phillips, R., & Dubow, E. (1983). Diabetic control in children and adolescents: Psychosocial factors and therapeutic efficacy. *Journal of Youth and Adolescents, 12*(2), 77–95.

Barkin, S. Z., Barkin, R. M., & Roth, M. L. (1977). Immunization status: A parameter of patient compliance. *Clinical Pediatrics, 16*(9), 840–841.

Barnes, K. E., Gunther, D., Jordan, I., & Gray, A. S. (1971). The effects of various persuasive communications on community health: A pilot study. *Canadian Journal of Public Health, 62*, 105–110.

Baum, D., & Creer, T. L. (1986). Medication compliance in children with asthma. *Journal of Asthma, 23*(2), 49–59.

Becker, M. H., Drachman, R. H., & Kirscht, J. P. (1972a). Predicting mothers' compliance with pediatric medical regimens. *Medical Care, 81*(4), 843–854.

Becker, M. H., Drachman, R. H., & Kirscht, J. P. (1972b). Motivations as predictors of health behavior. *Health Services Report, 87*(9), 852–862.

Becker, M. H., Drachman, R. H., & Kirscht, J. P. (1974). A new approach to explaining sick role behavior. *American Journal of Public Health, 64*(3), 205–216.

Becker, M. H., Maiman, L. A., Kirscht, J. P., Haefner, D. P., & Drachman, R. H. (1977). The health belief model and prediction of dietary compliance: A field experiment. *Journal of Health and Social Behavior, 18*, 348–366.

Becker, M. H., Nathanson, C. A., Drachman, R. H., & Kirscht, J. P. (1977). Mother's health

beliefs and children's clinic visits: A prospective study. *Journal of Community Health, 3*(2), 125–135.
Becker, M. H., Rosenstock, I. M., Radius, S. M., Drachman, R., Schuberth, K. C., & Teets, K. C. (1978). Compliance with a medical regimen for asthma: A test of the health belief model. *Public Health Reports, 93*(3), 258–276.
Belmonte, M. M., Gunn, T., & Gonthier, M. (1981). The problem of cheating in the diabetic child and adolescent. *Diabetes Care, 4*(1), 116–120.
Bennett-Johnson, S., Silverstein, J., Rosenbloom, A., Carter, R., & Cunningham, W. (1986). Assessing daily management in childhood diabetes. *Health Psychology, 5*(6), 546–563.
Blotcky, A. D., Conaster, C., Cohen, D. G., & Klopovitch, P. (1985). Psychosocial characteristics of adolescents who refuse cancer treatment. *Journal of Consulting and Clinical Psychology, 53*(5), 729–731.
Blount, R. L., Dahlquist, L. M., Baer, R. A., & Wuori, D. (1984). A brief effective method for teaching children to swallow pills. *Behavior Therapy, 15,* 381–387.
Brown, R. T., Borden, K. A., Clingerman, S. R. (1985). Adherence to methylphenidate therapy in a pediatric population: A preliminary investigation. *Psychopharmacology Bulletin, 21*(1), 28–36.
Buchanan, N., & Mashigo, S. (1977). Problems in prescribing for ambulatory black children. *South African Medical Journal, 52,* 227–229.
Carney, R. M., Schechter, K., & Davis, T. (1983). Improving adherence to blood glucose testing in insulin-dependent diabetic children. *Behavior Therapy, 14,* 247–254.
Carstenson, R., & O'Grady, L. F. (1980). A breast self-examination program for high school students. *American Journal of Public Health, 20*(12), 1293–1294.
Cipes, M. H. (1985). Self-management versus parental involvement to increase children's compliance with home fluoride mouthrinsing. *Pediatric Dentistry, 7*(2), 111–118.
Cipes, M. H., & Miraglia, M. (1985). Monitoring versus contingency contracting to increase children's compliance with home fluoride mouthrinsing. *Pediatric Dentistry, 7*(3), 198–204.
Cluss, P. A., & Epstein, L. H. (1984). A riboflavin tracer method for assessment of medication compliance in children. *Behavior Research Methods Instruments & Computers, 16*(5), 444–446.
Cluss, P. A., Epstein, L. H., Galvis, S. A., Fireman, P., & Friday, G. (1984). Effect of compliance for chronic asthmatic children. *Journal of Consulting and Clinical Psychology, 52*(5), 909–910.
Cohen, E. A., Gelfand, D. M., Dodd, D. K., Jensen, J., & Turner, C. (1980). Self-control practices associated with weight loss maintenance in children and adolescents. *Behavior Therapy, 11,* 26–37.
Colcher, I. S., & Bass, J. W. (1972). Penicillin treatment of streptococcal pharyngitis. *Journal of the American Medical Association, 22*(6), 657–659.
Daneman, D., Epstein, L. H., Siminerio, L., Beck, S., Farkas, G., & Figuero, J. (1982). Effects of enhanced conventional therapy on metabolic control in children with insulin-dependent diabetes mellitus. *Diabetes Care, 5*(5), 472–478.
Dawson, K. P., & Jamison, A. (1971). Value of blood phenytoin estimation in management of childhood epilepsy. *Archives of Diseases in Children, 46*(247), 386–388.
Deaton, A. V. (1985). Adaptive noncompliance in pediatric asthma: The parent expert. *Journal of Pediatric Psychology, 10*(1), 1–14.
Dickey, F. F., Mattar, M. E., & Chudzik, G. M. (1975). Pharmacist counseling increases drug regimen compliance. *Hospitals, 49,* 85–86.
Dolgin, M. J., Katz, E. R., Doctors, S. R., & Siegel, S. E. (1986). Caregivers' perceptions of medical compliance in adolescents with cancer. *Journal of Adolescent Health Care, 7*(1), 22–27.
Durant, R. H., Jay, M. S., Linder, C. W., Shoffitt, T., & Litt, I. (1984). Influence of psychosocial factors on adolescent compliance with oral contraceptives. *Journal of Adolescent Health Care, 5*(1), 1–6.
Eisen, M., Zellman, G. L., & McAlister, A. L. (1985). A health belief model approach to adoles-

cents' fertility control: Some pilot program findings. *Health Education Quarterly, 12*(2), 185–210.
Eney, R. D., & Goldstein, E. O. (1976). Compliance of chronic asthmatics with oral administration of theophylline as measured by serum and salivary levels. *Pediatrics, 57*(4), 513–517.
Epstein, L. H., Beck, S., Figueroa, J., Farkas, G., Kazdin, A. E., & Daneman, D. (1981). The effects of targeting improvements in urine glucose on metabolic control in children with insulin dependent diabetes. *Journal of Applied Behavior Analysis, 14*(4), 365–375.
Finklestein, S. M., Budd, J. R., Warwick, W. J., Kujawa, S. J., Wielinski, C. L., & Ewing, L. B. (1986). Feasibility and compliance studies of a home measurement monitoring program for cystic fibrosis. *Journal of Chronic Diseases, 39*(3), 195–205.
Fosarelli, P., DeAngelis, C., & Kaszuba, A. (1985). Compliance with follow-up appointments generated in a pediatric emergency room. *American Journal of Preventative Medicine, 1*, 23–29.
Friedman, I. M., Litt, I. F., King, D. R., Kramer, C., Henson, R., Holtzman, D., & Halverson, D. (1986). Compliance with anticonvulsant therapy by epileptic youth. *Journal of Adolescent Health Care, 7*(1), 12–17.
Frieman, J., & Buchanan, N. (1978). Drug compliance and therapeutic considerations in 75 black epileptic children. *The Central African Journal of Medicine, 24*(7), 136–140.
Gross, A. M. (1982). Self-management training and medication compliance in children with diabetes. *Child and Family Behavior Therapy, 4*(2), 47–55.
Gross, A. M., Delcher, H. K., Snitzer, J., Bianchi, B., & Epstein, S. (1984). Personality variables and metabolic control in children with diabetes. *The Journal of Genetic Psychology, 146*(1), 19–26.
Gross, A. M., Magalnick, L. J., & Richardson, P. (1985). Self-management training with families of insulin-dependent diabetic children: A controlled long-term investigation. *Child and Family Behavior Therapy, 7*(1), 35–50.
Hamburg, B. A., & Inoff, G. E. (1982). Relationships between behavioral factors and diabetic control in children and adolescents: A camp study. *Psychosomatic Medicine, 44*(1), 321–339.
Harris, M. B., Sutton, M., Kaufman, E. M., & Carmichael, C. (1980). Correlates of success and retention on a multifaceted long-term behavior modification program for obese adolescent girls. *Addictive Behaviors, 5*, 25–34.
Jamison, R. N., Lewis, S., & Burish, T. G. (1986). Cooperation with treatment in adolescent cancer patients. *Journal of Adolescent Health Care, 2*(3), 162–167.
Jones, F. A., & Caldwell, H. S. (1981). Factors affecting patient compliance with diagnostic recommendations. *American Journal of Orthopsychiatry, 51*(4), 700–709.
Kaplan, R. M., Chadwick, M. W., & Schimmel, L. E. (1985). Social learning intervention to promote metabolic control on Type I Diabetes Mellitus: Pilot experimental results. *Diabetes Care, 8*(2), 152–155.
Killam, P. E., Apodaca, L., Manella, K. J., & Varni, J. W. (1983). Behavioral pediatric weight rehabilitation in myelomeningocele: Program description and therapeutic adherence factors. *The American Journal of Maternal Child Nursing, 8*(4), 280–286.
Korsch, B. M., Fine, R. N., & Negrete, V. F. (1978). Noncompliance in children with renal transplants. *Pediatrics, 61*(6), 872–876.
Korsch, B. M., & Negrete, V. F. (1972). Doctor–patient communication. *Scientific American, 227*(2), 66–74.
Kruger, S., & Rawlins, P. (1984). Pediatric dismissal protocol to aid the transition from hospital care to home care. *Image, 16*(4), 120–125.
Lisk, D. R., & Greene, S. H. (1985). Drug compliance and seizure control in epileptic children. *Postgraduate Medical Journal, 61*, 401–405.
Litt, I. F. (1985). Know thyself-Adolescents' self-assessment of compliance behavior. *Journal of Pediatrics, 75*, 693–696.

Litt, I. F., & Cuskey, W. R. (1981). Compliance with salicylate therapy in adolescents with rheumatoid arthritis. *American Journal of Diseases of Childhood, 135,* 434–436.
Litt, I. F., & Cuskey, W. R. (1983). Satisfaction with health care: A predictor of adolescent's appointment keeping. *Journal of Adolescent Health Care, 5,* 196–200.
Litt, I. F., Cuskey, W. R., & Rosenberg, A. (1982). Role of self-esteem and autonomy in determining medication compliance among adolescents with juvenile rheumatoid arthritis. *Pediatrics, 69*(1), 15–17.
Litt, I. F., Cuskey, W. R., & Rudd, S. (1980). Identifying adolescents at risk for noncompliance with contraceptive therapy. *The Journal of Pediatrics, 26*(4), 742–745.
Lund, A. K., & Kegeles, S. S. (1982). Increasing adolescents' acceptance of long-term personal health behavior. *Health Psychology, 1*(1), 27–43.
Magrab, P. R., & Papadopoulou, Z. L. (1977). The effect of a token economy on dietary compliance for children on hemodialysis. *Journal of Applied Behavior Analysis, 10*(4), 573–578.
Maiman, L. A., Becker, M., Liptak, G. S., Nazarian, L. F., & Rounds, K. A. (1988). Improving pediatrician's compliance-enhancing practices. *American Journal of Diseases of Childhood, 142,* 773–779.
Marteau, T. M., Johnston, M., Baum, J. D., & Bloch, S. (1987). Goals of treatment in diabetes: A comparison of doctors and parents of children with diabetes. *Journal of Behavioral Medicine, 10*(1), 33–48.
Mattar, M., Markello, J., Sumner, J. Y., & Yaffe, J. (1975). Pharmaceutic factors affecting pediatric compliance. *Pediatrics, 55*(1), 101–107.
McCaul, K. D., & Glascow, R. E. (1983). *Relationships among psychosocial variables. Regimen adherence and diabetes control.* Paper presented at the American Psychological Association, Anaheim, CA.
McLean, J. C., & McLorie, G. A. (1984). Improving patient compliance in pediatric outpatient surgery. *Association of Operating Room Nurses Journal, 40*(5), 676–680.
Meyers, A., Dolan, T. F., & Mueller, D. (1975). Compliance and self-medication in cystic fibrosis. *American Journal of Diseases of Childhood, 129,* 1011–1013.
Miller, C. A., Fine, A., & Adams-Taylor, S. (1989). *Monitoring Children's Health* (2nd ed.). Washington, DC: American Public Health Association.
National Center for Health Statistics. (1983). *Patterns of Ambulatory Care in Pediatrics: The National Ambulatory Medical Care Survey, United States, January 1980–December 1981* (DHHS Publication No. PHS 84-1736). Washington, DC: U.S. Government Printing Office.
National Center for Health Statistics. (1986). *Current Estimates from the National Health Interview Survey: United States, 1985* (DHHS Publication No. PHS 86-1588). Washington, DC: U.S. Government Printing Office.
Neel, E. U., Jay, S., & Litt, I. F. (1985). The relationship of self-concept and autonomy to oral contraceptive compliance among adolescent females. *Journal of Adolescent Health Care, 6*(6), 445–447.
Neinstein, L. S. (1982). Lowering broken appointment rates at a teenage health center. *Journal of Adolescent Health Care, 2*(2), 110–113.
Office of Assistant Secretary for Health and Surgeon General. (1979). *Healthy people: The Surgeon General's Report on Health Promotion and Disease Prevention, 1979* (DHHS Publication No. 79-55071). Washington, DC: U.S. Government Printing Office.
Parrish, J. M., Charlop, M. H., & Fenton, L. R. (1986). Use of a stated waiting list contingency and reward opportunity to increase appointment keeping in an outpatient pediatric psychology clinic. *Journal of Pediatric Psychology, 11*(1), 81–89.
Public Health Service. (1988). *Promoting Health/Preventing Disease: Objectives for the Nation.* Washington, DC: U.S. Government Printing Office. (Original work published in 1980)
Radius, S. M., Becker, M. H., Rosenstock, I. M., Drachman, R. H., Schuberth, K. C., & Teets, K.

C. (1978). Factors influencing mother's compliance with a medication regimen for asthmatic children. *The Journal of Asthma Research, 15*(3), 133-149.

Rapoff, M. A., Lindsley, C. B., & Christophersen, E. R. (1984). Improving compliance with medical regimens: Case study with juvenile rheumatoid arthritis. *Archives of Physical and Medical Rehabilitation, 65,* 267-269.

Rapoff, M. A., Lindsley, C. B., & Christophersen, E. R. (1985). Parent perception of problems experienced by their children in complying with treatments for juvenile rheumatoid arthritis. *Archives of Physical and Medical Rehabilitation, 66,* 427-429.

Rapoff, M. A., Purviance, M. R., & Lindsley, C. B. (1988). Educational and behavioral strategies for improving medication compliance in juvenile rheumatoid arthritis. *Archives of Physical and Medical Rehabilitation, 69,* 439-441.

Schafer, L. C., Glasgow, R. E., & McCaul, K. D. (1982). Increasing the adherence of diabetic adolescents. *Journal of Behavioral Medicine, 5*(3-362).

Schafer, L. C., Glasgow, R. E., McCaul, K. D., & Dreher, M. (1983). Adherence to iddm regimens: Relationship to psychosocial variables and metabolic control. *Diabetes Care, 6*(5), 493-498.

Sergis-Deavenport, E., & Varni, J. W. (1983). Behavioral assessment and management of adherence to factor replacement therapy in hemophilia. *Journal of Pediatric Psychology, 8*(4), 367-377.

Shenkel, R. J., Rogers, J. P., Perfetto, G., & Levin, R. A. (1986). Importance of significant others in predicting cooperation with diabetic regimen. *International Journal of Psychiatry in Medicine, 15*(2), 149-155.

Shmarak, K. L. (1971). Reduce your broken appointment rate: How one children and youth project reduced its broken appointment rate. *American Journal of Public Health, 61*(12), 2400-2404.

Shope, J. T. (Third Quarter/1980). Intervention to improve compliance with pediatric anticonvulsant therapy. *Patient Counselling, and Health Education, 2,* 135-141.

Smith, N. A., Seale, J. P., & Shaw, J. (1984). Medication compliance in children with asthma. *Australian Pediatric Journal, 20,* 47-51.

Smith, N. A., Seale, L. P., Ley, P., Shaw, J., & Bracs, P. U. (1986). Effects of intervention on medication compliance in children with asthma. *The Medical Journal of Australia, 144,* 119-122.

Smith, S. D., Rosen, D., Trueworthy, R. C., & Lowman, J. T. (1979). A reliable method for evaluating drug compliance in children with cancer. *Cancer, 43,* 169-173.

Sublett, J. L., Pollard, S. J., Kadlec, G. J., & Karibo, J. M. (1979). Non-compliance in asthmatic children: A study of theophylline levels in a pediatric emergency room population. *Annals of Allergy, 43,* 95-97.

Summey, P. (1978). Compliance of schoolage children in getting and wearing glasses. *The Sightsaving Review, 48*(2), 59-69.

Tebbi, C. K., Cummings, M., Zevon, M. A., Smith, L., Richards, M., & Mallon, M. (1986). Compliance of pediatric and adolescent cancer patients. *Cancer, 58,* 1179-1184.

Tinkleman, D. G., Vanderpool, G. E., Carroll, M. S., Page, E. G., & Spangler, D. L. (1980). Compliance differences following administration of theophylline at six and twelve hour intervals. *Annals of Allergy, 44,* 283-286.

Trostle, J. A., Hauser, A., & Susser, I. S. (1983). The logic of noncompliance: Management of epilepsy from the patient's point of view. *Culture, Medicine and Psychiatry, 7,* 35-56.

Warren-Boulton, E., Anderson, B. J., Schawartz, N. L., & Drexler, A. (1981). A group approach to the management of diabetes in adolescents and young adults. *Diabetes Care, 4*(6), 620-623.

Waszak, L. (1987). *The effects of parent education on adherence and metabolic control of children with insulin-dependent diabetes mellitus.* Unpublished doctoral dissertation, University of Pittsburgh, PA.

Weinstein, A. G., Cuskey, W. (1985). Theophylline compliance in asthmatic children. *Annals of Allergy, 54,* 19–24.

Williams, C. A., & Forehand, R. (1984). An examination of predictor variables for child compliance and noncompliance. *Journal of Abnormal Psychology, 12*(3), 491–504.

Williams, R. L., Maiman, L., Broadbent, D. N., Kotok, D., Lawrence, R. A., & Webb, S. (1986). Educational strategies to improve compliance with an antibiotic regimen. *American Journal of Diseases of Childhood, 140,* 216–220.

Yokley, J. M., & Glenwick, D. S. (1984). Increasing the immunization of preschool children: An evaluation of applied community interventions. *Journal of Applied Behavior Analysis, 17,* 313–325.

II THEORIES OF HEALTH COMPLIANCE BEHAVIOR

Norman A. Krasnegor

This section of the book contains four chapters. Each of these focuses on theoretical approaches for understanding health compliances behavior. The first two works offer specific viewpoints for characterizing developmental aspects of compliance. The third contribution is a more general theory of health compliance that has meaningful implications for compliance behavior in adolescents. The fourth offers a bridge between theoretical considerations and the issues of measurement and intervention.

The chapter by Ronald Iannotti and Patricia J. Bush, "Toward a Developmental Theory of Compliance," addresses three domains that the authors posit must be understood to achieve an insight into the factors that are responsible for health compliance behavior in children as they develop. The three domains are, respectively, (a) memory and causality, (b) development of personal control, and (c) social, cultural, and socioeconomic factors. The authors introduce their Children's Health Belief Model (CHBM) to help illustrate the relevance of these domains for health compliance behavior.

Iannotti and Bush stress that appropriate developmental levels of cognitive processes are essential for carrying out behaviors that relate to adherence to medical regimens. They point out that children must not only be able to remember to recall but must be able to remember what to recall. Further, they suggest that an essential ingredient in compliance is the understanding by a child of causal relationships and the consequences of engaging in or failing to engage in certain behaviors. Personal control in the view of Iannotti and Bush is essential because it subsumes the ideas of self-regulation, self-efficacy, autonomy, and locus of control. These factors are conceptualized as the source of motivation to be compliant or noncompliant. Because personal control has a developmental trajectory, it can help to explain why children at different periods of their life are more or less likely to comply with medical regimens. The authors also make a strong case for studying social, cultural, and socioeconomic factors to understand compliance behaviors of children. They point to the family, neighborhood environment, cultural differences, and socioeconomic conditions as being important determinants of compliance behavior.

Iannotti and Bush's perspective about integrating developmental and compliance theories has value in that common mechanisms are shown to be operative in both domains. Thus, if one is interested in gaining a deep understanding of children's compliance behaviors, borrowing of concepts from developmental theory should help illuminate why and how children do or do not adhere to medical regimes.

The next chapter by Barbara J. Anderson and James C. Coyne, "Family Context and Compliance Behavior in Chronically Ill Children," has as its focus compliance behavior of chronically ill children in the context of the family. The authors employ a theory, the Miscarried Helping Model, to characterize and explain the "interactive context of family behavior around compliance tasks." The theory uses social psychological and family therapy concepts to analyze and study how families cope with the medical regimens required of parents and their children who are afflicted with an illness that is chronic in nature. Anderson and Coyne are interested in exploring the roles of parent as helper and child as recipient of such aid. The major issue discussed, in the context of the Miscarried Helping Model, is what happens when help proferred by a parent to their chronically ill child backfires, and a power struggle ensues around the issue of the child taking care of him or herself. This struggle reduces to the issue of autonomy (see Iannotti & Bush, this volume).

In the context of the theory, miscarried helping is defined as parental behaviors carried out to aid the child that, over time, lead to interactions that may be inimical to the desired well-being and adjustment of their child. The major problems seem to arise when a well-intentioned parent seeks to help but becomes "overprotective" and demanding to insure the well-being of the child. Such behaviors, in the parent, conflict with an ill child's emerging competencies associated with taking care of him or herself. If such behavioral interactions become a pattern, they may lead ultimately to a condition in which the "illness-related problems become reconstructed as relationship problems." In the extreme case, the conflicting needs of parent and chronically ill child lead to a deterioration of the helping process. On the one hand the parent may become authoritarian and directive, and on the other the child struggles against the requests to comply under these conditions.

Anderson and Coyne posit that two sets of factors might influence miscarried helping. These are developmental or age-related factors and disease-related ones. The authors point out that compliance to a medical regime for chronically ill young children is usually the responsibility of the parent. However, parental involvement in compliance is often challenged around the time of puberty. It is at that point in development when a child becomes more independent. This point of transition to adolescence is typically the time when conflicts arise between parents and offspring over issues of independence, authority, and responsibility.

The illness itself may contribute to miscarried helping in at least three or four ways: (a) If, for example, a child does carry out the regimen but due to imprecision of the testing or worsening of the disease the child has a setback, recriminations and accusations may arise; (b) also, parents may be under false assumptions about how much control the child may have over the disease. Thus fluctuations in the disease process may occur and be erroneously attributed to lack of compliance by the child; (c) because chronic diseases are not cured and the child may show deterioration over time due to the pathology, parents may overly focus on the child's well-being due to their own frustration at not being able to insure their child's health; (d) a final factor has to do with the problems arising with the interaction of the parent/child dyad and the health care system. There may be a lack of communication between health care professionals and the family about what can be realistically expected in terms of following a medical regimen.

The theory described is of great importance because it identifies behavioral mechanisms that may go awry vis-à-vis compliance in the chronically ill child and has implications concerning ways to intervene that could be undertaken to maximize effective compliance.

The next chapter in this section, "Theories of Compliance, and Turning Necessities into Preferences: Applications to Adolescent Health Action," is written by Howard Leventhal. Leventhal is well known as both a theoretician and a researcher in the field of health compliance behavior. The chapter provides an historical overview of compliance research in terms of the dominant models that have been employed to gain both an understanding of the mechanisms underpinning the concept and produce the most efficient way to engender and maintain desired health behaviors. Leventhal indicates that the data support the conclusion that compliance is a multivariate problem. His review further demonstrates that change in compliance is best produced using behavioral approaches. But, initial gains are not maintained over the long haul (not more than 1 year in duration).

Leventhal examines the issue of motivation, a theme that is prominent in the theories described in the previous two chapters. He concludes that investigators "have given too little attention to the maintenance of motivation for change and have put too much emphasis on lack of self-efficacy and behavioral skills to account for maintenance failures." Leventhal also points out that few interventions to enhance compliance take into account subjects' personal knowledge base. He suggests that one should use such information to design a tailored approach to influence health compliance.

Leventhal posits a self-regulation framework for studying and understanding adherence. This model implies that the patient establishes goal-concerning health threats that guide behavior. The behavior is influenced by perceptions of self and resources in the environment. Shifts in the environment and the self-system can alter the individual's perception, affect, behavior, and appraisals that relate to the disease threat. Leventhal indicates that "the net result will be changes in the perceived effectiveness of specific behaviors selected to meet these goals."

Leventhal introduces the concept of framing. He suggests that how a problem is posed can influence the way a person will decide to solve it. By manipulating the framing of health threats, he suggests, one can motivate people to more effectively deal with the threat or promote health behaviors (e.g., brushing of teeth or taking showers). The author next addresses health compliance behavior of adolescents. Leventhal indicates that in order to initiate and maintain health-related behaviors in teenagers one must understand three domains: (a) the rapid physical changes that ensue around puberty, (b) the social and physical environment of the adolescent, and (c) the behaviors that are targeted for change. Leventhal concludes that the self-regulation model, combined with framing and a detailed understanding of what teenagers know about themselves, are the necessary ingredients for formulating effective health interventions that can be meaningfully maintained.

The last chapter in this section, "Why do Adolescents have Difficulty Adhering to Health Regimes," by Jeanne Brooks-Gunn, is not, strictly speaking, a theoretical treatise. Rather, it can best be thought of as a segue or bridge between the preceding work by Leventhal and the chapter that follows by Suzanne Johnson. Leventhal's work relates to Brooks-Gunn's contribution because his thesis relates to metalevel analytic principles that may help to answer the questions raised by the author. Also, Brooks-Gunn and Leventhal both focus their attention on the developmental period of adolescence. Brooks-Gunn relates to Johnson's chapter because both authors have in common, at least in part, an interest in the issues of assessment and measurement of the concept of health compliance.

Brooks-Gunn discusses the vulnerability and resistance of teenagers regarding their compliance in connection with two important health behaviors, practicing safe sexual behavior and dietary intake in relation to eating disorders and obesity. The author makes the essential point that health behaviors of adolescents must be understood in the context of a biopsychosocial framework. Brooks-Gunn along with others in this volume (see Johnson) agree that compliance is a multidimensional construct.

Brooks-Gunn posits that compliance is influenced by cultural, environmental, and individual processes. These latter processes (individual) consist of biological constraints (e.g., pubertal changes in girls associated with body changes and distribution of fat), emotional factors (increase in negative affect in adolescence), and social and social-cognitive processes (e.g., perceived costs and benefits of adherence, self-efficacy, and perception of risk). Brooks-Gunn relates the relevance of understanding the importance of future consequences (theory of formal operations) and the capacity to employ decision-making rules by teenagers as keys for acquiring compliance behaviors. She highlights the significant others in the social environment that influence health compliance of teenagers. These individuals are peers and parents.

Brooks-Gunn reviews the intervention approaches she feels have relevance for influencing health compliance. These are education, fear arousal, problem solving, skills training and employment, and continuing education programs. Brooks-Gunn similarly reviews the methods for assessing health compliance behavior in adolescents. These are various types of surveys, self-reports, and multiple respondents (see Johnson, this volume). This part of her discussion leads directly into the issue of measurement detailed in the next section on measurement in the respective chapters of Johnson and Rudd.

3 Toward a Developmental Theory of Compliance

Ronald J. Iannotti
Patricia J. Bush
Georgetown University School of Medicine

Compliance of children with health prescriptions implies different things at different ages. In the toddler it simply may mean assenting to the administration of medications or treatments by a parent or physician. In early childhood it may mean complying with parents' and physicians' recommendations for adherence to healthful behaviors, such as following a prudent diet and avoiding risky behaviors, or cooperating with treatment regimens, including treatment of chronic disorders such as asthma as well as acute problems such as bacterial infections. It is not until the age of 10 years or so, however, that the average parent expects a child to begin to take a more active role in areas such as hygiene, dressing properly, getting enough sleep, taking medicines, and following a treatment regimen prescribed by a physician. By the middle teen years, most adolescents are expected to take major responsibility for their health care and to require only occasional monitoring by a parent or other authority figure. The expectations for adults are actually quite similar to those for adolescents with increased self-responsibility accompanied by occasional monitoring by a significant other, usually a spouse. In old age the pattern begins to reverse, with increasing responsibility for health care falling on others. This chapter focuses on childhood, particularly the period from 5 years of age to early adolescence.

There are a number of excellent reviews of theories of compliance in this volume (Dunbar, Dunning, & Dwyer; Leventhal; Karoly) and in the literature (Christensen, 1985; Karoly, 1981; Leventhal & Cameron, 1987; Leventhal, Zimmerman, & Gutmann, 1984; Svarstad, 1986). Therefore, current theories are not reviewed in this chapter. Instead, selected developmental research in three domains is presented that may contribute to a better understanding of compliance behavior across the life span, but particularly in childhood and early adolescence. These domains are not exclusive of other developmental areas; however, they have been given insufficient consideration in theoretical models that are almost entirely adult oriented. It is suggested that a theory of compliance that applies to children as well as adults must account for developmental changes in these three domains. First, changing developmental processes that have implications for compliance, such as memory and understanding of causality, are reviewed. The development of personal control as a general concept and as it applies to compliance with prescriptions for health promotion and treatment is then presented. Finally, the unique influence on children of social, cultural, and socioeconomic contexts is discussed. To illustrate some of these issues, a Children's Health Belief Model (CHBM), which may have some utility in explaining children's health compliance behaviors, is introduced. The CHBM was developed for children's expectations to take action in response to illness but demonstrates the kind of adaptations necessary for adult models to become developmental models for compliance.

CHANGING DEVELOPMENTAL PROCESSES

Developmental processes that influence compliance include memory, perception of time, understanding of causality and consequences, and the social and physiological changes that accompany stages of development, particularly adolescence. Age, or developmental stage, is a crude measure of processes that change throughout the life span.

COGNITIVE PROCESSES

Memory

Essential to compliance behavior is whether the patient, regardless of age, remembers to perform the prescribed behavior. Much of the existing developmental research on memory focuses on the ability to recall or recognize prior information (Walsh, 1983). Limitations that affect compliance and memory have been identified by Levy and Loftus (1984). Children may not comply with physicians' instructions because of the use of abstract rather than concrete, specific instructions, the number of statements being presented, the children's limited medical knowledge, or a level of anxiety that is either too high or too low to facilitate action. These elements, though particularly important for children, affect compliance at any age. It is not unusual for pediatric patients and their parents to misunderstand their prescriptions (Ley, 1977) and yet not ask questions that would clear up misunderstandings (NCPIE, 1989). Age and intelligence do not systematically relate to recall, and the use of reinforcement, memory aids, and rehearsal that has provided some success for increased compliance in adults may work in children as well.

Many children skip their doses of medicine because they or their parents have forgotten (Tebbi et al., 1986). Another problem is forgetting to shake liquid medicines designed for pediatric use. The area of memory research that is most relevant to compliance is prospective memory, or remembering to take action in the future (Harris, 1984; Meacham, 1982). This research differentiates remembering *to* recall from remembering *what* to recall. Remembering to keep appointments and remembering to take medicines are two relevant examples of prospective memory. Remembering to take medicines may simply be remembering to take a specific action, or it may involve remembering to engage in a sequence of actions (e.g., taking a medicine before a meal). Prospective memory improves with incentives, external prompts, other memory aids, and increased commitment (Harris, 1984). Increased commitment may be a function of locus of control, self-efficacy, and readiness factors (illness concern, perceived severity, and perceived benefits). A number of the interventions designed to facilitate compliance (e.g., reminders, drug calendars, schedules, and simplifying procedures) are directed toward enhancing prospective memory. Meacham (1982) also notes the importance of the social context for executing planned actions such as compliance. Research on prospective memory could help to identify the most efficient and effective means of gaining compliance at different ages.

Understanding of Causality and Consequences

As presented later, in the CHBM taking action in response to a health problem is motivated by children's perception of the severity of the illness, the benefit of the action, concern regarding having the illness, and vulnerability to the illness. Complex cognitive processes are required to understand the multiple causes of an illness that contribute to one's vulnerability, the varied aspects of an illness that contribute to its severity and one's concern about contracting it, and the consequences of taking an action that contribute to an evaluation of its benefits and risks. Pediatric patients differ considerably in these cognitive skills as they develop from preoperational through formal operational thinking (Inhelder & Piaget, 1964), and even as adult patients may not have the health knowledge or the logical operations necessary to arrive at similar conclusions as a physician when deciding on a course of treatment. Understanding causality (which contributes to understanding the consequences of compliance or noncompliance and how a sequence of events facilitates recovery), perception of time (which permits understanding of long-term vs. short-term consequences), and formal operations (being able to consider multiple abstract causes and consequences) are processes that need to be considered in terms of developmental progression and individual differences.

Conclusions

Attempts at increasing compliance should be individualized to the patient's level of cognitive awareness and understanding of causal sequences with consideration of social and physiological influences as well. Physicians should determine whether patients understand the instructions before the patient leaves their office, asking the patient to repeat or summarize the instructions and to make a verbal commitment to comply with those instructions. The child's role in therapy and that of the parent should be adjusted to reflect their ability to understand disease processes and the function of treatment. In some cases, a greater emphasis on the child's decision making and treatment monitoring is appropriate, whereas in others greater reliance on parents is necessary. When the complexity of treatment or monitoring is beyond the capabilities of parent or child, responsibility for treatment may have to be reorganized to take advantage of those skills already acquired and to recruit the most salient social support systems for that individual.

PERSONAL CONTROL

Personal control is at the heart of the compliance issue. If compliance to medical prescriptions were not subject to individual control and variation, it would not be an area of such intense interest. Physicians would prescribe and patients would behave accordingly. There would be no need for a volume such as this on patient compliance. Instead, treatment efficacy would be the only concern.

If the individual, child or parent, expresses personal control over the treatment regimen, then an understanding of the individual's perception of that regimen is important. This includes understanding the perspective of the individual (i.e., for children particularly there is a need to identify their perspective or their understanding of illness severity and the benefits and efficacy of treatment). In their review of the literature, Burbach and Peterson (1986) conclude that the development of children's understanding of health and illness is consistent with Piaget's theory (Inhelder & Piaget, 1964), suggesting that there is systematic development in a predictable sequence of stages similar to those proposed by Bibace and Walsh (1980). The six stages parallel the preoperational, concrete operational, and formal operational stages of development. The six stages described by Bibace and Walsh are phenomenism, contagion, contamination, internalization, physiological, and psychophysiological conceptions of illness. In early childhood, children interpret the world in terms of familiar events and experiences. Causality is not understood in traditional terms. A mixture of physiological, social, and mechanical explanations are combined in novel ways in middle childhood. Children in this stage connect cause, illness, and treatment but do not always grasp the sequence or the internal processes necessary to bring about health or cure. In early adolescence, children are willing to speculate on the necessary processes, dealing with them in increasingly more complex ways, until something approaching a majority of adolescents arrive at somewhat scientific explanations of illness etiology and treatment. This level of understanding is that usually assumed in adult models of compliance. There is no evidence of gender differences in any of these studies. Complex cognitive and affective processes are also involved in the development and operation of self-regulatory actions (Bandura, 1989).

Several theorists, coming from different perspectives, have suggested that personal control or self-regulation may be the motivating factor in health promotion efforts (Leventhal & Cameron, 1987; Leventhal, Zimmerman, & Gutmann, 1984; Peterson & Stunkard, 1989; Rosenstock, Strecher, & Becker, 1988; Strecher, DeVellis, Becker, & Rosenstock, 1986). This position is perhaps best articulated by Peterson and Stunkard (1989), who incorporate Bandura's (1977, 1989) concept of self-efficacy into a theory of personal control. But personal control may also motivate noncompliance or resistance to the recommendations of an authority figure such as a physician. Personal control has been broadly defined to include the influence of (a) self-efficacy, (b) locus of control, and (c) autonomy. Whereas perceptions of personal efficacy, internal locus of control, and autonomy are usually viewed positively in development, personal control is not inherently good. These perceptions may also reflect the patient's beliefs that personal control, not physician control, produces health. Noncompliance is indeed one source of evidence for personal rather than physician control.

Self-efficacy and locus of control are usually conceptualized as beliefs, but autonomy reflects behaviors and opportunities to behave. Most of the research on self-efficacy has focused on adult populations. Health locus of control has been measured in children as young as 3 years but more frequently in school-age children. Although autonomy begins to develop in the toddler years, most of the research on autonomy relative to health behaviors is with school-age children.

Self-Efficacy

Self-efficacy, or, according to Bandura (1977), the perception "that one can successfully execute the behavior required to produce the outcomes" (p. 193), has been the focus of much of the recent interest in personal control and compliance. Rosenstock et al. (1988) recognize the importance of locus of control in the existing elements of the Health Belief Model (HBM) but suggest a modification to the HBM to include self-efficacy. In their reviews of the literature, both O'Leary (1985) and Strecher et al. (1986) conclude that self-efficacy may have mediated compliance in several successful health behavior interventions. Self-efficacy may be enhanced through intervention with subsequent improvement in health behaviors.

Locus of Control

A related construct is children's health locus of control. Internal control reflects a belief that one has influence or control over one's health, and that one's behavior affects the incidence or prognosis of a disease. External control is the belief that one's health is predominantly under the control of powerful others, chance, or a social system or institution. Individuals with internal locus of control are more likely to exhibit recommended health behaviors (Tinsley & Holtgrave, 1989). Health locus of control was one of the most important personal factors in the CHBM, significantly influencing those motivational factors having a direct effect on the child's expectation to take medicines in response to health problems (Bush & Iannotti, 1990). Hamburg and Inoff (1982) report that locus of control was related to metabolic control, not degree of compliance, in child and adolescent diabetics. Similar findings reported by Rappaport, Landman, Fenton, and Levine (1986) indicate that, for treatment of encopresis in children, locus of control was related to outcome but not to compliance. They conclude that locus of control may be useful for identifying children at risk for poor outcomes.

Cognitive development and the understanding of causality and long-term consequences may affect locus of control. Although it is difficult to measure health locus of control in young children, internal health locus of control appears to increase with age and to have some stability throughout the school years (the relative rank of children within an age group remains somewhat constant over time).

There are socioeconomic influences on locus of control (Bush, Parcel, & Davidson, 1983; e.g., children growing up in a lower socioeconomic environment are more likely to believe in fatalism, helplessness, and external control, as well as familial influences; e.g., children who experience approval, trust, and a nurturing family environment are more likely to develop an internal locus of control). Children's health locus of control is related to the health locus of control of the primary caretaker (Bush & Iannotti, 1988; O'Brien, Bush, & Parcel, 1989).

Autonomy

Autonomy relative to health behaviors has been measured as behaviors that indicate the child has control or responsibility for some aspect of health promotion, disease prevention, or treatment. Because a parent or guardian usually has control of the resources for these behaviors, or at least has responsibility for structuring the home environment to moderate the level of autonomy permitted, autonomy reflects both a child's independent behaviors and a parent's independence granting. Autonomy, as defined in this chapter, is those behaviors indicating that the child cooperates in, takes the initiative for, has the capability for, or has responsibility for health promotion or treatment.

In their research Lewis and Lewis (1982, 1983) clearly demonstrate the role of the child in making health-related decisions. Our own research suggests that children perceive themselves as having considerable autonomy in taking health action (Bush & Iannotti, 1985; Bush, Iannotti, & Davidson, 1985; Iannotti & Bush, 1992). Two samples of children were interviewed about medicine use and use of abusable substances. The first sample included 420 children stratified on socioeconomic status, gender, and grade in elementary school. Three years later 300 children in Grades 3 through 7 were interviewed, including 142 children from the first sample. The responses of these subjects have implications for compliance of children, particularly preadolescent children.

Results suggested that children perceive themselves as active in the treatment process. Most of the children demonstrated familiarity with treatment options; they could name medicines including brand names. Knowledge relating to medicine efficacy was generally low, however. There were significant age differences on a number of responses relating to the children's role in their own and other's use of medicines. Some of the results from both of these studies are displayed in Table 3.1.

Children's involvement in the medicine taking of others was significantly greater in the older children. Children who had purchased medicines without an adult present increased from 2% in kindergarten to 29% in Grade 7. Picking up prescription medicines increased from 0 to 44%. Lower socioeconomic urban neighborhoods presented more opportunities for children to buy medicines. A majority of the children responded that they had brought medicines to others and one-fourth of the seventh graders had independently given medicines to another child. The influence of children on the medicine taking of others was evident.

TABLE 3.1
Percentage of Positive Response to Medicine Autonomy Items

Child's Autonomy Items	K	3	7	Study 1 Mean K-3	Study 2 Mean 3-7
Had access to household meds*	70	76	100	76	88
All household meds were accessible*		45	78		63
Asked for the med	22	43	78	21	76
Got household meds for self*		73	89		84
Got household meds for self independently*		22	45		34
Got household meds for others*	30	62	71	54	67
Got household meds for others independently*		9	36		25
Took med independently*	20	23	51	15	36
Took med independently for headache*		20	45		31
Took med independently for sore throat*		17	33		28
Gave med to another child independently*		9	25		15
Purchased med independently*	2	10	29	7	25
Picked up prescription independently	0	21	44	2	37
Took medicine to school		6	9		8

*Significant positive association with grade, $p < .05$.

The implications of these findings for compliance, particularly the potential influence of children on other children's compliance behaviors, have not been investigated.

The involvement of children in their own responses to illness is even more evident. Most children said they had access to household medicines, with significantly more older children than young, ranging from 70% of kindergarten children to 100% of seventh graders. Physical access to selected medicines was restricted in some homes, but they were still accessible to a majority of children, 63%. Many children took medicines without participation of adults, increasing from 20% at third grade to 45% at seventh. When children were sick, they influenced their treatment. They asked for medicines, got medicines for themselves, and took medicines on their own.

Autonomy behaviors were somewhat stable in the 142 children who were retested 3 years later ($r = .17$, $p < .05$). As might be expected, children with asthma and allergies had significantly more autonomy in medicine use than other children. Parental attitudes or behavior differences did not appear to account for individual differences in autonomy. The significant positive predictors of autonomy were age, family size, risk taking, and autonomy in related areas (e.g., substance use—cigarettes or alcohol).

The primary caretaker (person who had primary responsibility for taking care of the child—93% mothers) of 90% of the children in Study 2 also were interviewed about their health and illness behaviors and attitudes and the health behavior and attitudes of their children. Primary caretakers did not always agree with their children's perceptions of themselves as autonomous medicine users, but primary caretakers and children generally agreed on the age at which autonomy behaviors were first exhibited. The average age at which primary caretakers thought most children were ready to take a medicine without asking an adult was 12.7 years. Even those primary caretakers whose children had already done so at a younger age believed that the average child was not ready until approximately age 12. More of the children (35.7%) reported they had taken medicine independently than reported by primary caretakers (18%), although the average age for the first occurrence reported by primary caretakers and children was the same (9.1 years). Primary caretakers reported that, at an average age of 9.1 years, 45.5% of the children used a topical medicine without first asking permission. The ages for autonomous behaviors indicated by primary caretakers and children were generally not significantly different. Although the measures of agreement between primary caretakers and children were frequently significant, they were quite small, Kappa statistics ranging from .02 to .22. The most notable disagreement reflecting children's independence in medicine use was for potential medicine use in school. Few primary caretakers (21.7%) reported that their children ever took medicines to school, but 8.3% of children had medicines with them at school on the day they were interviewed. Yet primary caretakers rarely confirmed their children's reports, and the list of medicines possessed by the children whose primary caretakers indicated their children never took a medicine to school included medicines that could have caused problems if taken too frequently or if taken by other children.

There is evidence that autonomy facilitates compliance in adolescence (Friedman & Litt, 1987). Yet there must be communication between parent and adolescent. Lack of agreement between parent and child about who is responsible for following the treatment is one correlate of noncompliance (Tebbi et al., 1986) and shared responsibility may be necessary (Beck et al., 1980).

Conclusions

Physicians might do well to include children in their discussions of treatment plans and to provide children with rationales for compliance with the treatment plan. Korsch, Gozzi, and Francis (1968) found that few pediatric interactions were child directed and only .8% of child-directed statements were health oriented rather than social. Physicians usually seek information from the child and provide information to the parent (Pantell, Stewart, Dias, Wells, & Ross, 1982). Physicians may need to consider the autonomy and personal control of a child before deciding on a treatment plan that would include the child's participation. Brief assessments of health locus of control, self-efficacy, and autonomy could contribute to planning interventions designed to enhance compliance and to individualizing treatment and intervention. Further research is needed on the relationship of autonomy and health locus of control to self-efficacy and compliance.

SOCIAL, CULTURAL, AND SOCIOECONOMIC CONTEXT

Each of the developmental processes discussed previously needs to be placed within its social, cultural, and socioeconomic context. For example, parental health beliefs and attitudes have been shown to be correlated with their children's health beliefs and attitudes, although the direct effect on children's behavioral expectations appears to be limited (Bush & Iannotti, 1988, 1990). Children, more than adults, are limited in their opportunities for displaying independence and personal control. Parental expectations for their child affect the opportunities provided for independent health actions and the role assigned to the child in maintaining compliance to health prescriptions. Parents provide both the motivation for displaying self-control and compliance and the context to practice these behaviors. Socialization into schools and religious institutions also provides both direction and opportunities for developing self-control, compliance, and independence.

The social dynamics of family, peers, and institutions (school, church, and work) may have strong influences on compliance that vary with age. It is not unusual for compliance to decrease during the adolescent years (e.g., Jacobson et al., 1987). Changing social and physiological processes are most evident at this stage of development. Peer influences increase while the adolescent is establishing independence from family and school, and rapid physiological changes may complicate the intended effects of treatment.

Family Context

In research on nonhealth-related behaviors, it is evident that parental style and parent–child interactions influence the early development of compliance. Self-control develops rapidly through 8 or 9 years of age and may continue to increase more slowly until young adulthood or later. Parental behaviors that foster self-control are warmth and reasoning in discipline (Baumrind, 1971; Kuczynski, 1978; Pitkanen-Pulkkinen, 1979). Children treated with warmth and reasoning are more likely to exhibit self-control by making more mature choices when not under the direct guidance of their parents. Kuczynski (1984) demonstrated that mothers changed their parent–child interaction styles and disciplinary techniques when long-term versus short-term compliance was the goal. These changes in parental style (i.e., more use of reasoning and nurturance) facilitated compliance and reduced negativism in the children.

The direct effect of parents on children's compliance with medical treatment is well accepted. Parental involvement and support improves compliance in adolescence, particularly when there is low conflict or tension in the relationship (Friedman & Litt, 1987). The family environment affects opportunities for children to develop self-reliance and self-control. For example, single parents grant more autonomy to children for health self-care than two-parent families, and there is greater autonomy in larger families (Iannotti & Bush, 1992). Family conflict and disequilibrium also increase noncompliance (Tebbi et al., 1986). Christiaanse, Lavigne, and Lerner (1989) examined compliance, measured as mean and percentage of therapeutic theophylline levels, in 7- to 17-year-old children with chronic asthma. Regression analyses including family environment, self-variables, and psychological adjustment as predictors of compliance, suggested that family cohesion may interact with psychological adjustment to contribute to compliance in children and adolescents. A balance between parental support and adolescent autonomy is probably optimum (Beck et al., 1980; Pratt, 1973).

Cultural and Socioeconomic Context

The family and neighborhood environment reflect differences in the value placed on compliance. Urban neighborhoods provide greater opportunities for children to be involved in the process of medicine taking because of the easier access to medicines at neighborhood stores, and the greater likelihood that urban children assist in the purchase of medicines (Bush & Davidson, 1982). But, as already indicated, autonomy does not assure compliance. Compliance is usually greater in cultures and families that are achievement oriented, are educationally advanced, are in the middle to upper social class, and include self-control in their definition of maturity (Whiting & Whiting, 1975). Cultural values for the particular behavior are also important. For example, Ekstrand and Ekstrand (1986) compared the perceptions of "good" behavior of Swedish and Indian children and their parents. Indian parents emphasized manners and obedience whereas Swedish parents stressed independence, assertiveness, and emotional development. When asked to define "bad" behavior, Indian parents clearly stated behaviors that were the opposite of those defined as good, but Swedish parents exhibited more vague, abstract, and contradictory expectations, indicating that assertiveness could be bad as well as good. The majority of Indian children said good behavior was doing well in school, but this was mentioned by less than 3% of Swedish children. Most Swedish children (66%) said that independent behavior was good behavior, but this was not mentioned by the Indian children. Compliance with treatment recommendations would have very different meanings for children in these two cultures, one valuing independence and the other valuing obedience. Cultural differences such as these have implications for the meaning of compliance within a culture, normative expectations regarding compliance, and the likelihood that members of that culture will comply.

Conclusions

Interventions directed at improving compliance must consider these social and environmental influences. Cultural differences must be considered in designing interventions. Just as the research on autonomy argues for including the child in the treatment process, the research on family and cultural dynamics argues for interventions that take into account these differences. Involvement of parent and child in health education and in the treatment process is necessary. Efforts to improve compliance need to include parent education, parent counseling, and use of social support networks. Physicians need to become familiar with the cultural expectations of their pediatric patients if they are not already attuned to these differences.

A CHILDREN'S HEALTH BELIEF MODEL

The original conception of the Health Belief Model (HBM) focused on preventive health behaviors (Rosenstock, 1966) and included the following major "readiness to take action" elements: (a) the level of threat posed by the health problem as determined by the individual's perception of the problem's severity and perception of vulnerability to it; (b) the individual's perception of benefit to be derived from engaging in a behavior to reduce the threat, weighed against his or her perception of barriers (psychological, physical, social, economic) to performing the behavior; and (c) some type of external or internal trigger or cue to action. Becker and his associates reformulated the HBM to predict compliance with physician directives, placing greater emphasis on motivations, prior experiences, and interpersonal relationships (Becker, 1974; Becker & Maiman, 1975; Becker, Maiman, Kirscht, Hefner, Drachman, 1977; Maiman & Becker, 1974). The HBM has been criticized for excluding social elements, such as the influence of significant others (Christensen, 1985).

The Children's Health Belief Model (CHBM)

Bush and Iannotti (1985, 1988, 1990) adapted the HBM to include some developmental processes central to compliance. The resulting CHBM places children's health behavior within its personal and social context. Compared to the adult model, that does not account for the development of the readiness factors that directly influence health behaviors, the CHBM readiness factors have their origin in personal attributes and social environmental influences. The personal attributes include personality characteristics (e.g., risk taking), the developing self-system (e.g., locus of control, self-esteem, self-efficacy, self-control), personal competencies (e.g., health knowledge, health autonomy), and demographic markers of other social and environmental influences (e.g., gender, socioeconomic status). The influence of others (e.g., family, peers, and social groups) is introduced in this developmental model; however, these social influences should be recognized in models of adult compliance behaviors as well. A good developmental model reflects changing personal, social, and environmental influences and is applicable across the life span; it is not limited to a particular stage of life. The model should include the elements of developmental processes, personal control, and the social and cultural context described earlier that are likely to influence the development of compliance or to have different effects at different developmental stages.

The CHBM was initially developed on the sample of 420 elementary schoolchildren, described earlier. The children were individually interviewed to assess modifying, readiness, and behavior factors including health beliefs and attitudes, previous illness experiences, and expectations to take action in response to minor health problems (actual health behaviors were not observed). The model was then expanded to include additional modifying factors, such as parental influences, and was tested on the sample of 270 urban preadolescents, stratified by socioeconomic status, grade level, and gender, and their primary caretakers. This version of the CHBM (Fig. 3.1) was very successful in predicting children's expectation to take action in response to common health problems (Bush & Iannotti, 1988, 1990), accounting for 63% of the variance. In this application of

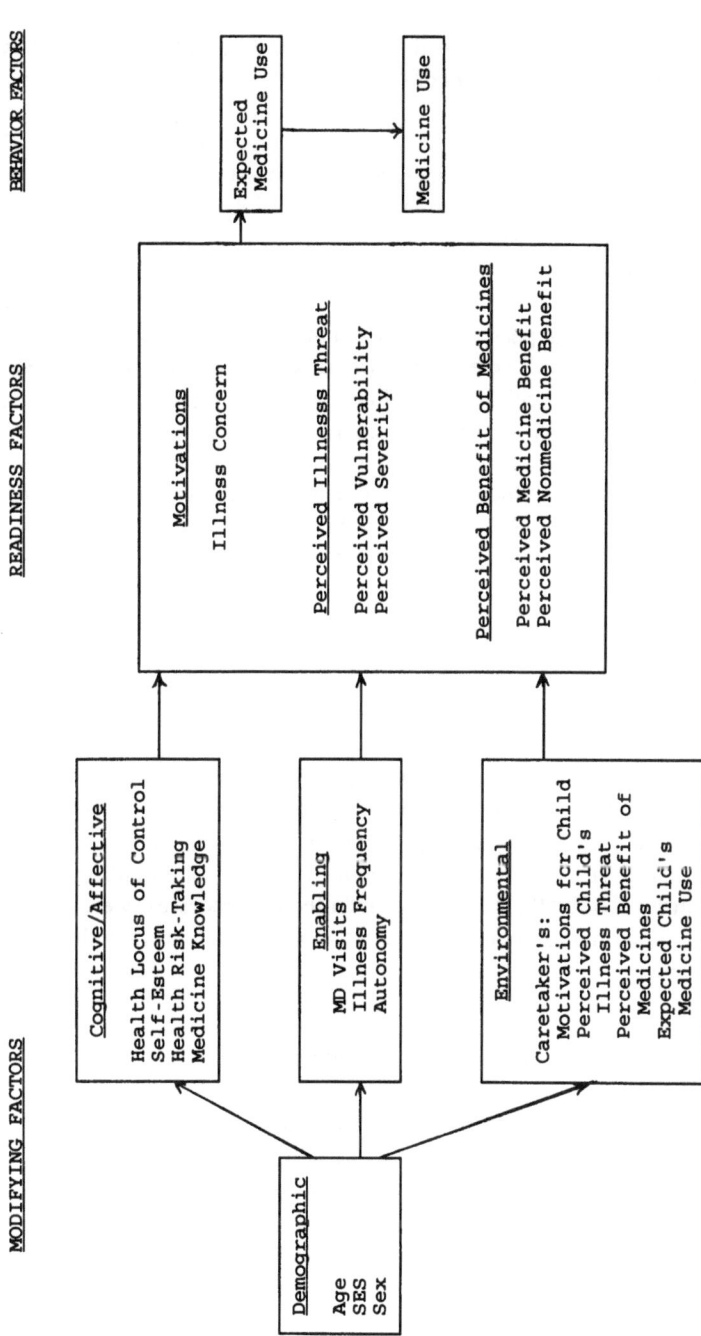

FIG. 3.1. The children's health belief model as applied to medicine use.

the CHBM, family influences were limited to that of the primary caretaker, and peer influences were measured as perceived by the child. Severity of the illness ($\beta = 0.46$) and benefit of taking medicines ($\beta = 0.39$), both as perceived by the child, were the two best predictors of children's expectations to take action. Two other variables also in the original HBM, illness concern ($\beta = 0.11$) and perceived vulnerability ($\beta = 0.17$), had weaker but significant relationships. These elements of the HBM have been included in successful interventions in adults (Jones, Jones, & Katz, 1987; Maiman, Becker, Liptak, Nazarian, & Rounds, 1988) and have been associated with compliance in adolescence and adults (Edwards & Montgomery, 1989; O'Connell, Price, Roberts, Jurs, & McKinley, 1985).

From a developmental perspective, two findings from our test of hypothesized causal paths in the CHBM were particularly noteworthy: (a) Primary caretakers' attitudes influenced their children's readiness and expectations to take medicines (Sum of paths = -0.10), but the children's own cognitions and attitudes had a stronger influence (Sum of paths = -0.25); and (b) significant correlations were observed between many of the primary caretakers' readiness, cognitive/affective, and enabling variables in the model and the corresponding variables for their children. There are two messages here. One is that parents do indeed influence their children's health beliefs and behaviors. The other is that this effect is small when compared to other developmental influences on children's attitudes and behaviors.

Conclusions

The CHBM suggests that children's health orientations may develop somewhat independently of their parents' influence. Developmental cognitive and affective variables were not strongly related to parents' motivational beliefs and yet played a significant role in children's health belief systems. Children's motivational variables, influenced by their cognitive and affective processes, were much more important in determining their expectations to use medicines than their parents' values or beliefs.

RESEARCH QUESTIONS

A number of research questions present themselves: What is the influence of different parental styles on development of health locus of control, self-efficacy, personal control, and autonomy? There is some evidence that parents can encourage personal control and influence autonomy. The family environments and the parenting styles that facilitate this development should be examined.

What are the determinants of long-term versus short-term compliance at different ages? Do self-regulation skills generalize across domains? Most of the research in this area focuses on compliance with parental directives. In addition to this basic research, further study of compliance with health directives is needed.

What is the role of cognitive development and children's understanding of long-term versus short-term consequences on compliance? How can prospective memory be enhanced and how can the social context of memory facilitate this process? There have been few studies of the relationship of cognitive development with compliance. Cognitive skills should be assessed prior to compliance interventions and, when possible, efforts at enhancing compliance should match the intervention with the cognitive level of the child.

What are the ethnic and cultural influences on these relationships? Perhaps the most difficult challenge is to assess ethnic and cultural influences on compliance. More information is needed about the cultural characteristics of samples in compliance studies and diverse samples should continue to be encouraged.

The answer to these questions should contribute to a better understanding of the development of compliance as a process that includes personal, social, and cultural dimensions. There is a serious need for more research with children, to complement that being done with adolescents and adults. The CHBM offers a possible framework, but in its current conceptualization it is cross-sectional and does not sufficiently reflect hanging developmental processes or the reciprocal effect of health and illness experiences on the beliefs and attitudes that influence compliance.

Other research efforts need to focus on the pediatric interaction between child, parent, and physician (NCPIE, 1989). How can communication among child, parent, and health care professional be improved? How can health professionals be encouraged to communicate effectively with children at their own level as well as with parents at theirs? What are appropriate roles for children in their own treatment? How can health professionals enlist the child's and adolescent's extended social network to improve compliance?

SUMMARY

There is a clear need to integrate developmental theories and processes into theories of compliance. The challenge to researchers in developmental aspects of compliance is to apply the developmental literature in these areas to their theoretical and clinical approaches to compliance. The challenge to developmental and social researchers is to consider the practical applications of their theoretical and empirical advances to health promotion, disease prevention, and, the domain that is the focus of this volume, compliance with physician recommendations and treatment.

ACKNOWLEDGMENTS

Portions of this chapter were presented at the National Institute of Child Health and Human Development Workshop on Developmental Aspects of Health Compliance Behavior, Bethesda, Md., July 1989. The work presented in this chapter was supported by grants from the National Institute on Drug Abuse (DA 02686, DA 04497) and the National Heart, Lung, and Blood Institute (HL 35261).

REFERENCES

Bandura, A. (1977). Self-efficacy: Toward a unifying theory of behavioral change. *Psychological Review, 84,* 191–215.

Bandura, A. (1989). Human agency in social cognitive theory. *American Psychologist, 44,* 1175–1184.

Baumrind, D. (1971). Current patterns of parental authority. *Developmental Psychology Monographs, 4,* 1–20.

Beck, D. E., Fennell, R. S., Yost, R. L., Robinson, J. D., Geary, D., & Richards, G. A. (1980). Evaluation of an educational program on compliance with medication regimens in pediatric patients with renal transplants. *Journal of Pediatrics,* 1094–1097.

Becker, M. H. (Ed.). (1974). *The Health Belief Model and personal health behavior.* Thorofare, NJ: Charles B. Slack.

Becker, M. H., & Maiman, L. A. (1975). Sociobehavioral determinants of compliance with medical care recommendations. *Medical Care, 13,* 10–24.

Becker, M. H., Maiman, L. A., Kirscht, J. P., Hefner, D. P., & Drachman, R. H. (1977). Predictions of dietary compliance: A field experiment. *Journal of Health and Social Behavior, 18,* 348–365.

Bibace, R., & Walsh, M. E. (1980). Development of children's concepts of illness. *Pediatrics, 66,* 913–917.

Burbach, D. J., & Peterson, L. (1986). Children's concepts of physical illness: A review and critique of the cognitive developmental literature. *Health Psychology, 5,* 307–325.

Bush, P. J., & Davidson, F. R. (1982). Medicines and "drugs": What do children think? *Health Education Quarterly, 9,* 209–224.

Bush, P. J., & Iannotti, R. J. (1985). The development of children's health orientations and behaviors: Lessons for substance use prevention. In C. L. Jones & B. J. Battjes (Eds.), *Etiology of drug abuse: Implications for prevention* (pp. 45–74) (DHHS Publication No. ADM 85-1335). Washington, DC: U.S. Government Printing Office.

Bush, P. J., & Iannotti, R. J. (1988). Origins and stability of children's health beliefs relative to medicine use. *Social Science and Medicine, 27,* 345–352.

Bush, P. J., & Iannotti, R. J. (1990). A children's health belief model. *Medical Care, 28,* 69–86.

Bush, P. J., Iannotti, R. J., & Davidson, F. R. (1985). A longitudinal study of children and medicines. In D. D. Breimer & P. Speiser (Eds.), *Topics in pharmaceutical sciences 1985* (pp. 391–403). Amsterdam: Elsevier.

Bush, P. J., Parcel, G. S., & Davidson, F. R. (1983). *Reliability of a shortened children's health locus of control scale.* (ERIC No. ED 223 354). Boulder, CO.

Christensen, D. B. (1985). Understanding patient drug-taking compliance. *Journal of Social and Administrative Pharmacy, 32,* 70–77.

Christiaanse, M. E., Lavigne, J. V., & Lerner, C. V. (1989). Psychosocial aspects of compliance in children and adolescents with asthma. *Developmental and Behavioral Pediatrics, 10,* 75–80.

Edwards, M. M., & Montgomery, S. B. (1989, October). *An application of the health belief model*

to college students' health protective strategies with regard to aids transmission. Presented at the American Public Health Association, Chicago.
Ekstrand, L. J., & Ekstrand, G. (1986, July). *Children's perceptions of norms in two cultures.* Presented at the Eighth International Conference Association for Cross-Cultural Psychology, Istanbul, Turkey.
Friedman, I. M., & Litt, I. F. (1987). Adolescents' compliance with therapeutic regimens. *Journal of Adolescent Health Care, 8,* 52–67.
Hamberg, B. A., & Inoff, G. E. (1982). Relationships between behavioral factors and diabetic control in children and adolescents: A camp study. *Psychosomatic Medicine, 44,* 321–339.
Harris, J. E. (1984). Remembering to do things: A forgotten topic. In J. E. Harris & P. E. Morris (Eds.), *Everyday memory, actions and absent-mindedness* (pp. 71–92). New York: Academic Press.
Iannotti, R. J., & Bush, P. J. (1992). The development of autonomy in children's health behaviors. In E. J. Susman, L. V. Feagans, & W. Ray (Eds.), *Emotion, cognition, health, and development in children and adolescents* (pp. 53–74). Hillsdale, NJ: Lawrence Erlbaum Associates.
Inhelder, B., & Piaget, J. (1964). *The early growth of logic in the child* (E. A. Lunzer & D. Papert, Trans). London: Routledge & Kegan Paul.
Jacobson, A. M., Hauser, S. T., Wolfsdorf, J. I., Houlihan, J., Milley, J. E., Herskowitz, R. D., Wertlieb, D., & Watt, E. (1987). Psychologic predictors of compliance in children with recent onset of diabetes mellitus. *Journal of Pediatrics, 110,* 805–811.
Jones, P. K., Jones, S. L., & Katz, J. (1987). Improving compliance for asthmatic patients visiting the emergency department using a health belief model intervention. *Journal of Asthma, 24,* 119–206.
Karoly, P. (1981). Self-management problems in children. In E. J. Mach & L. G. Terdal (Eds.), *Behavioral assessment of childhood disorders* (pp. 79–126). New York: Guilford Press.
Korsch, B. M., Gozzi, E. K., & Francis, V. (1968). Gaps in doctor–patient communication: Interaction and patient satisfaction. *Pediatrics, 42,* 855–871.
Kuczynski, L. (1978). *Intensity and orientation of reasoning: Motivational determinants of children's compliance.* Paper presented at the meeting of the American Psychological Association, Toronto.
Kuczynski, L. (1984). Socialization goals and mother–child interaction: Strategies for long-term and short-term compliance. *Developmental Psychology, 20,* 1061–1073.
Leventhal, H., & Cameron, L. (1987). Behavioral theories and the problem of compliance. *Patient Education and Counseling, 10,* 117–138.
Leventhal, H., Zimmerman, R., & Gutmann, M. (1984). Compliance: A self-regulation perspective. In W. D. Gentry (Ed.), *Handbook of behavioral medicine* (pp. 369–436). New York: Guilford Press.
Levy, R. L., & Loftus, G. R. (1984). Compliance and memory. In J. E. Harris & P. E. Morris (Eds.), *Everyday memory, actions and absent-mindedness* (pp. 93–112). New York: Academic Press.
Lewis, C. E., & Lewis, M. A. (1982). Children's health-related decision making. *Health Education Quarterly, 9,* 129–141.
Lewis, C. E., & Lewis, M. A. (1983). Improving the health of children: Must the children be involved? *Annual Review of Public Health, 4,* 259–283.
Ley, P. (1977). Psychological studies of doctor–patient communication. In S. Rachman (Ed.), *Contributions to medical psychology.* New York: Oxford.
Maiman, L. A., & Becker, M. H. (1974). The health belief model: Origins and correlates in psychological theory. *Health Education Monographs, 2,* 336–353.
Maiman, L. A., Becker, M. H., Liptak, G. S., Nazarian, L. F., & Rounds, K. A. (1988). Improving pediatricians' compliance-enhancing practices. *American Journal of Diseases of Children, 142,* 773–779.

Meacham, J. A. (1982). A note on remembering to execute planned actions. *Journal of Applied Developmental Psychology, 3,* 121–133.

National Council on Patient Information and Education. (1989). *Children and America's other drug problem: Guidelines for improving prescription medicine use among children and teenagers.* Washington, DC: Author.

O'Brien, R. W., Bush, P. J., & Parcel, G. S. (1989). Stability in a measure of children's health locus of control. *Journal of School Health, 59,* 161–164.

O'Connell, J. K., Price, J. H., Roberts, S. M., Jurs, S. G., & McKinley, R. (1985). Utilizing the health belief model to predict dieting and exercising behavior of obese and nonobese adolescents. *Health Education Quarterly, 12,* 343–351.

O'Leary, A. (1985). Self-efficacy and health. *Behaviour Research and Therapy, 23,* 437–451.

Pantell, R. H., Stewart, T. J., Dias, J. K., Wells, P., & Ross, A. W. (1982). Physician communication with children and parents. *Pediatrics, 70,* 396–402.

Peterson, C., & Stunkard, A. J. (1989). Personal control and health promotion. *Social Science and Medicine, 28,* 819–828.

Pitkanen-Pulkkinen, L. (1979). Self-control as a prerequisite for constructive behavior. In S. Feshbach & A. Fraczek (Eds.), *Aggression and behavior change* (pp. 250–270). New York: Praeger.

Pratt, L. (1973). Child rearing methods and children's health behavior. *Journal of Health and Social Behavior, 14,* 61–69.

Rappaport, L., Landman, G., Fenton, T., & Levine, M. D. (1986). Locus of control as predictor of compliance and outcome in treatment of encopresis. *Journal of Pediatrics, 109,* 1061–1064.

Rosenstock, I. (1966). Why people use health services. *Milbank Memorial Fund Quarterly, 44,* 94–124.

Rosenstock, I. M., Strecher, V. J., & Becker, M. H. (1988). Social learning theory and the health belief model. *Health Education Quarterly, 15,* 175–183.

Strecher, V. J., DeVellis, B. M., Becker, M. H., & Rosenstock, I. M. (1986). The role of self-efficacy in achieving health behavior change. *Health Education Quarterly, 13,* 73–91.

Svarstad, B. (1986). Patient–practitioner relationships and compliance with prescribed medical regimens. In L. Aiken & D. Mechanic (Eds.), *Applications of social science to clinical medicine and health policy* (pp. 438–459). New Brunswick, NJ: Rutgers University Press.

Tebbi, C., Cummings, K. M., Zevon, M. A., Smith, L., Richards, M., & Mallon, N. (1986). Compliance of pediatric and adolescent cancer patients. *Cancer, 58,* 1179–1184.

Tinsley, B. J., & Holtgrave, D. R. (1989). Maternal health locus of control beliefs, utilization of childhood preventive health services, and infant health. *Developmental and Behavioral Pediatrics, 10,* 236–241.

Walsh, D. C. (1983). Age differences in learning and memory. In D. S. Woodruff & J. E. Birren (Eds.), *Aging: Scientific perspectives and social issues* (pp. 149–177). Monterey, CA: Brooks/Cole.

Whiting, B., & Whiting, J. W. M. (1975). *Children of six cultures.* Cambridge, MA: Harvard University Press.

4 Family Context and Compliance Behavior in Chronically Ill Children

Barbara J. Anderson
Harvard University Medical School

James C. Coyne
University of Michigan Medical School

From a theoretical perspective, we know very little about family contributions to the development of compliant behavior patterns in children and adolescents with chronic physical illnesses. Theories of family functioning with respect to the development of children with chronic physical illnesses have not focused on responses over time to the tasks of compliance with medical treatment regimen that face both parents and child *nor on the interactive context of parental helping* with these tasks in the family.

Over the past two decades, three major theories of family functioning with respect to chronic childhood disease have been presented: Pless and Pinkerton's Integrated Model of Adjustment (1975), Minuchin, Baker, and Rosman's Psychosomatic Family Model (1978), and McCubbin and McCubbin's Family Adjustment and Adaptation Response Model (1988). These theories have not focused on compliance with the medical regimen as a central task facing children and families. After briefly discussing the lack of attention to this area in theories of families with chronically-ill children, we introduce the application of a theory that directly addresses the interactive context of family behavior around compliance tasks, the Miscarried Helping Model (Coyne, Wortman, & Lehman, 1988).

THEORIES OF FAMILY FUNCTIONING WITH RESPECT TO FAMILY INTERACTION AND CHILDREN'S COMPLIANCE BEHAVIOR

The major theories of family functioning that have been applied to chronic illness in childhood have not taken a *family interaction* or *family process* perspective on coping with illness. A family perspective on coping with illness involves a shift from viewing the family and other relationships from the perspective of patients to viewing patients in terms of their involvement in these relationships (Ransom, 1989). A family perspective underscores that coping with chronic illness is not simply a matter of just what the individual does, but of the organization of relationships in the family. We briefly identify three major theories that are often presented as addressing a family perspective. However, these models do not address the context of family interactions around compliance behavior nor do they focus on the process and organization of relationships in the family. Constructs in Pless and Pinkerton's Integrated Model of Adjustment (1975) do not directly focus on the family's contributions to compliance behavior or how the child adjusts to compliance demands. Such constructs are at a much more molecular, interactive level than the constructs in this model. The more molar constructs in this model, such as "Response of Family" and "Coping Style," potentially address parental responses to treatment demands and to their child's cooperation with treatment as well as potentially speak to how the child adjusts to the demands of treatment. However, the theory does not specifically address family interactions around compliance behaviors or help dilemmas faced by parents of chronically ill children and adolescents. . . Pless and Pinkerton (1975) acknowledge that the family does react to the disorder per se as well as "to the behavior of the child in relation to his illness" (p. 30). In summary, Pless and Pinkerton's Integrated Model of Adjustment made important contributions to the study of the child with chronic disease by giving central focus to the family. However, the family context surrounding compliance behavior was not directly addressed in this theory.

Other theories have taken family functioning, rather than child adjustment, as their primary focus. Clearly, the best known of these theories is the Psychosomatic Family Model first presented by Minuchin, Baker, and Rosman in 1978. In this model, Minuchin and colleagues report that, for a subgroup of children with "psychosomatic" diabetes, asthma, or anorexia nervosa, the child's symptoms both play a key role in maintaining family homeostasis and are triggered from physiological arousal activity stimulated by distressing dysfunctional family interactional patterns. As we have recently argued in several papers critiquing the Psychosomatic Family Model (Coyne & Anderson, 1988, 1989), this theory was built on a data base that has never been scientifically presented nor reviewed and depends on an outmoded view of how psychosocial and family factors are involved in illness (i.e., psychosomatic models of illness, which assume that *arousal* is the only or primary means by which psychosocial factors influence illness). *The key outcome variables in the Psychosomatic Family Model are somatic symptoms, not compliance behaviors,* and this theory does not address inadequate self-care behavior as an "interactional tactic" in chronically ill children who are not functioning within an acceptable medical level. The "psychosomatic" chronically ill child is seen as a "conflict defuser" playing an active role in maladaptive family interactions. Likewise, the parents are said to use the ill child to detour around conflict especially marital issues. Yet, whereas conflict is central to the model of the psychosomatic family, conflict is decontextualized from the real illness-related conflicts that face chronically ill children and families, such as negotiating symptom monitoring and following treatment prescriptions (Coyne & Anderson, 1988). Thus, from the Psychosomatic Family Model we cannot identify how conflict develops or is expressed around treatment-related issues, or how families influence the development of compliance behavior in their ill child.

In fact, when we examine theories concerning the family and chronic childhood disease, the closest we get to addressing family interactive behavior with respect to compliance with treatment is McCubbin and McCubbin's Family Adjustment and Adaptation Response Model. This model focuses on the family's efforts to manage the demands imposed by an illness in terms of demands of the illness, the family's capabilities for meeting the demands (resources and coping style), and situational and global (subjective) meanings. This model does distinguish between the two phases of Adjustment and Adaptation, separated by a period of crisis (Patterson, 1989). However, this theory is not process oriented and does not directly address how the family adjusts and adapts to the sharing of treatment tasks. Although this model does identify treatment demands as a stress and chronic strain on the child *and family,* this theory does not speculate about the development or importance of parent–child interactions around compliance with treatment tasks.

THE MISCARRIED HELPING THEORY

There is a body of literature at the intersection of social psychology and family therapy that provides a theoretical and process-oriented approach to how families cope with the compliance tasks facing parents and their chronically ill children. Coyne, Wortman, and Lehman (1988) have suggested:

> in contrast to the dominant themes of the social support literature, the family therapy literature has contributed an understanding of how people involved with an ill person, or person in distress—particularly those closest to that person—may become emotionally overinvolved, critical and hostile to the stressed person, and become psychologically distressed themselves. The family therapy literature suggests that both underinvolvement (which can be seen as a lack of support) and overinvolvement of family members can lead to negative adaptational outcomes. Apparently contradicting the social support literature's assumption that the distressed or ill person will benefit from greater involvement with others, family therapists often seek to disengage or individuate the distressed person from a destructive overinvolvement in close relationships. (p. 3)

Various aspects of a possible miscarried helping process in adults have been discussed in the context of chronic pain, disability, and illnesses such as Alzheimer's, renal failure, and stroke (Coyne et al., 1988). The specific issues, coping tasks, and appropriateness of various forms of involvement by family members vary across these chronic illnesses, but there is a basis for postulating a general underlying process, whereby efforts to be helpful to persons who are ill or under stress can become miscarried, particularly in close relationships. Without denying the benefits of positive involvement, Coyne et al. point to some potential pitfalls in the process of overinvolvement on the part of helpers and identify this as the key variable in the miscarried helping process. Their theoretical paper illustrates from diverse literatures how a support provider's investment in being helpful and achieving a positive outcome may ironically lead to behavioral transactions that are detrimental to the patient's well-being and successful adaptation to treatment.

Based on this original miscarried helping model described by Coyne and colleagues (1988), in this chapter we describe an interactional approach to understanding the development of compliance behavior in chronically ill children and adolescents, a model in which the perspectives of both *the parent as helper* and *the child, as the recipient of the help* are taken into account. We focus on help that fails (i.e., parental efforts to achieve appropriate compliance behavior in their children that are *unsuccessful*) in our efforts to understand parental help that *works*.

In this chapter, we examine what happens when parental efforts to help their chronically ill child or adolescent backfire, and the motivation of chronically ill youngsters to take care of themselves gets sidelined by the power of another struggle—that of preserving individual autonomy in the face of parental helping. This is the process of "Miscarried Helping," described by Coyne, Wortman, and Lehman (1988), with reference to spouse interactions, as the failure of "well-intentioned support attempts because they are excessive, untimely, or inappropriate" (p. 2). We examine this process of miscarried helping as it sometimes occurs between parents and chronically ill children and adolescents around compliance tasks. First, we describe the *interactive processes* by which well-meant helping behaviors on the part of parents can, over time, come to undermine the very adaptive illness-related behavior they were attempting to foster in their child. Second, we identify disease-related and developmental factors that contribute to miscarried helping in the relationships between chronically ill children and their parents. Finally, we argue that theories of compliance behavior in chronically ill children must extend their focus to include the interactive context of parental involvement in treatment tasks.

"Miscarried Helping" Defined

Miscarried helping in the parent–child relationship refers to a process by which a parent's investment in being helpful and in achieving a positive outcome for his or her child paradoxically leads to interactions, over time, that are constraining and detrimental to the child's well-being and successful adaptation. The two essential components of this process—a parent's emotional investment in being helpful and in assuring a positive, healthy outcome for his or her chronically ill child—are ones frequently valued and encouraged in parents. But over time, in some relationships, these supportive behaviors become self-defeating and disabling to the child.

It is important to look at miscarried helping in families with chronically ill youngsters because the genetic component involved in many chronic childhood diseases as well as the complex medical regimen that often must be implemented at home, and the omnipresent threat of a life-threatening medical crisis, create a special vulnerability to miscarried helping in the interactions between parents and their ill child.

Overprotectiveness

Overprotection of chronically ill youngsters, especially by mothers, has been reported to occur across a range of chronic childhood illnesses (Sabbath, 1984). Overprotectiveness in families with chronically ill children has been discussed at length by Minuchin et al. (1978) as the excessive nurturing and sensitivity of family members to one another's distress. *Overprotective* has become a label of blame that carries no information about its origin or about the behavior of a child or the characteristics of the illness or treatment that might contribute to such a parental response. As discussed by Fiske, Coyne, and Smith (in press), "Family theorists have been biased toward viewing family members with suspicion and as likely negative influences on patient adaptation. In the absence of data, they have presumed both a high prevalence of wives' and mothers' overprotectiveness and conceptualized it as a cover for hostility. Yet, some degree of protectiveness is both normative and necessary to assist vulnerable and dependent patients and forestall catastrophic outcomes" (Gillis, 1984).

Similarly, as we discussed in our critique of Minuchin's classic text, *Psychosomatic Families*, "overprotectiveness" in families with diabetic children could be viewed as an inevitable response to repeated metabolic crises in a child, rather than a deficiency in the parent that instigates these crises (Coyne & Anderson, 1988). Indeed, "overprotectiveness" is not an attribute of behavior but a judgment about the fit of behavior to the context. Whether behavior is best viewed as "overprotective" rather than as reflecting appropriate vigilance and concern depends on the threat inherent in a situation and the alternative means of dealing with it. Close parental scrutiny is sometimes warranted by the chronically ill child's age, disease status, and regimen complexity. A high degree of parental involvement in their chronically ill child's life is sometimes unavoidable, as parents struggle with unpredictable short-term illness dilemmas, all the while continuing to carry out multiple daily treatment requirements. Research with families in which the patient with a chronic disease is an adult has documented that hostile critical exchanges are frequently more destructive than overprotectiveness (Fiske, Coyne, & Smith, in press).

We suggest an alternate *interactional model* for understanding "overprotectiveness" in which the helper, here the parent, is not singled out as the locus of the problem. Instead, we examine how *developmental* and *disease-related* factors may create miscarried helping out of initially well-intentioned investment and supportive behavior on the part of the parent.

As discussed by Coyne et al. (1988), *helping behavior has both a content as well as a context* that it creates, surrounding the interactions between the helper and the recipient of help. In providing help, the helper—here the parent—is also providing a statement about his or her own commitment, competencies, and feelings—and about those of the child. Constructs like overprotectiveness and enmeshment overlook the context of the protective behavior—the messages communicated about the participants that serve to perpetuate the problem.

The Evolution of "Miscarried Helping" in the Parent–Child Relationship

Helping youngsters with a chronic illness can take many forms—encouraging them to be strong and persistent in the face of painful, uncomfortable, or inconvenient treatments, and assisting them with injections or other self-administered therapies. Inevitably, there is ambiguity and potential conflict between the need to foster initiative and self-efficacy in the ill child and to protect him or her from harm and unnecessary suffering. Similarly, there are tradeoffs between the parents' handling situations in ways that insure their children's health and efficacy, and their provision of opportunities for the children to develop their own competencies, even in the face of possible failure and medical risk. In attempting to help, parents also express messages that can be as salient as their instrumental acts. By helping and verbally encouraging their chronically ill children, parents may at times create in the child feelings of remorse, incompetence, resentment, or feelings of being forced to comply with demands. Probably most importantly, children and adolescents may at times feel that their autonomy to decide to perform the needed therapy has been stripped away. Over time, parental involvement in the helping process may become overinvolvement, as parental investment in being helpful and in achieving a desirable outcome for their child grows. For most chronic diseases, children face dilemmas about how best to adapt to the illness and treatment—how to negotiate their world with an imperfect body; how to accommodate to painful or inconvenient treatments; and how to fit special diets or medications into their efforts to live as normal a life as possible; how to take care of themselves. Parental *help* with these personal challenges may be replaced, over time, by *demands* as parental urgency for the desired behavior and commitment to the treatment goal increases. When this occurs, a reframing of the original situation occurs, much as that described by Coyne and colleagues (1988) in discussing miscarried helping among spouses:

over time the helper and recipient may accumulate issues about their relationship that take precedence over other concerns. For instance, demands and intrusiveness on the part of the overinvolved support provider may confront the recipient with an unfortunate choice between preserving autonomy by resisting these efforts or doing what is adaptive. If someone is too insistent in suggesting their suggestions that a person not eat between meals, then "refusing to be pushed around" may take precedence over "cheating on my diet" as a label for snacking, and snacking becomes more justifiable. Over time, the initial dilemma of whether or not to snack can be suppressed by the more general disagreements over the support provider's right or need to make such suggestions and the recipient's commitment to the diet plan and ability to comply with it. (p. 5)

An interactive cycle is set in motion. Increased doubts about the child's motivation and behavior, demands, and criticisms by a caring parent who is invested in the well-being of the child often lead to increased child dysfunction and maladaptive choices with respect to self-care. The parents fail to see that there is a limit to what they can do directly for their child. The parent increases demands and expectations and, meeting with failure, often begins to feel distressed. Feeling distressed, the parent tries even harder to achieve a successful outcome in the child's behavior and meets a reciprocal resistance. The parents in turn may become quick to personalize any lapses or ineptitude on the part of the child, increasing the child's sense of helplessness and beliefs that he or she is confronting implacable and unreasonable foes. Both the parent's and child's senses of fairness and justice may be offended in ways that justify each one's insensitivity to the needs and feelings of the other.

In examining how this miscarriage of the helping process becomes established in some families with chronically ill children, we can discuss five somewhat arbitrary phases. First, the chronic illness is presented to the family at diagnosis as a shared problem, a "family affair." For many chronic childhood diseases there is an inherited component that contributes to initial parental feelings of guilt and responsibility. Second, fueled by sincere efforts to help and cope, parents often are shocked when they realize the toll that managing the illness and simultaneously fulfilling other parental roles and adult responsibilities has on their life. Third, the child also realizes, sooner or later, that the illness-related attention and support have a "darker" side—and that he or she sometimes feels coerced, intruded upon, and robbed of the autonomy to make the decisions that are in his or her own best interest.

The fourth phase occurs when issues other than health take over (i.e., when illness-related problems become reconstructed as relationship problems). As parents increase their expectations and focus more and more on the child's performance, all in the name of the "child's best interests," the child's need to master the illness becomes waylaid by feelings of lack of autonomy in the face of these increasing demands and expectations. Some older children who have successfully moved from doing things because their doctor or parent wanted them to, an external attribution, to a more internal attribution of taking care of themselves because they want to, may again revert to the earlier stance of choosing—or not choosing—adaptive behavior for its impact on their parents. Further, as parents and children suffer frustrations and setbacks a cycle of mutual distrust may set in, with the parents doubting their children's commitment to preserving their own well-being and the children doubting their parents' respect and concern for them. A growing divergence between parents and children in their perspective on what is taking place and why may preclude any efforts to resolve their differences by discussion or negotiation.

The endpoint of this miscarried helping process occurs when both parent and child have escalated their demands and resistance until the helping process has deteriorated. Parents rely heavily on what Patterson and Reid (1970) call *coercive control,* in which desired outcomes are achieved only by aggressive, threatening acts. And we know from the work of Patterson that this is a self-defeating posture, for the victories claimed are short-lived. The compliance or concessions that are obtained in the short term are at the expense of a decreasing receptivity and sense of cooperation. Moreover, parents may begin to perceive the child as "spiteful, uncooperative, and ungrateful." By attributing the problem to the child's character, the parent may feel relieved of any responsibility for the child's failure to comply with the treatment plan. At this point, the child uses resistance or incompetence in response to parental coercion in an effort to get the parent to lower the demands. The youngster may gain some sense of control from his or her successful efforts to frustrate the parent's demands and intrusions, to get them off his or her back. In the extreme the youngster may come to feel absolved of any need for self-responsibility, given the perception the parent is utterly unfair and unreasonable. Most often, neither parent nor child can see the situational and interactional factors that have debilitated their relationship and removed them from their original goals.

FACTORS AFFECTING MISCARRIED HELPING IN CHRONIC CHILDHOOD ILLNESS

Developmental Factors

Two sets of factors that may influence the likelihood of a miscarried helping process are developmental or age-related factors, and disease or treatment-related factors. When a very young child has a chronic physical illness, the parent is, in reality, the "patient." The helplessness and dependency of infants and preschool-aged children are magnified by the need for parents to monitor symptoms and to be responsible for complex, intrusive treatments. For many chronic diseases, during early childhood, parent involvement and cooperation are required in every area of the child's treatment. For example, with an illness that has a complex treatment regimen that involves many aspects of the child's behavior, such as insulin-dependent diabetes mellitus, parents of young children are responsible for around-the-clock monitoring of their child's behavior and physical symptoms and clinical decision making concerning therapy changes (e.g., insulin dosage; timing or amounts of food the child needs to eat). As clinical responsibilities for monitoring and maintaining life are transferred from physician to parents, parental vigilance is also prescribed. In summary, by definition, the parental role is intense, and high involvement is demanded during early childhood when a young child has a chronic disease.

Parental involvement in treatment is challenged when the child's skills and dependency needs shift at puberty. Across chronic childhood diseases, it has been shown that responsibilities for treatment shift gradually from parent to a shared status with the child during middle childhood, 8–11 years (McCollum, 1981). As youngsters normally acquire increased cognitive, physical, and interpersonal skills, they are more competent participants in the treatment process. At puberty, any parental involvement is frequently challenged. The transition from parent to child in responsibility for treatment increases abruptly during early adolescence, and young teenagers' needs for privacy, for peer acceptance, and for control sharply change the pattern of "shared" family responsibility for the disease and its treatment. Significant attention must be given to relearning the parental helping role during the adolescent years.

Illness and Treatment Factors

There are several illness and treatment factors that contribute to "miscarried helping" interactions. As suggested by Coyne et al. (1988), whenever ambiguity about treatment outcomes and reasons for treatment setbacks exist, family members are "set up" to consider the child's motivation and behavior as partly responsible when treatment fails. In many situations it is easier for parents and children to blame themselves or each other than it is for them to doubt the repeated assurances that they have received from medical personnel that the outcome is entirely dependent on what they do, and that if they do the right thing a positive outcome is assured. Too often such assurances set them up for the mutual accusations and recriminations when the inevitable crises occur that are best attributed to the imperfect tools and inadequate information with which they must confront their situation. Moreover, when the reasons for setbacks in the child's disease progress are ambiguous, as is the extent to which progress can be influenced by supportive efforts of the parent, the parent's desire to control the outcome reinvests them in the helping process and in achieving a successful outcome. For example, when 5-year-old Jason who has diabetes began consistently having high blood sugars at noon, his mother increased his home blood sugar monitoring to 8–10 times per day, despite Jason's protests over so many finger-sticks. Suggestions by health care professionals that she was overdoing the testing angered and offended Jason's mother, who felt she was doing what she could to try to understand and correct his worrisome high blood sugars.

A second and related illness factor affecting miscarried helping interactions concerns unrealistic assumptions that parents may develop that the child has more control over the disease course than is actually the case. With an illness such as IDDM in which treatment outcomes cannot be projected precisely, a climate is created in which unrealistic expectations flourish. In addition, when symptoms fluctuate or are ambiguously tied to the prescribed treatment regimen, the parent may assume that the diabetic child has control over the symptoms and may automatically blame the high blood sugar readings on the child's noncompliance. Furthermore, symptoms that are difficult to validate externally such as pain or depression, symptoms that frequently co-occur with a wide range of chronic childhood diseases, may lead to suspicion on the part of the parent that the child is exaggerating the problem.

A third disease-related factor that contributes to the evolution of miscarried helping in families is the unchanging, chronic nature of the child's situation that leaves many parents feeling drained and trapped. When the disease trajectory is prolonged and downward, as is often the case with chronic childhood illnesses, parents inevitably feel drained by their continuous investment in the process and trapped by the unending caregiving role they face. This frustration can lead the parent to focus more and more single-mindedly on the child's disease state. To relieve their own distress, parents may get more desperate in their efforts to insure a successful outcome for their child.

A final disease-related factor affecting "helping" with treatment tasks in families lies in the relationship of the parent and chronically ill child to the medical system. Too often what appears to be the neurotic concern of the parent or the stubbornness and self-destructiveness of the child is best understood in terms of the adequacy of their contact with the medical system. Too little attention is given to whether basic information has been provided, whether what has been said has been accurately heard by each family member, or how the sometimes abstract and vague admonitions of health care professionals are to be implemented realistically into daily routines within the family.

SUMMARY AND CONCLUSIONS

In conclusion, in this chapter we have argued for an interactional and situational approach for understanding parental helping that does not blame the parent or the child but looks at how the context of helping may interact with age-related and illness-related issues to create "miscarried helping" out of initially well-intentioned investment and helping behavior on the part of the parent. In the text, *Compliance: The Dilemma of the Chronically Ill,* Gervasio (1986) reports in her chapter on family relationships that most health practitioners "are only intuitively aware of the potential impact of the family on compliance" (p. 124). The next step is formulating "a well-integrated theoretical framework leading to specific and reliable treatments amenable to empirical research" (p. 124). As pointed out in the introduction of this chapter, the family and chronically ill children have been viewed from several different theoretical perspectives. However, the focus has never been on the development and impact of family interaction patterns concerning helping the child with treatment or compliance tasks. In contrast to these previous theoretical approaches, the "well-integrated theoretical framework" for compliance behavior in children and families called for by Gervasio must begin to appreciate that "helping the child with treatment tasks" has both an instrumental aspect, or *content,* as well as an expressive aspect, or larger *context* or framework around the helping interaction. The "miscarried helping" model discussed in this chapter has the potential *to identify successful helping efforts* in families and show how these impact over time on the motivation and compliance of the chronically ill child, as illustrated in the following case example:

B.J. was a bright, attractive 14-year-old girl with diabetes of 6 years duration, who until puberty had always had stable and excellent blood sugar levels. Recently, after months of poor blood sugar control, decreased energy, and increased school absences, all in the context of much extra blood sugar monitoring on the part of B.J. and her parents, their endocrinologist recommended that B.J. add an additional injection of insulin to her regimen to help stabilize her control and return to "feeling good again." B.J. was furious with her doctor's recommendation and refused to attempt another shot each day. The parents were equally furious with B.J. for resisting this professional advice and tried to pressure her to take the extra shot. The doctor left the decision up to B.J.

The parents became increasingly frustrated, escalated their pressures on B.J. to add the shot to her treatment plan (threatened with dating privileges, etc.). B.J. felt increasingly misunderstood, picked on, and controlled. The doctor finally suggested that they seek the help of a family therapist. Although the mother said that B.J. would just "spit at a therapist" or be ugly and rebellious, the mother and daughter after several more of increasing weeks of family conflict did sit with a therapist to review the problem.

The therapist met with mother and B.J. together and then with each separately. With very little effort the therapist was able to get B.J. to agree to try this change in her regimen for 3 weeks with no strings attached—if she did not feel better physically and feel that this extra shot was something she could "live with" after 3 weeks, B.J. could return to her current regimen. B.J.'s mother agreed to cease any discussion of the benefits or importance of an additional shot and promised not to discuss this topic in the next 3 weeks. The therapist advised the parents that there was a risk involved in this approach—that B.J. might still not make the choice they wanted her to. However, it was the only path by which B.J. could experience any choice and potential positive benefit from the added burden of treatment.

After 3 weeks (and now after 6 months), B.J. did feel better and did have more energy with this more complex regimen and was agreeable to making the recommended changes. B.J.'s mother and father are relieved and are able to see now that their concern and pressure removed their daughter's focus from the issue of her own health to the issue of her autonomy.

The Miscarried Helping Theory addresses the reality that parents with chronically ill children are faced with two sometimes conflicting sets of tasks: first, taking responsibility for implementing a regimen at home and warding off the immediate threat of medical crises; and second, establishing a context in which the child takes developmentally appropriate strides in assuming self-responsibility. In meeting the first set of tasks, particularly when driven by a sense of urgency and impending disaster or not adequately informed about their limits of influence over the disease, the child may be seen as an object or obstacle. The parent may resort to coercive or hostile–critical responses that achieve immediate compliance but make it more difficult to achieve compliance in the long run or to develop the child's self-responsibility. Baron (1988) has discussed how destructive hostile criticism can be in families:

> Criticism leaves recipients feeling badly not only about themselves, but about the providers of criticism. It can derail efforts at problem-solving and reconciliation. Once introduced into an ongoing disagreement, hostile criticism and the resulting rebuttals and counter-accusations can replace what has been the topic at hand. Such criticism serves to initiate or intensify conflict and strengthen patterns of avoidance or defiance. More generally, destructive criticism increases family members' reliance on ineffective ways of dealing with their conflicts and negative feelings. (p. 199)

The Miscarried Helping theory clarifies how parental hostility and criticism can evolve out of initially well-intentioned behavior to help the child and directly addresses issues of how and when to intervene in compliance struggles in families.

REFERENCES

Baron, R. A. (1988). Negative effects of destructive criticism: Impact on conflict, self-efficacy, and task performance. *Journal of Applied Psychology, 73,* 199–207.

Coyne, J. C., & Anderson, B. J. (1988). The "Psychosomatic Family" reconsidered: Diabetes in context. *Journal of Marital and Family Therapy, 14*(2), 113–123.

Coyne, J. C., & Anderson, B. J. (1989). The "Psychosomatic Family" reconsidered II: Recalling a defective model and looking ahead. *Journal of Marital and Family Therapy, 15*(2), 139–148.

Coyne, J. C., Wortman, C. B., & Lehman, D. R. (1988). The other side of support: Emotional overinvolvement and miscarried helping. In B. Gottlieb (Ed.), *Social support: Formats, processes, and effects* (pp. 305–33). New York: Sage.

Fiske, V., Coyne, J. C., & Smith, D. A. F. (in press). Couples coping with myocardial infarction: An empirical reconsideration of the role of overprotectiveness. *Journal of Family Psychology.*

Gervasio, A. H. (1986). Family relationships and compliance. In K. E. Gerber & A. M. Nehemkis (Eds.), *Compliance: The dilemma of the chronically ill* (pp. 98–127). New York: Springer.

Gillis, C. L. (1984). Reducing family stress during and after coronary artery bypass surgery. *Nursing Clinics of North America, 19,* 1103–1111.

McCollum, A. (1981). *The chronically ill child.* New Haven, CT: Yale University Press.

McCubbin, M. A., & McCubbin, H. I. (1988). Family stress theory and assessment. In H. I. McCubbin & A. I. Thompson (Eds.), *Family assessment inventories for research and practice* (pp. 3–34). Madison: University of Wisconsin.

Minuchin, S., Rosman, B. L., & Baker, L. (1978). *Psychosomatic families: Anorexia nervosa in context.* Cambridge, MA: Harvard University Press.

Patterson, G. R., & Reid, J. B. (1970). Reciprocity and coercion: Two facets of social systems. In C. Neuringer & J. Michael (Eds.), *Behavior modification in clinical psychology* (pp. 274–306). New York: Appleton–Century–Croft.

Patterson, J. M. (1989). A family stress model: The family adjustment and adaptation response. In C. N. Ramsey (Ed.), *Family systems in medicine* (pp. 95–118). New York: Guilford Press.

Pless, I. B., & Pinkerton, P. (1975). *Chronic childhood disorder: Promoting patterns of adjustment.* New York: Year Book Medical Publishers.

Ransom, D. C. (1989). Development of family therapy and family theory. In C. N. Ramsey (Ed.), *Family systems in medicine* (pp. 18–35). New York: Guilford Press.

Sabbath, B. (1984). Understanding the impact of chronic childhood illness on families. *Pediatric Clinics of No. America, 31*(1), 47–58.

5 Theories of Compliance, and Turning Necessities Into Preferences: Application to Adolescent Health Action

Howard Leventhal
Rutgers—The State University of New Jersey

The first part of this chapter presents a synopsis of the history of compliance theory and reviews key findings in several of the areas in which compliance research has flourished. My objective in conducting this review is to identify successes and failures of prior and current research programs and to highlight the theoretical additions and instrumental actions already taken to overcome the failures. As the great majority of studies have been conducted with adults, the data does not focus on special features of compliance for adolescents, nor do the data provide one with a developmental view of compliance problems. The review does, however, set the stage for Part two in which I present a self-regulation view of treatment adherence. Self-regulation models represent a significant step away from the "normative," authoritarian framework implicit in the definition of compliance and provide an effective framework both for the analysis of compliance among adolescents and for a life-span perspective on compliance/adherence problems. Within the self-regulatory framework I address the specific issue of converting necessities, acts that one must do, into preferences, or acts that one wishes or has an urge to do. Finally, I close with a brief discussion regarding the application of these ideas to health actions in adolescents and their implications for a life-span perspective on compliance/adherence issues.

THE HISTORY OF COMPLIANCE RESEARCH

Compliance is a word that appears to have defined a complete theory of behavior and generated a substantial body of empirical research. Psychological theory suggests that we can compute a match between prescribed standards for health-promotive (and health-damaging) behavior and actual or observed behaviors of patients (Sackett & Haynes, 1976). Sociological theory, on the other hand, suggests that compliance represents an hierarchical social system in which the practitioners' role is to provide accurate diagnoses and treatment regimens, and the patients' role is to listen and follow instructions (Leventhal, Zimmerman, & Gutmann, 1984; Stimson, 1974).

There are at least two distinct negative aspects to viewing the practitioner/patient relationship in terms of compliance, or prescribed actions the patient "must do." First, the link between adherence and outcome is uncertain. As can be seen by examining the diagonal defined by cells b and c of Fig. 5.1, nonadherence may be medically advantageous when diagnosis and prescription are less than optimal (cell b), and patients often get better without treatment (cell c). Second, even when a diagnosis is correct and the medical regimen is appropriate, the patient may find it difficult or impossible to execute the desirable behavior in his or her environment. Thus, the patient's life situation can be as important as the facts of the disease in determining the possibility for adherence. At the very least, therefore, the matrix suggest that treatment may be improved if the physician tries to identify the problems patients may have in performing prescribed regimens and takes into account the patients' observations regarding treatment outcomes, modifying the regimens to facilitate performance and alleviate negative effects. Medical sociologists and psychiatrists (Szasz & Hollander, 1956) have instead substituted a less authoritarian term, adherence, for the term, compliance, with the hope that a more productive view of the practitioner/patient relationship would emerge.

In sum, the conceptual shift from compliance to adherence represented an important first step in moving away from models emphasizing obedience to instructions toward models emphasizing the independence, or self-regulatory activity, of the patient. The adherence concept did not, however, identify specific features of the environment and the person that might be involved in the process of active participation in diagnosis and treatment. Thus, there was continued

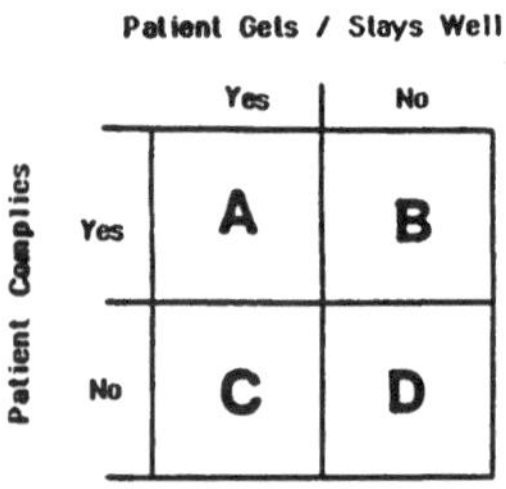

FIG. 5.1. Outcomes represented by cells A (adhere & get well) and D (nonadherent and remain ill) provide information that support becoming and remaining adherent. Experiences matching cells B and C, common during illness episodes, contradict becoming and remaining adherent. After Sackett & Haynes (1976).

	Patient Gets / Stays Well	
Patient Complies	Yes	No
Yes	A	B
No	C	D

pressure to elaborate behavioral models to better understand the adherence process and improve health outcomes.

Synopsis of Existent Models of Patient Adherence

Personality and Situational Hypotheses. Early compliance research attempted to identify patient characteristics that might be associated with compliance or noncompliance (Leventhal, Meyer, & Gutmann, 1980). This atheoretical search was driven by the assumption that patients failed to comply with medical prescriptions because they were resistant or incompetent. Failure to comply was the fault of the patient, and blaming the patient probably was a natural consequence of regarding treatment as necessary and beneficial.

Given the extraordinarily high estimates of rates of noncompliance, 20% to 80% depending on the regimen and/or study (Sackett & Snow, 1979), it is no surprise that studies failed to reveal a characteristic personality pattern of the noncompliant patient. Consequently, some practitioners re-examined the adherence problem and reframed it as a situational rather than a personal problem, a step that led them to introduce changes in the *situations* in which noncompliance occurred. For example, Finnerty, Shaw, and Himmelsbach (1973) introduced individualized appointments to the patients using their inner city clinic rather than assigning them a common appointment time and observed a dramatic increase in compliance, failures to keep appointments declining from over 50% to under 5%. Alderman and Schoenbaum's (1975) innovative work-site hypertension clinic reflected a similar approach to enhancing adherence by bringing screening and treatment to the patient. When the target is a complex health behavior such as weight change or smoking cessation, situational changes have not produced the same impressive outcomes. This limitation aside, the concern with situations has been of clear benefit as it encouraged investigators and practitioners to focus upon specific, observable actions and encouraged the application of behavioral models to adherence problems. At least two broad classes of behavioral models that have been influential in the compliance arena, operant and cognitive, merit discussion.

Operant Behavioral Models. Operant models focus on the environmental stimuli or cues that elicit behavior, the rewards that reinforce the behavior, the gradual shaping or patterning of behavior, and its automation with repetition (see Henderson, Hall, & Lipton, 1979, for a review). Behavioral cues include reminders, follow-up phone calls, and booster sessions and rewards ranging over all types of incentives including social approbation for the "correct" response. An intriguing application of this Skinnerian approach can be seen in Wooley, Blackwell, and Winget's (1978) development of a total, in-hospital, environment for the treatment of chronic illness behavior. The ward staff was trained to ignore patient complaints about physical problems and to respond to patients only when they talked about daily activities such as socializing, taking a walk, and so on. Marked reductions occurred in illness behaviors during hospitalization, and these changes were maintained in the patient's home environments if the family sustained the same reward structure as received in the hospital.

There is an important aside to the preceding study. Prior to its conduct, the investigators instructed patients to deliver rewards (tokens) to staff persons or visitors whenever that person discussed a topic the patient found of interest. The data generated in this preliminary study were clear in showing that patients preferred inquiries and conversations that focused on their purported (and medically unsubstantiated) ills. In short, the investigators used a simple phenomenological approach to establish that the existent reward system favored the discussion of illness behavior. Thus, whereas radical behaviorism motivated the construction of the controlled environment, the investigators used a cognitive or phenomenological method to identify reinforcers and to instantiate the environment (see, Locke, 1971).

Cognitive Behavioral Models. At least two factors were important for the development of cognitive behavioral models. First, the great majority of adherence problems cannot be resolved by creating special environments to control schedules of reinforcements. Second, conscious self-appraisal and verbal report play a central role in human social behavior, and they play a key role in establishing the focus for the controlled environment just described. Given these facts, it was natural for investigators and practitioners to reach for models that would help them construct and assess techniques for behavioral changes based on linguistic and pictorial communication.

Three classes of cognitive-behavioral analysis emerged, each of which offers a rich array of procedures for research and practice. The first, *communication models,* focuses on the steps (McGuire, 1985) from message generation through reception, comprehension, retention, acceptance (attitude change) to compliance in action and the processes underlying movement along these steps. For example, the movement from attitude to action requires messages that create motivation to act and messages that generate plans that define where, when (cues for action), and how actions can be performed (Leventhal, 1970; see also Fazio, 1986). These models have had their major impact upon media programs in the public health arena and in the development of educational materials for use in clinical practice settings (Ley, 1977).

The second, *social learning* models, posits that learning is a product of "pictorial and verbal" communications that occur during actual performance and/or the observation of others (Bandura, 1969), and that performance depends on the individual's belief in his or her ability (self-efficacy) to perform the promotive behavior that he or she has practiced and/or observed (Bandura, 1977). The approach has been influential in promoting research on prevention of risk behaviors such as cigarette smoking (Flay, 1985; Flay & Cook, 1981) and adherence to regimens prescribed for recovery from serious chronic disease.

The third set, *cognitive/decision models*, includes the health belief model and the reasoned action model. The former, developed in the 1950s (Hochbaum, 1958; Rosenstock, 1974; Rosenstock, Hochbaum, & Leventhal, 1960), applies a normative decision model to preventive and treatment behavior (Becker, 1974; Becker & Maiman, 1975). Motivation for health action is hypothesized to be a product of perceived vulnerability (the probability of a negative outcome) and perceived severity (utility) of a health threat, and the selection and performance of a specific response is a function of the costs and benefits of each of the actions available for coping with the perceived threat. The model has been used to account for adherence to a wide range of both preventive and treatment behaviors (Janz & Becker, 1984).

The reasoned action model's emphasis on conscious intention and behavioral norms distinguishes it from the health belief model. It assumes that behavior is a product of a conscious intention or decision to act, and that intentions are a product of the perceived instrumentality or the association of a specific action with the individual's values (Fishbein & Ajzen, 1975). The reasoned action model also emphasizes normative perceptions, that is, the individual's belief respecting the attitude of important reference groups toward the specific action.

The preceding models have tended to produce nonoverlapping bodies of empirical research. For example, the literature for social learning theory tends to be separate from that of communication theory, as the former developed from the application of learning theory to clinical and personality psychology and focused the investigators on developing skills for the performance of specific responses. Communication theory, on the other hand, originated in social psychology (Hovland, Janis, & Kelley, 1953) and focused investigators on informational factors involved in altering attitudes, values, and motives (Petty & Cacioppo, 1986) and has been less attentive to skill development.

Domains of Adherence Research

How have the aforementioned theories fared in attempting to account for and influence adherence to health promotive and treatment behaviors? Research on these issues falls into three broad domains: prevention, treatment, and rehabilitation (e.g., Sackett & Haynes, 1976; Sackett & Snow, 1979), and each domain can be further subdivided with respect to the specific diseases, the particular behaviors associated with these diseases (see Table 5.1), and changes in these behaviors over the natural history of each disease. For example, the treatment of a cardiac problem such as hypertension requires a number of behaviors, each of which can be seen as a target to measure adherence, for example, keeping medical appointments, medication use (e.g., diuretics, beta-blockers), and

TABLE 5.1
Prevention and Treatment of Disease by Reducing Risk Behaviors and Increasing Health Behaviors

Prevention Risk Behaviors	Diseases				
	CHD	Stroke	Cancer	Diabetes	Hypertension
Quit Smoking	X	X	X		X
Weight loss	X	X		X	X
Exercise	X			?	X
High Fiber Diet			X		
Treatment Regimens and Measures					
Appointment keeping	X	X	X	X	
Beta blockers	X	X			X
Insulin				X	
Weight loss	X			X	X
Surgery	?		X		
Noxious medication			X	X	

weight loss, etc. Although adherence at an early point (e.g., appointment keeping) is a necessary antecedent to later steps such as medication adherence, it does not insure adherence to the later criterion.

Adherence issues may also differ for acute and chronic illnesses. Indeed, one suspects that no single theory will be adequate to address the various problems that emerge given the multiple dimensions defining the adherence domain, though a single model may go far toward resolving these problems if its variables are convincingly related to the different cells of this multidimensional matrix. The definition of the dimensions for such a matrix is a demanding task that calls for a well thought out taxonomy of adherence responses and the context in which they occur.

Outcomes. Three of the many conclusions that can be drawn from the vast array of adherence studies merit special attention. First, adherence is clearly a multivariate problem; many factors affect it and different factors may affect adherence for different behaviors. Indeed, even when we confine our view to data for the domain of a single disease, we may find inconsistency in adherence as we move from one dependent variable to another, for example, from appointment keeping to medication taking.

Second, many studies show that behavioral approaches are highly successful in producing initial change, for example, in getting people to quit smoking and/or lose weight (Leventhal, Baker, Brandon, & Fleming, 1989; Leventhal & Cleary, 1980; Leventhal, Zimmerman, & Guttmann, 1984). In general, behavioral change is far more likely with behavioral than with communication approaches. This may reflect the greater intensity of contact between behavior therapist (i.e., communicator) and subject for behavioral interventions and the focus of behavioral interventions on specific responses.

Third, regardless of the specific action targeted for change, and regardless of the intervention procedure, virtually all studies report a sharp decline in adherence subsequent to initial, high levels of success. For example, at the end of an intensive behavioral intervention, it is not unusual to find 90% to 100% of individuals quitting smoking, stopping drinking, losing weight, or taking medication as prescribed, the percentage adherent dropping to the 30% to 50% range 3 to 6 months and to 15% to 30% 1-year postprogram. The 20-year-old curves published by Hunt and Matarazzo (1973) still provide a reasonably accurate summary of adherence over the long term (see Fig. 5.2).

Response to Failures. Failure to maintain change has clearly been the major deficit of behavioral interventions, and efforts to overcome this deficit a major focus of research. Investigators have examined the effects of environmental cues and reinforcers such as reminder phone calls and booster sessions in an effort to overcome this deficit. Recent efforts focusing on social support via buddy systems, spousal involvement, and so forth, to provide stable cues and rewards for the maintenance of healthful action have unfortunately shown minimal to no benefit (Cohen et al., 1988).

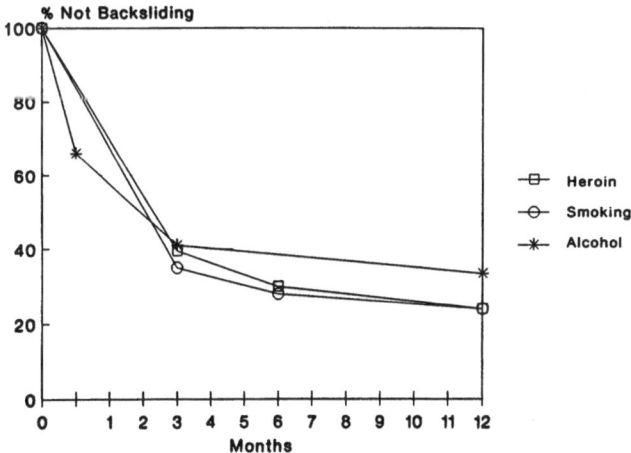

FIG. 5.2. Proportion of participants remaining in withdrawal following cessation of smoking and the use of alcohol and heroin. From Hunt and Materazzo (1973).

In an innovative effort to deal with the apparent "collapse of will" and the return to addictive smoking and/or drinking following a lapse in a newly acquired abstinence pattern, Marlatt and Gordon (1980) formulated the concept of the abstinence violation effect. This concept refers to the sense of despair and guilt that can follow a lapse and undermine the individual's sense of self-efficacy. Lapses are common when the individual is unprepared to anticipate, recognize, and cope with the urges to eat and/or smoke that are stimulated by both internal and external cues. To avoid such setbacks, behavioral counseling was developed that incorporated self-monitoring and coping skills training to help individuals to recognize and cope with threat cues and deal with the regulation of their own emotional responses to lapses (Curry, Marlatt, & Gordon, 1987). One way to ameliorate the guilt and despair of a lapse is to prepare people for setbacks; by making lapses seem commonplace, we might prevent attributions of weakness to the self. This may entail some risk, however, as the preparation may be permissive of and/or encourage lapses. Early results are only moderately promising (Curry, Marlatt, Gordon, & Baer, 1988).

Components Essential For Prior Successes

At this point in time it seems fair to conclude that the very great majority of studies testing behavioral strategies show effective maintenance of behavioral change for 6 months to 1-year postintervention, with an occasional study showing strong effects at 1-year and moderate effects at 2-year follow-ups (Stunkard, Craighead, & O'Brien, 1980; Tiffany & Baker, 1988). Whereas this conclusion may seem overly negative, it can serve a positive function if it leads to a careful re-examination of our basic goals and theoretical constructs and discourages the blind repetition of studies that do nothing more than use the same intervention strategies with somewhat more elegant experimental designs and more precise methods to measure outcomes. If we trust the talents and integrity of our colleagues, as we should, there is little reason to expect extraordinary gain from minimal improvements on what has been already done. This clearly appears to be the case in studies of smoking prevention in schoolchildren (see Flay, 1985; Leventhal et al., 1989). This is not to say that we should denigrate or ignore prior successes. Both communication and behavioral strategies produced substantial short-term behavioral changes in different contexts. A careful examination of the conditions associated with these successes may help us to move forward and resolve the maintenance problem.

Motives, Skills, and Appraisals. The examination of models and empirical literature we have discussed brings us to focus on two broad sets of factors: *motivational variables* responsible for the desire to adopt healthy behaviors and stop health-damaging ones, and *skill factors* responsible for the selection and execution of specific responses. The importance of the combining factors from both sets was seen with clarity in early studies of the impact of fear communications upon health action (Leventhal, 1979; Leventhal, Singer, & Jones, 1965) which showed that a motivating threat message was necessary but not sufficient for the occurrence of a behavioral change such as taking a tetanus inoculation or quitting smoking. To go beyond attitude change, that is, to elicit action as well as to convince people that protective action is good and smoking is bad, it was necessary to include an action plan along with the threat message. The plan spelled out the necessary sequence of behaviors for successful action, asked the recipient to review his daily routine and locate a place in that routine to incorporate the action, and then asked for a decision to act. Thus, both a threat message and a plan were necessary for a behavioral effect, but the intensity of the threat seemed of little consequence.

A similar picture emerged from studies of smoking cessation. Both rapid smoking or rapid puffing were necessary for change, that is, they were used to condition or establish a motive for cessation (Tiffany, Martin, & Baker, 1986), but neither was sufficient. A complex counselling package consisting of identification of threats to cessation and coping strategies for threat management was necessary to maintain the change beyond the initial months, though it too was insufficient to promote quitting.

Data from both the communication and therapy paradigms also converge in identifying a third factor, the individual's *appraisal of outcomes,* for the maintenance of behavioral change. Sustained change seems more likely when lapses are attributed to external factors and successful management is attributed to personal skill and competence (Abramson, Seligman, & Teasdale, 1978; Curry, Marlatt, & Gordon, 1987; Rosen, Terry, & Leventhal, 1982). Lack of knowledge respecting what is an appropriate outcome may lead to inappropriate attributions and undermine the maintenance of effective change. For example, patients who are following a diet and shedding 2 pounds a week to control their blood pressure may be doing very well by medical standards but regard themselves as failing if they expect to lose 5 or more pounds a week and have not been told how rapidly they can and should lose weight. Failure to detect and modify this inaccurate appraisal could lead to treatment termination.

Regulating the External and Internal (Feelings) Environment. Finally, it is clear that failure to adhere to recommended health promotive practices may reflect inability to manage feelings of anxiety and distress. These feelings may be evoked by negative life events, by efforts to stop a health risk behavior such as smoking (Leventhal & Watts, 1966), or by feelings of distress and guilt evoked by lapses in successful control of a health risk behavior such as smoking (Marlatt & Gordon, 1980). Bolstering the individual's belief in his or her ability to manage feelings may allow him or her to undertake health-promotive actions (Rosen, Terry, & Leventhal, 1982). A pharmacologic intervention such as the nicotine patch may be an important step in this direction.

Sustained Motivation: A Missing Ingredient

In my judgment, investigators have given too little attention to the maintenance of motivation for change and have put too much emphasis on lack of self-efficacy and behavioral skills to account for maintenance failures. This is particularly true when one examines the development and maintenance of healthy behaviors and the avoidance of risky behaviors by adolescents, as the rapid changes in biological and psychological development during adolescence lead to major shifts in motivation and interest in continuing health activities. Marlatt and Gordon's (1980) effort to control the abstinence violation effect is an exception.

Two types of data on smoking cessation support the need to focus on motivation. The first is the great advantage in the magnitude of observed quitting achieved via behavioral therapies in comparison to the effect observed after antismoking communications. Whereas the therapies clearly have an advantage in intensity of client contact, a potentially more important advantage is that therapy is conducted with volunteers who want to quit. Studies of antismoking communications typically present their messages to audiences of randomly selected smokers many of whom may have little or no desire to quit, that is, they are at a different stage or mental "set" respecting quitting (Prochaska & DiClemente, 1983).

The second set of data is from studies of physician-based smoking interventions. A meta analysis by Kottke, Battista, De Frieses, and Brekke (1988) shows that physician interventions produce on average a very modest increase in cessation, in intervention groups relative to controls, for example, 12% versus 7.5%. A careful examination of these studies reveal, however, a very much higher range of success rates, for example, a 20% to 40% or more, when the trial is conducted on patients with significant pulmonary or cardiac disease (Ockene, 1987; Pederson, 1982). Those suffering from illness are more receptive to the intervention.

Both the sizable effects seen with volunteers and the physically ill point to the importance of the individual's prior motivational state for achieving change. The knowledge that one is at risk and the emotions associated with this knowledge are likely to be the key factors involved in producing the sizable effects seen in both cases. That one can make use of individual motivation in developing a health-promotive intervention is seen in a final example drawn from studies of the prevention of smoking in schoolchildren. Most studies (e.g., Best et al., 1984; Botvin et al., 1990; Botvin, Renick, & Baker, 1983; Murray, Leupker, Johnson, & Mittelmark, 1984) in this area show a small-to-modest-sized effect in preventing the onset of smoking for adolescents exposed to experimental programs teaching skills for coping with peer pressures in comparison to adolescents in control conditions. These effects require, however, very intense exposure, the experimental programs using as many as 20 or more classroom sessions during an initial program year and as many as 5 to 8 booster sessions in subsequent years. By contrast, exposure to but 3 sessions of antismoking information designed to enhance existent *personal motives* for avoiding smoking showed a moderate reduction in rates of recruitment to smoking among 7th- and 8th-grade students 18 months after the program (Leventhal et al.). Although the program was unsuccessful in achieving longer term changes, as was the case with prior efforts, the 18-month data encourage a closer look at efforts to connect the antismoking message to *personal motivation*. To connect the antismoking message to the individual's existent motivational system, we asked our young participants to tell us about earlier, personal life experiences, such as the times they had ignored warnings and regretted doing so, and drew a clear parallel between these prior experiences and smoking (e.g., ignoring warnings such as the coughing and burning in initial smoking allows people to become addicted). Although it is unclear if the life skills training used by Botvin and his colleagues includes precisely this motivational component, I suspect it has similar effects. The findings also reinforce the idea that the type of exposure and not the mere amount may be critical for achieving effects.

The general point is that few adherence interventions have been preceded by a detailed examination of the personal knowledge base of their subjects and then proceeded to design their intervention to influence this knowledge base. Specifically, most studies ignore what people know and feel about themselves and about specific health threats, although this knowledge generates the motives that drive the skills needed to minimize risk. In addition, behavioral investigators have been slow to pay attention to the biological and social factors underlying the behaviors they wish to change or bring into being. This should be no surprise, as behavioral theories suggest one can use the same change procedures for all responses ignoring differences between behaviors and individuals, though it is well known that behavioral cues and reinforcers do not fall upon or stimulate an empty organism.

A SELF-REGULATION FRAMEWORK FOR ADHERENCE

In a search for new approaches to resolve the maintenance problem, a number of investigators are recasting the adherence problem in a *self-regulation framework*. Self-regulation models treat individuals as actively involved in attempts to reduce gaps between their perceived current status and immediate and longer term goals (Carver & Scheier, 1981; Kanfer, 1977; Lazarus & Folkman, 1984; Lazarus & Launier, 1978; Leventhal, 1970, Leventhal, Meyer, & Nerenz, 1980, Leventhal & Nerenz, 1983; Powers, 1973). As developed in the current area, these models postulate that health and illness behaviors reflect the individual's representation of current or anticipated health threats, and perceptions of the relevance of

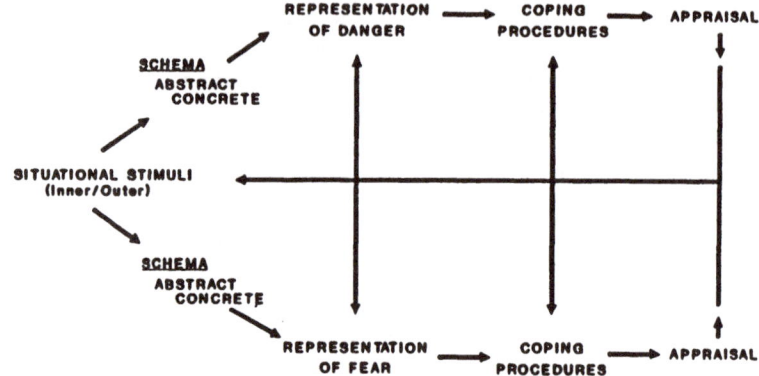

FIG. 5.3. Parallel Processing Model for adaptation to health threats: Internal and external stimuli make contact with and are processed elaborated upon by both conceptual (abstract) and concrete (perceptual) memory schemata to form representations (experience) of both disease threats (danger) and emotion (fear). The features of these representations initiate and shape procedures for coping. The effects of coping upon the representations are appraised in relation to expectations about the effectiveness of the coping response and the nature of the representation (e.g., is the symptom a sign of a transient or a serious, chronic condition). Appraisals feed back and update the representation, changing, for example, the identity of the problem, its controllability, etc., and changing expectations respecting the effectiveness of the coping procedure. Not shown but also appraised is the individual's perception of his effectiveness in performing these actions, and his perceptions of the effectiveness of his support (expert and nonexpert) system.

particular actions for managing or controlling these threats. Whereas these models conceptualize adherence issues from the perspective of the patient/subject, they also provide a framework for integrating cognitive and behavioral concepts.

Figure 5.3 presents a simple, self-regulation model developed by our group. Five characteristics of the model deserve comment:

1. It postulates a multicomponent, *interacting system* underlying the production of behavior.

2. The *interpretation* or *processing* of stimuli generates multiattribute representations of both health threats and treatments. Representations are generated by a multilevel processing system that is both abstract or propositional and concrete or experiential. For example, the act of smoking by someone who wishes to quit may generate abstract ideas about health risks and conflicting concrete experiences of reward from increased relaxation and mental alertness.

3. As the attributes of representations define the *goals* or *reference values* that are the targets for behavioral regulation, it is clear that both the choice of behavioral procedure and its execution are guided or shaped by the representation.

4. The *appraisal* of coping outcomes involves the ongoing monitoring of the gap between various reference values and perceived outcomes. This monitoring or check process generates assessments of the adequacy of specific actions, the appraisal of self-competence in executing these actions, the accuracy of the representation, and assessments of various contextual factors including features of the self and the support system. Representations, for example, their identity or label, time-lines, etc., are constantly being updated and changed in light of new evidence generated by the individual's acts to control and/or alter the experience of a current illness or protect against a prospective illness threat.

5. The information system is *hierarchically* structured in two ways. The first such hierarchy concerns the nesting of the problem-solving components, that is, the representation, coping, and appraisal processes in a contextual framework formed by cultural and institutional factors and by various aspects of the individual's self-system. For example, a middle-aged male's adaptation to a coronary infarction will be guided by his representation of this disease (i.e., its symptoms, presumed temporal course, imagined consequences, etc.) and his representation and procedures for managing its treatment. These factors are nested under his self-concept that may include a myriad of beliefs such as ideas about his hardiness and ability to resist disease, and beliefs about his ability to tolerate pain and distress and participate in rehabilitative exercise programs. If he discovers that several genetically related family members suffered serious coronary disease and early death from smoking, he may perceive himself at high risk of a second infarction and sudden death, a perception that may motivate him to quit smoking and to find a variety of preventive measures more attractive. His view of the disease will also be shaped by his experiences with health care institutions and their perceived ability to treat coronary disease. If these institutions ignore prevention and focus on medication and cure, he is likely to treat coronary disease as though it were another acute illness.

In summary, the self-regulation perspective construes the individual as actively constructing a representation of illness threats that establishes and sustains remote and proximal goals that guide coping and establish criteria for the evaluation of coping success. Second, the representation and coping procedures are influenced by ideas about the self and environmental resources. Changes in the environment and the self-system can alter the representation, emotional reactions, coping procedures, and appraisals related to a disease threat. The net result will be changes in motivation to avoid risk and or promote health, and changes in the perceived effectiveness of specific behaviors selected to meet these goals. It is my belief that strides will be made toward resolving the maintenance problem when we have a deeper understanding of two sets of complex interactions: (a) those between the individual's declarative (representations) and procedural knowledge (coping and appraisal) and (b) those between the declarative and procedural knowledge systems relevant to the health threat, and the way these cognitions and skills are sustained by the cultural, social, and self-systems. The changing self and social context of adolescence creates fascinating and difficult to manage problems for teaching the avoidance of risky behaviors and adherence to healthy ones.

Self-Regulation and Adherence to Medication Regimens

Before addressing the complex relationship between context and the representational processes involved in self-regulation, it is necessary to show how a self-regulation model describes the process of adherence to treatment. To do this, I briefly describe findings of studies on the way representations affect adherence to medication for hypertension and diabetes.

Commonsense Representations of Illnesses. Interviews of individuals with chronic high blood pressure revealed a major discrepancy between their medical and personal knowledge of its symptomatology (Meyer, Leventhal, & Gutmann, 1985). As an example, 80% of a group of 50 patients in treatment for high blood pressure agreed that hypertension is asymptomatic, but later in the very same interview, 92% of these respondents mentioned various somatic signs (palpitations, headache, face flushing) that allowed them to tell when their own blood pressure was elevated. The discrepancy between their asymptomatic medical view and their symptomatic personal one bothered them not at all, though many spontaneously suggested the interviewer should not pass on this information to their physicians. Moreover, patients who believed treatment had a beneficial effect on their symptoms were less likely to miss medications and were in better blood pressure control. Thus, contrary to their abstract knowledge that blood pressure is asymptomatic, concrete symptom experiences served as markers of high blood pressure, and changes in these experiences were used to evaluate treatment.

The preceding effect was replicated in a second group of 65 newly treated patients. At their first treatment visit, only 71% of these individuals believed they could monitor their blood pressure symptomatically, a figure that increased to 92% six months later. In addition, those patients who monitored their symptoms were more likely to drop out of treatment 6 months later than were patients who did not monitor (43% vs. 21%). And patients who reported telling their doctor about their symptoms at the initial visit dropped out at a much higher rate than did patients who did not report making this communication (61% vs. 24%). It is likely that the discrepancy between patient and practitioner, the former believing that symptoms were indicators of blood pressure, the latter not, may account for the high dropout rates among the symptom communicators. Patients new to treatment were also very likely to drop out if they believed hypertension was an acute rather than a chronic condition (58% vs. 17%).

The behavior of hypertensives as just described would be adaptive if the symptoms they reported were related to their blood pressure. Computation of the association between blood pressures and symptoms both across persons and within persons over time suggests there is little or no linkage between pressure and symptoms. For example, the average correlations between the presence of various symptoms and blood pressure in the Meyer et al. (1985) study ranged between $-.08$ and $+.11$. Correlations computed within subjects over multiple points in time are not more encouraging. Data from employees of a large insurance company (Baumann & Leventhal, 1985) and from students in a laboratory study (Pennebaker & Watson, 1988) also show that subjects judge their blood pressure to be elevated when they are symptomatic, but both symptoms and judgments are unrelated to objective indicators of pressure. A strong relationship can be obtained between symptom experiences and pressure by placing the subject in a situation that induces elevations in both, for example, intensive exercise (Pennebaker & Watson, 1988), but it appears to be maladaptive to use symptoms as indicators of blood pressure elevation and as guides to treatment in the typical workday environment.

Studies of insulin use by diabetics confirm the hypothesis that highly personal symptomatic views of illness serve as guides to treatment adherence. Because mild to moderate hyperglycemia may generate pleasant sensations whereas mild to moderate hypoglycemia can generate dysphoria and other unpleasant subjective signs, patients may regulate insulin use to achieve a positive affective balance (Gonder-Frederick & Cox, 1991). Self-regulation designed to achieve a positive affect balance may put the diabetic at risk for serious complications.

The findings for diabetics and hypertensives strongly suggest that symptoms and illness threats generally tend to be assimilated into and interpreted within an acute disease framework. As our language suggests, noxious symptoms and emotional distress is very likely to be seen as an indicator of dis-ease, and we expect treatments to ameliorate symptoms and the underlying condition. Moreover, we expect beneficial effects within a limited time frame and judge treatments effective if they meet these implicit criteria. The interpretation or assimilation of new illness episodes to an underlying acute illness schema may also be reinforced by the reassuring nature of such an interpretation, that is, it implies that the episode is benign and self-limiting (Cioffi, 1991). Croyle and Jemmott (1991) have amassed a considerable body of data suggesting that individuals are cognitively biased to minimize the apparent severity of health threats. This bias may interfere with or facilitate adherence to recommended regimens depending on the specific disease and treatment at issue.

Self-Regulation and Practitioner Communication. The behavioral consequences of the misattribution of somatic symptoms to hypertension and the misinterpretation of the somatic sensations of hyperglycemia as signs of well-being make clear that the representation of disease and treatment can have important effects upon adherence. As many biological processes lack clear somatic signs, the individual's formulation of these processes will be of critical importance for their behavior. Preparing people to accurately interpret somatic experiences will be an important part of both treatment and preventive practices and a critical addition to current educational practices that appear to focus on providing information about underlying disease processes, the medications needed for treatment, and very general behavioral advice (e.g., lose weight and/or quit smoking) for prevention. In the absence of information for the appropriate interpretation of concrete somatic experiences, the fundamental assumption that one is ill when one feels somatic distress and well when one does not will likely override the abstract information provided in treatment protocols and result in deterioration of adherence when the two types of information are in conflict.

The need for information to guide interpretations of both disease and treatment outcomes was made abundantly clear in an audit of tape-recorded interactions between patients new to hypertensive treatment and their practitioners. In virtually none of these tapes did we hear a practitioner provide clear expectations regarding either the magnitude or the time-line for treatment-induced changes. In the one case where such information was exchanged, the patient who was losing 1 to 2 pounds per week expressed distress at the poor results of her efforts at dieting and asked to abandon treatment because she was not losing 5 or more pounds per week. Had she not expressed distress at her rate of weight loss and failed to be reassured by her physician that 1 to 2 pounds per week was the right amount to lose, she might have abandoned treatment. The inappropriateness of the patient's expectations should come as no surprise given that she, and most other patients, are unaware that the body will reduce its metabolic rate in response to a restriction of caloric intake (Keesey, 1986), resulting in disproportionately low weight loss relative to the dietary change. If, however, metabolic rate is maintained with an exercise program, weight loss will be more rapid and sustainable (Epstein, Wing, Koeske, & Valoski, 1984). As Epstein et al. (1984) suggested, the sense of self-control could be enhanced by dual interventions such as diet and exercise if they create more visible effects and a closer match between expectations and weight loss. The enhanced sense of control could increase positive emotions and the sense of well-being that often accompany both exercise and weight loss.

Blood glucose awareness training (BGAT) may represent the most intensive efforts to enhance adherence via self-regulatory process (Gonder-Frederick & Cox, 1991). Insulin-dependent diabetics, faced with a life-long problem of regulating blood sugar levels, must achieve a delicate balance between food intake, activity level, and self-administration of insulin. Unlike hypertension where blood pressure appears to have little if any effect on the generation of somatic cues, variation in blood glucose produces a wide range of somatic experiences, some of which are unreliable and invalid as indicators of blood glucose and others of which are not. BGAT provides a series of experiences designed to wean the individual away from invalid cues, a difficult task, and replace them with reliable valid indicators. The first step in the training uses a series of exercise episodes to enhance awareness of somatic cues followed by a series of steps, diary keeping, and self-monitoring, to identify cues that are reliable and valid indicators of elevations and declines in blood glucose levels. Once the cues are identified, the individual is provided with appropriate skills for an effective response. In short, somatic cues are the on-line targets for self-medication and cues that are both sensitive and specific indicators of blood glucose are useful targets for the ongoing process of self-regulation.

Lessons From Self-Regulation Studies

The data reviewed previously suggest that attending to an individual's view of health problems may be extremely important for enhancing adherence. First, they indicate that an individual's view of representation of a health problem may differ markedly from that of medical experts. Second, the cognitive representation of a problem, particularly its experiential component, shapes action by setting goals and affecting the selection of responses for goal attainment. Thus, the symptomatic feature of the representation is a powerful cue to action. Third, appraisals based on these same experiential factors play a key role in updating the individual's view of the health problem, the adequacy of the treatment used to control it, and one's ability to perform the treatment regimen. These appraisals will affect the maintenance of motivation for a specific course of action.

Finally, our underlying schemata appear to cast our representations of specific illness episodes in the shape of acute disease. Whereas our individual histories have confirmed and will continue to confirm a link between sensations of somatic distress and illness, this image is unlikely either to promote vigilance or to sustain the necessary long-term preventive activity needed to deal with the threats of chronic diseases that are initially asymptomatic. This acute disease bias is also useful for enhancing our sense of safety and resistance to permanent and harmful bodily changes. Unless we are continually symptomatic and distressed, we may be less concerned about risks than we should, feel younger than we are, judge our bodies to be healthier and more durable than they are, and be less likely to adhere to long-term regimens to control or prevent asymptomatic conditions. The question that needs to be addressed is whether a self-regulation theory will provide a useful framework for generating messages and programs that can change the schemata that underlie our perceptions of health threats and encourage the adoption of healthy actions to promote well-being. This seems a particularly serious problem for adolescent education, as this subgroup seems most likely to view health problems as acute, self-limiting events that occasionally intrude on life but have no long-term implications respecting their health status or functional abilities.

MAINTAINING ADHERENCE BY TURNING NECESSITIES TO PREFERENCES

It is often claimed that constant, indeed obsessive, self-monitoring and regulation is required for the successful control of behaviors that are homeostatically regulated. For example, Kirschenbaum and Tomarken (1982) argue that self-regulation of weight requires constant vigilance and the obsessive generation of self-instructions to resist urges and sustain a reduced level of food intake. From this perspective, urges are controlled by stimuli processed at a preconscious level, and consciousness, like the wary jailer (or superego), must adopt a constant and rigid vigil ever ready to pronounce self-instructions to resist impulse expression. This unpleasant picture is especially grim with respect to self-control for the exploring, readily stimulated, adolescent. But the picture may be less grim if we can devise a way of enlisting the very same mechanisms that underly the urges to eat and/or smoke and use them to generate urges for self-regulation and restraint! In short, can we turn necessities, that is, conscious self-monitoring, self-instruction programs for healthful behaviors, into preferences, or automatic urge-driven impulses to avoid fatty and high calorie foods, to avoid smoking, to take prescribed medication, and to exercise on a daily basis? And will different procedures be needed to generate urges for health-promoting actions versus urges to desist health-damaging ones, and will the same or different procedures be needed to generate health-promotive urges in adolescents and adults? By moving beyond conscious self-regulated adherence toward automatic self-regulation, we may be able to resolve the maintenance problem and take another, and perhaps final step, away from the compliance framework.

The Changing Balance of Motives

As with all behaviors, health-promotive and health-risk behaviors involve both rewards and costs, and the relative balance of these factors determines whether an action is or is not taken. Moreover, this balance fluctuates over time, the relative salience of specific benefits and costs evolving with changes in the individual's attention, environment, biological state, and personal values; these factors may vary day by day as a function of work and home setting and vary with the social and biological changes that occur over the life span. It is also generally true that factors that are proximal and attached to concrete experience will have greater impact upon action than those that are abstract and remote. For example, when an individual is discussing his alcohol problem with a friend or counselor in an environment free of alcohol-related cues, the remote and abstract costs of alcohol abuse such as job loss and liver disease are likely more salient and powerful sources of behavioral control than the rewards of drinking. But when the same individual is at a party or in a bar, environments where alcohol cues are salient, the urge to drink is likely to dominate these abstract forces for restraint unless countered by an active coping strategy (Vuchinich & Tucker, 1988). How best can we go about altering the balance of forces to favor abstinence of controlled drinking? Are we more likely to succeed by creating restraints or removing incentives for drinking, or must we do both? And can cues for restraint be inserted into those situations encouraging drinking?

Adding Restraints Versus Subtracting Incentives. Lewin (1935) indicated that we are more likely to succeed in stopping a risky behavior if we delete a force favoring the action than if we add a barrier to discourage it. Similarly, if we wish to encourage a nonpreferred, health-promotive behavior, it is better to remove a barrier against it than to add a force to encourage it. In each case, the preferred intervention produces less conflict and a more favorable balance of forces for the desired outcome.

For example, let us assume we wish to motivate a late, middle-aged man to adopt an exercise program following coronary bypass surgery (see Fig. 5.4) and have identified three barriers to adherence: He lacks the time as he is an extremely busy executive; he will experience discomfort during his initial tries as he has been relatively sedentary; and there is a substantial gap in social status between himself and other program participants. If these negative motives are balanced by three motives for participation, such as pressure from his wife and physician, the wish to recover physical strength, and embarrassment if he failed to complete the program, we might try to add a new motive for participation to tilt the balance in favor of rehabilitation. We could, for example, suggest that continuing in the program will reduce the risk of a repeat heart attack; if this strategy is successful, it would change the balance to four motives for participation and three against. We could also tilt the balance in favor of participation by removing a barrier, for example, by placing him in a group with other chief executives or by demonstrating that participation raises his energy level and allows him to complete more work than he could if he did not participate. Either change would alter the balance of motives to three in favor of exercise and two against.

When we compare the preceding outcomes, it is clear that adding a motive for participation creates a narrower margin for exercise, 4 to 3, than that which results from subtracting a barrier, 3 to 2 ratio; hence the latter is more likely to lead to adherence. Moreover, narrow ratios typically involve a greater numbers of forces, increasing the likelihood of conflict and of a shifting balance on any single occasion when these forces are brought to mind. If the executive in our

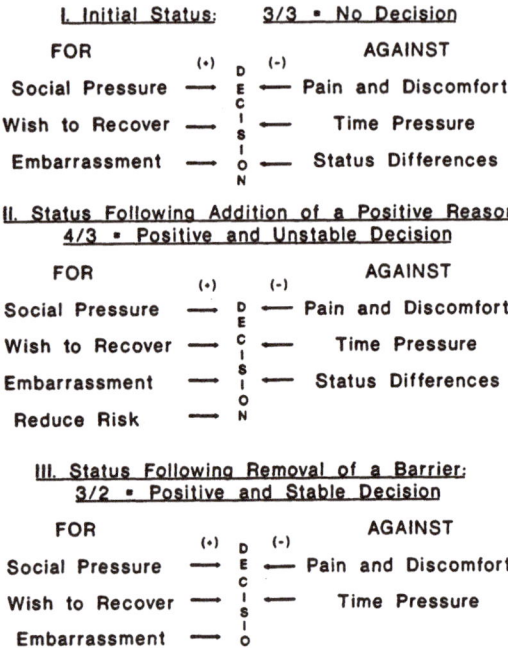

FIG. 5.4. A situation of decisional balance (panel I) i.e., equal number of factors for and against a health promoting action, can be changed by adding a motive for (panel II) or subtracting a motive against (panel III) the action. The ratio or differential promoting the health action is more favorable when a barrier is subtracted (3 to 2) than when one is added (4 to 3).

example had 9 reasons for participation and 8 against, in contrast to 3 in favor and 2 against, the vagaries of retrieval and the limitations in short-term memory may lead him to think of 4 in favor of participation and 3 against at one point in time, and 3 in favor and 4 against at another. The more elements involved in the decision, the greater the possibility if moment-to-moment change in the conscious array (Weinstein, 1988), and the more easily can the balance shift from participation to nonparticipation and back again, creating uncertainty and conflict.

Finally, the added motive for participation is all too often a promise for future gain, and future gains fare poorly in competition with immediate barriers. Thus, the decision or preference is more likely to favor continued participation in an exercise program following the removal of barriers than following the addition of a force for adherence. But can we alter the balance of motives to favor long-term adherence to healthy behaviors by removing forces encouraging risky behavior and removing barriers to healthy actions? And can we change factors that are concrete, "immediate," and most likely to influence action? Answers to these questions will vary with the age of the individual we are trying to influence. Adolescents may view attempts to reduce forces for risk taking as constraints on their independence and self-development rather than as efforts to insure their current and future well-being. Thus, the adolescents self-view as an individual moving toward autonomy and adulthood creates a context that can frame benign and health-promoting influences as restrictions that are responded to with hostility.

Altering the Balance of Motives By Message Framing

In a study designed to persuade college women to perform breast self-examination, Myerowitz and Chaiken (1987) found that subjects were more likely to perform such examinations when the communication was *framed* to emphasize loss from nonperformance than when it was *framed* to emphasize gains from performance. The idea of framing was borrowed from Kahneman and Tversky (1983), who had shown that individuals make contradictory decisions from the very same information depending on how that information is framed. Can framing be used to create schemata that will generate urges to initiate and sustain health-promotive behaviors? And is the concept relevant to shaping healthy behaviors and eliminating risky behaviors among adolescents?

Framing and the Automation of Behavior. The concept of framing, as used by Kahneman and Tversky (1983), refers to the organization of information in decision tasks where the individual is consciously engaged in considering and choosing among alternatives. Our goal is to adapt and use the framing concept to develop motives for healthy behaviors that are maintained over time. The objective is to develop motives in adolescents that are evoked automatically (i.e., without conscious effort) and experienced as urges and/or preferences for healthy actions.

Within the hierarchical context or our self-regulation model, framing can be seen as a procedure for directing attention to the cues and consequences for performing (gains) or not performing (losses) a recommended action. By directing attention, framing "biases" or organizes information, and the organization created by framing can be used to form associations that will generate new preferences and urges. Our hypothesis is that framing is a contextual factor that leads to the classical conditioning or automation of reactions by focusing attention to selected cues and linking these cues to desired reactions (Rachlin, 1989). Thus, whereas framing may use conscious involvement for the formation of associations, consciousness or deliberate attention can recede once conditioning takes place. The issue is what information to incorporate in our frame to form schemata that remove barriers and add forces for initiating and sustaining automatic healthy actions.

Framing Incentives for Health Actions. Toothbrushing and shower taking are two health actions with which we are all familiar, which though clearly learned are durable and have the properties of "urge-driven" preferences. What leads individuals to develop a ritual so that every morning upon rising and every night before retiring they squeeze paste on a brush and with more or less clumsy motions of the hands and odd grimaces of the face proceed to brush their teeth? And what history will motivate a tired adult to trade even momentarily the warmth and comfort of his bed for the cold tile of the bathroom floor and stand at the sink to repeat the toothbrushing ritual because ". . . his mouth feels dirty and he cannot remember whether he did or did not brush his teeth before retiring?" His movements are compulsive; he does not "wish" to rise, it is unlikely that he performed an elaborate mental calculus and decided to rise, but he must brush his teeth because he cannot lie in bed with a dirty mouth. And he will "feel" right and/or better after he does it!

Toothbrushing is an especially interesting response as it satisfies several of the properties needed to stimulate urges. First, the cues stimulating it are proximal, salient, and physically (if not psychologically) impossible to escape; they are in the individual's mouth. Second, the cues provoke an emotional reaction of discomfort and distress that has the properties of an *urge* that must and can only be alleviated by brushing. Third, the completion of the ritual brushing produces a positive affective response the intensity of which is totally incommensurate with the stimulus properties of the procedure. It may make sense to "feel" high and/or alert after inhaling nicotine or to experience a renewal of appetite after imbibing a tasty sweet, but it is somewhat of a puzzle as to why one should feel positive affect after completing a self-regulative toothbrushing ritual? One can hardly attribute it to the toothpaste, it rarely tastes that good, nor does it make sense to attribute it to a sadomasochistic desire for abuse elicited by the brushing. A more likely candidate is that the contrast between the "dirty" feel prior to brushing and the "clean" fresh feeling subsequent to brushing enhances the value of an otherwise trivial, positive incentive (Flaherty, 1991).

Framing for Motive Learning. How would you as a parent frame the toothbrushing tasks to make this morning and nighttime behavior a life-long ritual? Would you talk about the gains of healthy teeth in adulthood, link the act to the youngsters desire to grow up, or would you comment on the concrete sensations of cleanness after brushing? And if your child failed to brush, would you speak only of remote losses such as the cavities that will plague her in adulthood, or would you ask about immediate experience of loss and contrast it with the good feeling of a clean mouth and teeth (e.g., "Didn't your mouth feel yucky before and doesn't it feel nice and clean now that you brushed")? If you focused exclusively on remote gains and losses, it seems unlikely that toothbrushing would become a life-long practice motivated by the "urge" to have a clean mouth. Focusing on the concrete experiences before and after brushing links the former to a sense of loss and creates a discomfort or urge for change and makes the action of brushing the route for eliminating the discomfort and replacing it with a sense of cleanliness and freshness. The contrast of the "clean" feeling postbrushing with the feeling resulting from not brushing should create a tension between the two and enhance the positive reward of brushing. And if framing is done while you, the parent, are brushing your own teeth and commenting upon and sharing similar feelings, the result is a "fellowship of tooth brushing" that will further enhance the acquisition or conditioning of the urge to brush. The scenario is similar to that of a young child acquiring a taste for chili pepper, a food that is initially aversive but that he comes to prefer after repeated tastings in which its spicy quality is framed and linked with the pleasures he shares with the adults that surround him each day at the dinner table (Rozin, 1990).

PROMOTING HEALTHFUL ACTIONS IN ADOLESCENTS

Can we use framing to instill the urges and/or preferences that will initiate and maintain healthful actions by adolescents? An answer to this question requires careful analysis of factors in three domains: (a) the rapidly occurring physical changes occurring during adolescence, (b) the social and physical environment in which the adolescent lives, and (c) the behavioral domain targeted for intervention.

The Changing Adolescent. Rapid growth, sexual maturation, and the development and solidification of formal reasoning are among the many significant biological changes taking place during the 5 to 8 years marking adolescence (Paikoff & Brooks-Gunn, 1989). These changes create new impulses, new competencies (both physical and cognitive), and a rapidly changing physical and social self-presentation, which in our contemporary society propels the adolescent into new environments and new roles.

The Adolescent Environment. Adolescents are said to move out of the (presumably) protected environment of the home and into the more open environment of the society at large. Striving for independence and adult status, equipped with logical capacities useful for criticizing the absolutes accepted during childhood, and confronting the urges and capacities introduced by a maturing body, youngsters coming of age in the United States are concerned with integrating themselves into the peer culture and trying to define themselves as independent adults. The combination of maturational changes and access to a new and wider set of social relationships focuses attention on the immediate present and encourages experimentation with new social roles and new behaviors. As viewed through the framework of the peer culture, many traditional and family norms and values are transformed from goals for self-development to restraints on autonomy. An increase in risky and a decline in healthy behaviors is one possible outcome of this reevaluation.

Filling new roles and engaging in new behaviors involves the temporary acquisition, practice, and projection of self-"images" that can be responded to and validated by the peer audience as credible and acceptable or as foolish and out of step. Acceptance and reciprocity in role enactment validates the projected self and results in a sense of mutuality or intersubjectivity, that is, the sharing of feelings, of likes and dislikes, and of social values. *Mutuality is the core of friendship and it frames or brings together social cues, responses, and feelings to form new motivational structures.* As mutuality involves both participants, the similarity in social behavior in such relationships will be experienced as personal choice rather than as yielding to social influence, a consequence of the framing involved in motive acquisition. The sense of personal choice that pervades peer relationships may create a significant barrier to persuading the adolescent that he or she is a recipient or target of social influence.

There is reason to believe that youngsters are ill prepared for the biological and social changes that occur in adolescence. Schools and parents provide more or less realistic information about physical growth and environmental threats (e.g., watch out for drug pushers, etc.), but it is all too unlikely that adolescents will be told about and hear discussions of the new and intense emotional urges they will experience in association with their changing life situation (Fine, 1988). The absence of dialogue between adolescents and adults about sexual and aggressive urges and the fears and pleasures associated with these urges relinquishes the discussion and, therefore, the definition, evaluation, and modes of controlling these feelings to the peer group. Thus, the peer group becomes the major player in the interpretation and shaping of the adolescents' vague yet pressing internal states and it is the peer group that *defines the appropriate procedures for the evocation and control of these states.* In short, the peer group frames situations for the development of new motives. Moreover, role relationships are structured and given meaning in terms of adolescents' perceptions of their position in the community at large. Living in a dangerous community where life is cheap leads adolescents to associate toughness and ability to attack as critical elements for survival. These elements define the roles to be played and reciprocated, facilitate the formation of self-protective gangs and the use of cigarettes, alcohol, and illicit drugs as a way of defining the group and intensifying shared experiences.

The Behavioral Domain: Risk Behavior and Substance Use. It appears that there may be a dramatic reduction in healthy behaviors during the adolescent years. For example, there is a decline in attention to dental hygiene, diet (failure to eat breakfast), and reduction in hours and regularity of sleep, and an increase in risky behaviors such as smoking, alcohol and drug use (Leventhal, Prohaska, & Hirschman, 1985), and unprotected sexual activity. The generalized nature of these changes is somewhat surprising given the extremely low correlations observed between most health behaviors (Langlie, 1979). To understand these changes we must ask questions about the stimuli cuing and the incentives for acting and failing to act, the positive and negative emotional reactions associated with the act, and the conditions joining or framing these components. A similar analysis is necessary for potentially competing actions. As these questions and their answers tend to be specific to particular actions (e.g., smoking) I focus briefly on risky behaviors in one area, drug use and abuse.

The exploring attitude of adolescence encourages experimentation and risk taking with substances. Because youngsters lack accurate ways of defining their bodily experiences, they may err in their interpretation of risks and benefits associated with substance use and move with ease from use to abuse. Substances, ranging from legal (tobacco) to the illegal (marijuana, cocaine), have the potential for inducing strong, positive, affective reactions, that is, alert mental states and good feelings that create the illusion of benefit. These drugs can also create distinctly negative experiences, and their continued use appears to depend heavily on the relative balance of positive and negative effects over time. Peers can play a critical role in initiating adolescents to drug use by framing and providing interpretations and procedures for controlling the drug experience. Moreover, adolescent discourse about drugs is likely to provide the new experimental user with an accurate picture of his or her immediate and future subjective experiences with a substance. The congruity between peer communications and the adolescent experimenter's experience may generalize to and validate other peer communications about drugs and the meaning of the drug experience. Peers can focus the new smoker's attention on the pleasant components of smoking and encourage patience with its negative effects and alert the new user to the habituation of these unpleasant components. For example, it is well known that the aversive qualities of cigarettes such as coughing and burning adapt with repeated use (Hirschman, Leventhal, & Glynn, 1984). Less well known is that youngsters interpret this change as an indication they are safe from harm as adaptation to the noxious sensations is interpreted as resistance to damage (Leventhal, Glynn, & Fleming, 1987). When peers prepare one another for the occurrence and disappearance of the noxious side effects of a substance, they validate the groups belief that the behavior is harmless.

The belief that a risk behavior is harmless is also supported by the perception that a high proportion of individuals in one's immediate peer group engage in that behavior (Croyle & Jemmot, in press). As adolescents typically overestimate the prevalence of behaviors such as smoking, judging that half or more of their peers and two-thirds of adults are smokers (Chassin, Presson, Sherman, & McGrew, 1987; Leventhal, Glynn, & Fleming, 1987; Wills & Vaughan, 1989), these social misperceptions will create an illusion of safety and reduce the barriers to initial tries and early experimentation. These beliefs are probably related to the adolescents inability to imagine her or himself vulnerable to harm. Moreover, beliefs in one's resistance to harm and the development of skills while using apparently safe legal substances may facilitate experimentation with and transition to more potent illegal substances (Single, Kandel, & Faust, 1975). Thus, the adolescent's developing beliefs frame and give meaning to later experience with illegal drugs.

For the very great majority of youngsters, health risks are episodic; illnesses come and go. It is not surprising, therefore, to find that other risks are framed in this same way. Thus, youngsters expect to engage in risky behavior, for example, smoking, binge drinking, etc., on a temporary episodic basis emerging unscathed from these "bouts." Moreover, the experiences derived from high-risk actions are concrete, immediate, and experienced in a positive social context. The episodic framing of risky substance use and the positive mood and excitement accompanying use are consistent in supporting the adolescents' sense of invulnerability and minimizing the perception of risk taking that can have chronic or long-term consequences.

Finally, the perception of control can reduce the magnitude of threat associated with a particular risk and encourage risk-taking behavior (Weinstein, 1984). The fluctuations of mood and interests during adolescence and the sudden changes in behavior accompanying these shifts may make it seem as easy to stop as to start an action. Thus, it should not be surprising to find that adolescents think they will have no trouble quitting smoking whenever they might wish. Indeed, this belief is sufficiently strong that when asked about addiction many adolescents reply, "If I get addicted and can't stop I'll quit"!, and they seem insensitive to the contradiction inherent in this statement. Moreover, there are no perceptual cues for addiction; the only cue is the difficulty in quitting. The development of dependence is silent and insidious and not easily understood.

Although much of the argument outlined in this chapter is speculative, it is consistent with available observations. For example, data indicate differences in the initial experience with smoking among subgroups of youngsters, that is, adolescents prone to risk taking and having a very high level of substance use more frequently experiencing dizziness or apparent highs (Mosbach & Leventhal, 1988). It seems likely that the variation of subjective experience reflects differences in socialization, that is, what youngsters were led to expect rather than differences in physical temperament, though the question is clearly open to study. Studies also indicate that substance use and abuse is a likely outcome when the adult community relinquishes the adolescent to the peer group. Risky behavior is more common in the latchkey child, who, rather than heading home after school to wait for the parental phone call instead wanders about the shopping center with friends (Steinberg, 1986). In essence, adults have abrogated to the peer group the dialogue that defines subjective urges and develops stable motivational states.

Interventions for the Adolescent Period

The perspective on the drug abuse problem just outlined makes clear that a multilevel program is necessary for successful reduction of abuse. Programs need to target each layer of the environment in which the adolescent lives, starting with the remote physical and social environment through the neighborhood and family. These contextual factors define the goals or paths for individual development. They also establish the terms for friendship and gang formation, and the proximal objectives frame the immediate face-to-face interactions of the individual adolescent. The particular interventions that will prove to be effective at community, group, and individual level will likely vary as a function of the target group, for example, whether our objective is reducing drug abuse among inner city residents or reducing abuse among well-to-do suburbanites.

Whereas the well-to-do suburban dwellers may attribute the destructive plague of drug abuse to the personal characteristics of inner city residents, the extent of drug use may make both social and economic sense when viewed from within the framework of their inner city environment. Altering this framework would require extensive changes such as making models for alternative opportunities available for successful and productive lives, while providing evidence that effort and commitment to work will result in economic and social rewards and making clear that irresponsible behavior will consign one to a less desirable existence. The rewards given for alternative, nonabuse behaviors will be judged reasonable if they appear to be proportional to the rewards given for other tasks; perceived fairness will play a critical role in satisfaction with and the internalization of social norms and adult expectations. Thus, assuring the acceptance or internalization of alternatives to substance abuse requires major changes in the physical and social environment, including the empowerment of the adults who are to serve as models for these alternatives.

It is my belief that individually focused drug abuse prevention programs will be most effective when nested in the context of societal and community changes such as those outlined earlier. These programs will have two clearly distinct tasks: first, to frame or define the objectives and teach the skills needed to forge careers in life as alternatives to drugs; second, to establish stronger linkages between the adolescent and the formal and informal social contacts than can frame everyday experience and link affects to healthful life-promoting activities. A broad range of health-promotive behaviors can be incorporated in these programs, and engaging in these healthy action will make sense to the adolescent who is developing long-term commitments to future careers.

With respect to the first of these tasks, creating skills and motives, it appears that we are far more adept at skill training than at generating motives. Our theoretical analysis suggests, however, that generating innovative and powerful reasons (motives) for using skills to resist substances and substance abuse may be the key to long-term success. As the early section of this chapter suggested, the use of appropriately framed, personalized, threat information is clearly one possible source; threatening messages that present a *personal and realistic view* of threat and associate these feelings with highly available cues can induce a sense of vulnerability and change knowledge and attitudes and, on some occasions, change behavior (Bachman, Johnston, & O'Malley, 1990; Leventhal, 1970; Sutton, 1982).

Barriers, stimulated by threat or other means, are insufficient, however, for success over the long term. Barriers or motivation to avoid substance use and abuse must be complimented by alternative commitments. Alternative commitments reinforce old barriers to substance use and create new ones and do so to many forms of deviant behavior, both because they are distractors that remove the adolescent from high-risk settings and because drug use and abuse will threaten the rewards obtained from the social and work relationships involved with these alternative commitments. Involvement in such alternative valued goals must be initiated and sustained throughout the life span. Success in creating and maintaining alternative commitments will require that the social system recognize the changing needs and perspectives of the developing individual, communicate this recognition, and provide interpretations or meanings that make plausible particular ways of coping and/or adapting to these changing feelings and needs. Thus, socializing agents also must prepare the adolescent for the subjective feelings that motivate sexual activity and recognize the positive aspects of sexuality, and make clear the conflicts and psychological and physical damage to self that can follow sexual indulgence. Providing the skills needed to avoid pregnancy and sexually transmitted diseases is important but insufficient.

Once substance use is in place, that is, after initial use and experimentation have ended and dependency is driving abuse, whether of drugs or other emotionally stimulating and risky activities, interventions must confront the fact that risky behaviors may provide stronger positive rewards than do other life experiences. Programs designed to deal with dependence may first have to create motives that can undermine the positive rewards of use, that is, converting the experience of pleasure with the experience of threat before focusing on significant alternative involvements. It may also be necessary to create a system for skills training that is heavy on both the constraints and the social supports needed for initiating and sustaining abstinence. Both the individual's stage of substance use and the social context must be considered in any intervention program (Glynn, Leventhal, & Hirschman, 1986; Prochaska & DiClemente, 1983).

The second of these two tasks, the establishment of strong links between the adolescent and formal and informal social groups antagonistic to substance use, will be more difficult to achieve if our theoretical models do not address the way a changing context can affect the adolescent's behavioral domain. For example, community programs that attempt to reduce drug abuse by offering after-school or summer work may actually contribute to substance use by providing the resources for purchasing drugs. A program that defines new paths for personal development and foster the skills necessary to achieve substantial future rewards relating to these paths may prove more effective in creating barriers to drug abuse than work programs lacking a future orientation. The program would also focus on how substance use would interfere with such accomplishments. In summary, a theory for linking the adolescent to the social context needs to consider a wide range of issues ranging from the mundane (e.g., how to insure exposure to information) to the esoteric (that is, how to create realistic and concrete visions of future opportunities).

CONCLUSIONS

There are clear signs of theoretical and empirical advance in adherence research. Simpleminded models that viewed adherence as obedience to authority have been replaced by more elaborate cognitive-behavioral models that take into account person and situational factors in adherence to health, and avoidance of risky, behaviors. These models have been productive both in generating descriptive data to help explain adherence to health-promotive behaviors, and they have been useful in suggesting and generating interventions that have produced very substantial increases in adherence for the short term. The problems that remain, however, include failure to maintain behavioral change, weak "bottom-line" effects (i.e., small changes in weight, blood sugar, blood pressure, etc.), and weaknesses in creating healthy behaviors and eliminating risky behaviors among young people.

Adherence research appears to be entering a new era with the appearance of conceptual models focusing on the process of self-regulation. Studies based on the individuals' understanding of health threats, the relationship they perceive between the performance of recommended behaviors and specific targets or threat indicators, and the relationship between these more narrowly construed regulative systems and other life incentives and commitments may open the door to new advances. Self-regulation models nest the problem-solving domain, that is, the representation, coping, and appraisal process under the context of the self and the larger social system. These contextual systems can have direct effects on the specific components of the problem, altering its definition, the perceived possibilities and incentives for specific coping reactions, and the rules used for appraising coping outcomes. The individuals declarative and procedural knowledge, both that directly relevant to the problem and to the context, *frames* or gives meaning to and organizes experience. Recommendations for health-promotive and risk-reducing actions will be interpreted within this space, and, if properly framed, recommended actions and emotions can be linked with one another and with highly available environmental cues, such as somatic sensations. The result would be a consistent urge toward action and the experience of reward following action.

Our theoretical framework suggests that it will be of great value to carefully examine the texture of the adolescents' world if investigators and practitioners wish to encourage the development of healthy behaviors and the avoidance of risky behaviors in adolescents. There is a clear need to examine how adolescents perceive specific risks and how they perceive actions recommended to risk avoidance, for example, whether the risks and actions are seen as remote or immediate, whether they are supported by concrete evidence (the death of a basketball star) or by abstract verbalizations, and how they fit or conflict with the adolescent's rapidly changing physical and social self. In short, the new models suggest that education can be effective if information is framed and made relevant to the self as the self is manifest, here and now, and as at it will be manifested later on. It remains to be seen, however, whether the combination of the concepts of self-regulation and framing will provide new avenues for resolving the maintenance problem.

ACKNOWLEDGMENT

This research and manuscript preparation was supported by grant AG0351 of the National Institute on Aging.

REFERENCES

Abramson, L. Y., Seligman, M. E. P., & Teasdale, J. (1978). Learned helplessness in humans: Critique and reformulation. *Journal of Abnormal Psychology, 87*, 49–74.

Alderman, M. H., & Schoenbaum, E. (1975). Detection and treatment of hypertension at the worksite. *New England Journal of Medicine, 293*, 65–68.

Bachman, J. G., Johnston, L. D., & O'Malley, P. M. (1990). Explaining the recent decline in cocaine use among young adults: Further evidence that perceived risks and disapproval lead to reduced drug use. *Journal of Health and Social Behavior, 31*, 173–184.

Bandura, A. (1969). *Principles of behavior modification*. New York: Holt, Reinhart & Winston.

Bandura, A. (1977). Self-efficacy: Toward a unifying theory of behavioral change. *Psychological Review, 84*, 191–215.

Baumann, L. J., & Leventhal, H. (1985). "I can tell when my blood pressure is up, can't I?" *Health Psychology, 4*, 203–218.

Becker, M. H. (Ed.). (1974). The health belief model and personal health behavior. *Health Education Monograph, 2* (Whole No. 4).

Becker, M. H., & Maiman, L. A. (1975). Sociobehavioral determinants compliance with health and medical care recommendations. *Medical Care, 13*, 10–24.

Best, J. A., Flay, B. R., Towson, S. M. J., Ryan, K. B., Perry, C. L., Brown, K. S., Kersell, M. W., & D'Avernas, J. R. (1984). Smoking prevention and the concept of risk. *Journal of Applied Social Psychology, 14*, 257–273.

Botvin, G. J., Baker, E., Dusenbury, L., Tortu, S., & Botvin, E. M. (1990). Preventing adolescent drug abuse through a multi-modal cognitive-behavioral approach: Results of a three-year study. *Journal of Consulting and Clinical Psychology, 58*, 437–446.

Botvin, G. J., Renick, N. L., & Baker, E. (1983). The effects of format and booster sessions on a broad spectrum psychosocial approach to smoking prevention. *Journal of Behavioral Medicine, 6,* 359–379.

Carver, C. S., & Scheier, M. F. (1981). *Attention and self-regulation: A control-theory approach to human behavior.* New York: Springer–Verlag.

Chassin, L., Presson, C. C., Sherman, S. J., & McGrew, J. (1987). The changing smoking environment for middle and high school students: 1980–1983. *Journal of Behavioral Medicine, 10,* 581–594.

Cioffi, D. (1991). Beyond attentional strategies: A cognitive-perceptual model of somatic interpretation. *Psychological Bulletin, 109,* 25–41.

Cohen, S., Lichtenstein, E., Mermelstein, R., Kingsolver, K., Baer, J. S., & Karmarck, T. W. (1988). Social support interventions for smoking cessation. In B. H. Gottleib (Ed.), *Marshaling social support: Formats, processes, and effects* (pp. 211–2401). Newbury Park, CA: Sage.

Croyle, R. T., & Jemmott, J. B. III. (1991). Psychological reactions to risk factor testing. In J. A. Skelton & R. T. Croyle (Eds.), *The mental representation of health and illness* (pp. 85–107). New York: Springer–Verlag.

Curry, S., Marlatt, G. A., & Gordon, J. R. (1987). Abstinence violation effect: Validation of an attributional construct with smoking cessation. *Journal of Consulting and Clinical Psychology, 55,* 145–149.

Curry, S., Marlatt, G. A., Gordon, J. R., & Baer, J. S. (1988). A comparison of the alternative theoretical approaches to smoking cessation and relapse. *Health Psychology, 7,* 545–556.

Epstein, L. H., Wing, R. R., Koeske, R., & Valoski, A. (1984). The effects of diet plus exercise on weight change in parents and children. *Journal of Consulting and Clinical Psychology, 52,* 429–437.

Fazio, R. H. (1986). How do attitudes guide behavior? In R. M. Sorrentino & E. T. Higgins (Eds.), *The handbook of motivation and cognition: Foundations of social behavior* (pp. 204–243). New York: Guilford Press.

Fine, M. (1988). Sexuality, schooling, and adolescent females: The missing discourse of desire. *Harvard Educational Review, 58,* 29–53.

Finnerty, F. A., Shaw, L. W., & Himmelsbach, C. K. (1973). Hypertension in the inner city: II. Detection and follow-up. *Circulation, 47,* 76–78.

Fishbein, M., & Ajzen, I. (1975). *Belief, attitude, intention, and behavior: And introduction to theory and research.* Reading, MA: Addison-Wesley.

Flaherty, C. (1991). Incentive contrast and selected animal models of anxiety. In L. Dachowski & C. Flaherty (Eds.), *Current topics in animal learning: brain, emotion, and cognition* (pp. 207–244). Hillsdale, NJ: Lawrence Erlbaum Associates.

Flay, B. R. (1985). Psychosocial approaches to smoking intervention: A review of findings. *Health Psychology, 4,* 449–488.

Flay, B. R., & Cook, T. D. (1981). Evaluation of mass media prevention campaigns. In R. R. Rice & W. J. Paisley (Eds.), *Public communication campaigns* (pp. 239–264). Beverly Hills, CA: Sage.

Glynn, K., Leventhal, H., & Hirschman, R. (1986). *A cognitive developmental approach to smoking prevention.* NIDA Monograph Series ([pp. 130–152] Pub No. [ADM] 86-1334). Washington, DC: U.S. Government Printing Office.

Gonder-Frederick, L. A., & Cox, D. J. (1991). Symptoms perception, symptom beliefs, and blood glucose discrimination in the self-treatment of insulin-dependent diabetes. In J. A. Skelton & R. T. Croyle (Eds.), *Mental representations in health and illness* (pp. 220–246). New York: Springer-Verlag.

Gonder-Frederick, L. A., Cox, D. J., Bobbitt, S. A., & Pennebaker, J. W. (1989). Mood changes associated with blood pressure fluctuations in insulin-dependent mellitus. *Health Psychology, 8,* 45–49.

Henderson, T., Hall, J., & Lipton, T. (1979). Changing self-destructionist behavior. In G. Stone & F. Cohen (Eds.), *Health psychology: A handbook* (pp. 141–160). San Francisco: Jossey-Bass.

Hirschman, R., Leventhal, H., & Glynn, K. (1984). The development of smoking behavior: Conceptualization and supportive cross-sectional survey data. *Journal of Applied Social Psychology, 14,* 184–206.

Hochbaum, G. (1958). *Public participation in medical screening programs: A sociopsychological study* [DHEW Publication No. (PHS) 572]. Washington, DC: U.S. Government Printing Office.

Hovland, C. I., Janis, I. L., & Kelley, H. H. (1953). *Communication and persuasion.* New Haven, CT: Yale University Press.

Hunt, W. A. & Matarazzo, J. D. (1973). Three years later: Recent developments in the experimental modification of smoking behavior. *Journal of Abnormal Psychology, 2,* 107–114.

Janz, N., & Becker, M. (1984). The health belief model: A decade later. *Health Education Quarterly, 11,* 1–47.

Kahneman, D., & Tversky, A. (1983). Choices, values, and frames. *American Psychologist, 39,* 341–350.

Kanfer, F. H. (1977). The many faces of self-control, or behavior modification changes its focus. In R. B. Stuart (Ed.), *Behavioral self-management: Strategies, techniques, and outcomes* (pp. 1–48). New York: Brunner/Mazel.

Keesey, R. E. (1986). A set point theory of obesity. In K. D. Brownell & J. P. Foreyt (Eds.), *The physiology, psychology, and treatment of the eating disorders* (pp. 63–87). New York: Basic Books.

Kirschenbaum, D. S., & Tomarken, A. J. (1982). On facing the generalization problem: The study of self-regulatory failure. In P. C. Kendall (Ed.), *Advances in cognitive-behavioral research and therapy* (pp. 119–120). Englewood Cliffs, NJ: Prentice-Hall.

Kottke, T. E., Battista, R. N., De Frieses, G. H., & Brekke, M. L. (1988). Attributes of successful smoking cessation interventions in medical practice. *Journal of the American Medical Association, 259*(19), 2883–2889.

Langlie, J. K. (1979). Interrelationships among preventive health behaviors: A test if competing hypotheses. *Public Health Reports, 94,* 216–225.

Lazarus, R. S., & Folkman, S. (1984). *Stress, appraisal and coping.* New York: Springer-Verlag.

Lazarus, R. S., & Launier, R. (1978). Stress related transactions between person and environment. In L. A. Pervin & M. Lewis (Eds.), *Perspectives in interactional psychology* (pp. 287–327). New York: Plenum Press.

Leventhal, H. (1979). Findings and theory in the study of fear communications. *Advances in Experimental Social Psychology, 5,* 119–186.

Leventhal, H., Baker, T., Brandon, T., & Fleming, R. (1989). Intervening and preventing cigarette smoking. In T. Ney & A. Gale (Eds.), *Smoking and human behavior* (pp. 313–336). Oxford: Wiley.

Leventhal, H., & Cleary, P. D. (1980). The smoking problem: A review of the research and theory in behavioral risk modification. *Psychological Bulletin, 88,* 370–405.

Leventhal, H., Glynn, K., & Fleming, R. (1987). Is the smoking decision an "informed choice?": Effect of smoking risk factors on smoking beliefs. *Journal of the American Medical Association, 257,* 3373–3376.

Leventhal, H., Meyer, D., & Gutmann, M. (1980). The role of theory in the study of compliance to high blood pressure regimens. *Patient compliance to prescribed antihypertensive medication regimens: A report to the National Heart, Lung, and Blood Institute* (NIH Publication No. 81-2102). Washington, DC: U.S. Department of Health and Human Services.

Leventhal, H., Meyer, D., & Nerenz, D. (1980). The common sense representation of illness danger. In S. Rachman (Ed.), *Contributions to medical psychology* (Vol. 2, pp. 7–30). New York: Pergamon Press.

Leventhal, H., & Nerenz, D. R. (1983). A model for stress research with some implications for the control of stress disorders. In D. Meichenbaum & M. Jaremko (Eds.), *Stress reduction and prevention* (pp. 5–38). New York: Plenum Press.

Leventhal, H., Prohaska, T. R., & Hirschman, R. S. (1985). Preventive health behavior across the life-span. In J. C. Rosen & L. J. Solomon (Eds.), *Prevention in health psychology* (Vol. 8, pp. 191–235). Hanover, NH: University Press of New England.

Leventhal, H., Singer, R., & Jones, S. (1965). Effects of fear and specificity of recommendations upon attitudes and behavior. *Journal of Personality and Social Psychology, 2*, 20–29.

Leventhal, H., & Watts, J. C. (1966). Sources of resistance to fear-arousing communications on smoking and lung cancer. *Journal of Personality, 34*, 155–175.

Leventhal, H., Zimmerman, R., & Gutmann, M. (1984). Compliance: A self-regulation perspective. In W. D. Gentry (Ed.), *Handbook of behavioral medicine* (pp. 369–436). New York: Guilford Press.

Lewin, K. (1935). Environmental forces in child behavior and development. *A dynamic theory of personality* (pp. 66–113). New York: McGraw-Hill.

Locke, E. A. (1971). Is "behavior therapy" behavioristic? *Psychological Bulletin, 76*, 318–327.

Ley, P. (1977). Psychological studies of doctor–patient communication. In S. Rachman (Ed.), *Contributions to medical psychology* (Vol. 1, pp. 9–42). Oxford: Pergamon Press.

Marlatt, G. A., & Gordon, J. R. (1980). Determinants of relapse: Implications for the maintenance of behavior change. In P. O. Davison & S. M Davidson (Eds.), *Behavioral medicine: Changing health lifestyles* (pp. 410–452). New York: Brunner Mazel.

McGuire, W. J. (1985). Attitudes and attitude change. In G. Lindzey & E. Aronson (Eds.), *Handbook of social psychology* (Vol. 2, 3rd ed., pp. 233–246). New York: Random House.

Meyer, D., Leventhal, H., & Gutmann, M. (1985). Common-sense models of illness: The example of hypertension. *Health Psychology, 4*, 115–135.

Meyerowitz, B. E., & Chaiken, S. (1987). The effect of message framing on breast self-examination attitudes, intentions, and behavior. *Journal of Personality and Social Psychology, 52*, 505–510.

Mosbach, P., & Leventhal, H. (1988). Peer group identification and smoking: Implications for intervention. *Journal of Abnormal Psychology, 97*, 238–245.

Murray, D. M., Leupker, R. V., Johnson, C. A., & Mittelmark, M. B. (1984). The prevention of cigarette smoking in children: A comparison of four strategies. *Journal of Applied Social Psychology, 14*, 274–288.

Ockene, J. K. (1987). Physician delivered interventions for smoking cessation: Strategies for increasing effectiveness. *Preventive Medicine, 16*, 723–737.

Paikoff, R. L., & Brooks-Gunn, J. (1989). Physiological processes: What role do they play during the transition to adolescence? In R. Montemayor, G. Adams, & T. Gullotta (Eds.), *Advances in adolescent development: Vol. 2. The transition from childhood to adolescence* (pp. 63–84). Beverly Hill, CA: Sage.

Pederson, L. L. (1982). Compliance with physicians advice to quit smoking: A review of the literature. *Preventive Medicine, 11*, 71–84.

Pennebaker, J. W., & Watson, D. (1988). Blood pressure estimation and beliefs among normotensive and hypertensives. *Health Psychology, 7*, 309–328.

Petty, R. E., & Cacioppo, J. T. (1986). *Communication and persuasion: Central and peripheral routes to attitude change.* New York: Springer-Verlag.

Powers, W. T. (1973). *Behavior: The control of perception.* Chicago: Aldine.

Prochaska, J. O., & DiClemente, C. C. (1983). Stages and processes of self-change of smoking: Toward an integrative model of change. *Journal of Consulting and Clinical Psychology, 51*, 390–395.

Rachlin, H. (1989). *Judgment, decision, and choice: A cognitive behavioral.* New York: W. H. Freeman.

Rosen, T. J., Terry, N. S., & Leventhal, H. (1982). The role of esteem and coping in response to a threat communication. *Journal of Research in Personality, 16*, 90–107.

Rosenstock, I. M. (1974). The health belief model and preventive health behavior. *Health Education Monographs, 2,* 354–386.

Rosenstock, I. M., Hochbaum, G. M., & Leventhal, H. (1960). *The impact of Asian influenza on community life: A study in five cities.* (DHEW Publication No. 766). Washington, DC: U.S. Government Printing Office.

Rozin, R. (1990). Development in the food domain. *Developmental Psychology, 26,* 555–562.

Sackett, D., & Haynes, R. B. (1976). *Compliance and therapeutic regimens.* Baltimore: Johns Hopkins University Press.

Sackett, D. L., & Snow, J. C. (1979). The magnitude of compliance and noncompliance. In R. B. Haynes, D. W. Taylor, & D. L. Sackett (Eds.), *Compliance in health care* (pp. 11–22). Baltimore: Johns Hopkins University Press.

Single, E., Kandel D. B., & Faust, R. (1975). Patterns of multiple drug use in high school. *Journal of Health and Social Behavior, 15*(4), 344–357.

Steinberg, L. (1986). Latchkey children and susceptibility to peer pressure: An ecological analysis. *Developmental Psychology, 22,* 433–439.

Stimson, G. V. (1974). Obeying doctor's orders: A view from the other side. *Social Science and Medicine, 8,* 97–104.

Stunkard, A. J., Craighead, L. W., & O'Brien, R. O. (1980). Controlled trial of behavior therapy, pharmacotherapy, and their combination in the treatment of obese hypertensives. *The Lancet, November 15,* 1045–1047.

Sutton, S. R. (1982). Fear arousing communications: A critical examination of theory and research. In J. R. Eiser (Ed.), *Social psychology and behavioral medicine* (pp. 303–337). New York: Wiley.

Szasz, T., & Hollander, M. A. (1956). A contribution to the philosophy of medicine: The basic models of the doctor–patient relationship. *Archives of Internal Medicine, 97,* 585–592.

Tiffany, S. T., & Baker, T. B. (1988). The role of aversion and counseling strategies in treatments for cigarette smoking. In T. B. Baker & D. S. Cannon (Eds.), *Assessment and treatment of addictive disorders* (pp. 238–289). New York: Praeger.

Tiffany, S. T., Martin, E. M., & Baker, T. B. (1986). Treatments for cigarette smoking: An evaluation of the contributions of aversion and counseling procedures. *Behavioral Research and Therapy, 24,* 437–452.

Vuchinic, R., & Tucker, J. A. (1988). Contributions from behavioral theories of choice to an analysis of alcohol abuse. *Journal of Abnormal Psychology, 97,* 181–195.

Weinstein, N. D. (1984). Why it won't happen to me: Perception of risk and susceptibility. *Health Psychology, 3,* 431–457.

Weinstein, N. D. (1988). The precaution adoption process. *Health Psychology, 8,* 355–386.

Wills, T. A., & Vaughan, R. (1989). Social support and substance use in early adolescence. *Journal of Behavioral Medicine, 12,* 321–339.

Wooley, S. C., Blackwell, B., & Winget, C. (1978). A learning theory model of chronic illness behavior: Theory treatment and research. *Psychosomatic Medicine, 40,* 379–401.

6 Why Do Adolescents Have Difficulty Adhering to Health Regimes?

Jeanne Brooks-Gunn
Teachers College, Columbia University and Educational Testing Service

Adolescence is a challenging time in that adolescents begin engaging in so-called adult behaviors and are confronted with a plethora of interwoven and complex issues, such as autonomy, intimacy, and achievement. Often, adolescence is characterized by a series of developmental challenges that need to be mastered. These include the accommodation to pubertal changes, the alteration of childhood ties to parents, the regulation of moods, the reorganization of self-definitions, the acquisition of new academic and possibly work-related skills, and the management of sexual arousal and opposite-sex relationships (Brooks-Gunn & Petersen, 1983, 1991; Brooks-Gunn, Petersen, & Eichorn, 1985; Feldman & Elliott, 1990; Gunnar & Collins, 1988; Lerner & Foch, 1987; Montemayor, Adams, & Gullotta, 1990; Simmons & Blyth, 1987).

Additionally, adolescents must make decisions about whether, when, and how often to engage in a series of health-related behaviors. Whether examining adherence to regimes for controlling chronic illnesses, the maintenance of already established health regimes, or the acquisition of new health-promoting behavior, adolescents face a unique challenge; that is, they must learn to negotiate the transition from primarily parental regulation of behavior (or at least parental support, encouragement, and monitoring of health-related behaviors) to more self-regulation. If difficulties arise during this transition, they may turn to or otherwise be offered guidance from health professionals, peers, and/or school personnel. Families are affected by the necessity for more self-regulation. How well do adolescents negotiate this transition, and what are the circumstances that render the process difficult for them?

Promotion of Adolescent Adherence

It is my premise that health behaviors are likely to be affected by the transition to behavioral self-regulation during the first half of adolescence. Self-regulation difficulties are believed to arise at this time because of a convergence of many biological, emotional, cognitive, social cognitive, and social events. In this chapter, the genesis of such difficulties is explored using two domains of health behavior as exemplars—sexual behavior and dietary practices and attitudes. These two not only represent my research interests but focus on two somewhat different processes underlying health behavior, one in which health regimes exist prior to the transition to adolescence (dietary practices), and one in which new health regimes are developed during adolescence (sexual behavior).

Perhaps the most useful developmental model in which to frame adolescent health behavior employs the constructs of vulnerability and resilience, which have received the most attention in the field of developmental psychopathology. Vulnerability implies that a particular child or group of children who is at risk in a probabilistic sense for manifesting a certain behavior or set of behaviors is susceptible to decrements in well-being, in this case decrements in health-promoting behavior. Risk factors are those biological, psychosocial, and environmental conditions that are associated with low health promotion. The opposite of vulnerability and risk factors is resilience and protective factors. Both are predictive of behavior across a variety of ages and domains, some of which touch upon health promotion (Furstenberg, Brooks-Gunn, & Morgan, 1987; Garmezy, Masten, & Tellegen, 1984; Garmezy & Rutter, 1988; Werner & Smith, 1982). This framework has been applied to the study of sexual behavior, specifically the onset of sexual intercourse and use of contraceptives, and to dietary practices and attitudes, specifically those associated with eating problems and disorders (Attie & Brooks-Gunn, in press; Attie, Brooks-Gunn, & Petersen, 1990; Brooks-Gunn & Furstenberg, 1989; Brooks-Gunn & Paikoff, in press). Most of the examples in this chapter dwell on sexual behavior, given its link to compliance (abstention from sexual intercourse or contraceptive use), in order to avoid pregnancy and sexually transmitted diseases (STDs).

Using a general model of vulnerability and resilience, the health behaviors of young adolescents are explored in this chapter. First, the two health behaviors of interest in this chapter are described, both in terms of current research definitions and adolescent constructions of the two health behaviors. Additionally, three developmental issues in the study of adolescent health behavior are raised. Second, antecedents of vulnerability or resilience vis-à-vis health well-being are considered. The risk factors include those important during the transition towards adolescence generally—cultural context, individual factors (biological, emotional, cognitive, and social cognitive), and environmental factors (peers and parents). Evidence for each risk factor is briefly reviewed with respect to dietary practices and sexual well-being. Third, some of the current intervention initiatives associated with the promotion of sexual well-being are reviewed. These include educational, problem solving and skills training, and employment or continuing education strategies. Implications for future intervention strategies are also considered in this section. The fourth section touches on barriers to studying adolescents; these barriers include social and parental beliefs about the appropriateness of certain behaviors associated with sexuality. The fifth section raises several issues concerning the assessment of adolescent health behaviors, specifically, sample selection, reliability of self-reports, and use of multiple respondents. In the final section, difficulties with promoting healthy behaviors in adolescents are highlighted.

DESCRIBING ADOLESCENT HEALTH BEHAVIOR

Definitions of Health Behavior

Adolescent health behavior is more often discussed in terms of health prevention rather than health promotion, even though both are equally relevant (see the Surgeon General's 1979 *Report on Health Promotion and Disease Prevention*). With respect to the two domains of health behavior discussed in this chapter, this is particularly true for sexual behavior. Literature focuses on the onset of sexual intercourse and the use of contraceptives to prevent pregnancy and/or STDs. In an attempt to highlight health promotion, a definition of sexual well-being has been offered (Brooks-Gunn & Paikoff, in press). Four aspects of sexual well-being were identified and discussed—positive feelings about one's body and the acquisition of secondary sexual characteristics, feelings of sexual arousal and desire, the engagement in sexual behaviors, and, for those teenagers who are engaging in sexual intercourse, the practice of safe sex. All may be studied vis-à-vis antecedent risk factors and all may be the focus of intervention strategies. The point here is that most literature lacks such a health-promotion perspective, which has hampered our study of adolescent sexuality (Katchadourian, 1990).

Adolescent Constructions of Health Behavior

Adolescents may define health behavior differently from adults, although little information is available on this topic. If differences do exist, they may provide clues as to why young adolescents seem to have difficulty adhering to health regimes. For example, the overweight youth may perceive the necessity of following a reduced dietary intake plan more burdensome than an adult for a variety of reasons, including the importance of eating out with friends, the unavailability of appropriate food in school settings and fast food restaurants, the scarcity of time to procure or prepare food, inexperience with preparing one's own meals, and so forth. What is important here is that the meaning of food, and adherence to a regime that is different from that of one's friends, probably has different meanings for the young adolescent than for older persons. Additionally, the adolescent might perceive, for the first time, contradictions between what is valued as good eating habits and what most people actually consume.

With regard to sexual behavior, the persistence of prohibitions about youthful sexuality may place youth in a cultural double bind. At the same time that they are urged to avoid sex, adolescents also are told to act responsibly. From the teenager's perspective, being responsible for abstinence means that practicing birth control is a failure in responsibility (Brooks-Gunn & Furstenberg, 1990). Such contradictions may make it difficult for young teenagers to practice birth control reliably.

How youth perceive sexuality is almost never studied, possibly because it assumed that their constructions are similar to those of adults (Brooks-Gunn & Furstenberg, 1990).[1] We do not know how youth feel about their first experiences, with whom they share and withhold information, nor how they decide to have sex the first time. Instead, we know about the age of first intercourse, the relationship with the first partner, and use of contraceptives (see Brooks-Gunn & Furstenberg, 1989; Hayes, 1987; Hofferth & Hayes, 1987, for reviews of this literature). More detailed looks at the actual experience of sexual behavior and the feeling engendered, the context in which it occurs, the negotiation strategies used (and differences in strategies used by boys and girls), and the experience and management of sexual arousal are sorely needed (Brooks-Gunn & Paikoff, in press).

Youth also must construct the meaning of adherence to a health regime more generally. Even if health education is adequate (which is unlikely), youth may probably define adherence differently than do adults. Although little data exist, I suspect that many youth believe they are practicing good health-promoting behavior at levels of adherence that adults might define as less than adequate. For example, in a recent study of Philadelphia teenagers, the vast majority indicated that they had altered their sexual behavior as a result of the HIV epidemic. About two thirds said that they were using condoms as a consequence. However, of these youth, only about half reported using condoms the last time that they had intercourse (Brooks-Gunn & Furstenberg, 1990). It seems as though a significant proportion believed they had made a change; however, the change is not adequate protection against HIV, let alone against an unwanted pregnancy. Much more work on what youth believe is appropriate adherence to health regimes is urgently needed.

---

[1]In contrast, the meaning of puberty, at least in girls, has been extensively investigated (Brooks-Gunn, 1984; Brooks-Gunn & Reiter, 1990).

Developmental Issues in the Study of Adolescent Health Behavior

Several developmental issues must be raised in the study of adolescent health behavior—age trends in the expression of a behavior or compliance to a health regime, the co-occurrence of the health behavior in question with other behaviors, and the timing of individual behaviors.

It is believed that young adolescents exhibit less health-promoting behaviors than do older individuals.[2] Although literature from several sources supports this contention, surprisingly little frank developmental research exists, in the sense of making direct comparisons among children, younger adolescents, older adolescents, and young adults. With respect to the two health domains of interest here, research indicates that the dietary intake of some young adolescents is altered in the direction of a less healthy diet (Sallis, in press), and the percentage of children classified as obese increases after puberty is complete (Stunkard, d'Aquili, Fox, & Filion, 1982). Such increases may be due in part to eating and exercise habits that become less under parental control during adolescence. In the sexual behavior domain, youth are less likely to use contraceptives in the first than the second half of adolescence (Brooks-Gunn & Furstenberg, 1990; Hofferth & Hayes, 1987; Zelnik & Kantner, 1978).

Particular health behaviors tend to co-occur with other behaviors. For example, eating problems and disorders are often accompanied by depressive symptoms (Attie & Brooks-Gunn, 1989; Attie et al., 1990; Lancelot, Brooks-Gunn, & Warren, 1991). Early sexual intercourse (before age 14 or 15) tends to co-occur with smoking and drinking, use of illegal substances, and school dropout (Ensminger, 1987; Furstenberg et al., 1987; Jessor & Jessor, 1977). It is believed that such patterns of behavior render adolescents more vulnerable for long-term problem behavior (Jessor, in press).

Timing typically addresses the issue of where an individual is placed vis-à-vis his or her peer group with respect to a particular behavior (Brooks-Gunn, Petersen, & Eichorn, 1985). The peer group may refer to friends, classmates, or schoolmates as well as to neighborhood, regional, or national youth. Most often, timing is studied as a biological marker of puberty (Brooks-Gunn, 1988; Brooks-Gunn & Reiter, 1990). For example, being an early maturer renders girls vulnerable to eating problems and disorders (Attie et al., 1990). Early-maturing boys and girls experience sexual arousal earlier, given links between hormonal levels and

---

[2]Although these issues are explored in this chapter, I hasten to add that very few developmentally oriented comparative studies of health behaviors exist. Consequently, much of what is said about the differences and similarities of children, adolescents, and adults is speculative. Luckily, more definite statements may be made about younger versus older adolescents, as some studies have included a broad age range of youth.

arousal (Udry, 1988). Additionally, having a more mature body seems to result in earlier requests for independence from parents and embeddedness in peer groups comprised of more mature youth (Simmons & Blyth, 1987; Stattin & Magnusson, 1990). Both increased sexual arousal and peer group interaction probably contribute to earlier dating and sexuality, although by middle adolescence later maturers usually have caught up to their more precocious peers (Gargiulo, Attie, Brooks-Gunn, & Warren, 1987; Magnusson, Stattin, & Allen, 1985).

BIOPSYCHOSOCIAL RISK FACTORS INFLUENCING ADOLESCENT HEALTH BEHAVIOR

Cultural, environmental, and individual processes all influence adolescent health behavior. Adherence is multidimensional, and any one factor alone is not expected to explain significant amounts of variation. In addition, the context in which health behaviors are expected to be executed is influential. Finally, a different set of antecedent risk factors probably influence different health behaviors. With these caveats in mind, several of the prime candidates for influencing adolescent health behavior are briefly reviewed—cultural context, individual factors, and environmental factors.

Cultural Context

Cultural constructions of any particular health behavior in part determine the nature of debates about whether (and when) participation in the behavior or adherence regime is a problem and how one should go about promoting healthy behavior. Cultural beliefs about eating and weight problems abound. Those who do not keep their weight within normal ranges are often thought to be "weak," to have no self-discipline, or to have a personality problem. Individuals who are obese are believed to have no self-control and to be lazy, even though all the research evidence suggests that these generalizations are not true (Attie & Brooks-Gunn, 1987; Brownell & Wadden, 1984). These beliefs exist for children, youth, and adults alike. Indeed, even children in the first years of school rate their overweight peers more negatively than their classmates who are not overweight (Lerner, 1969, 1982). On the other hand, being thin is often reified as indicative of goodness and discipline, particularly for women (Attie & Brooks-Gunn, 1987; Rodin, Silberstein, & Striegel-Moore, 1984). That weight is highly heritable is not considered in most cultural constructions.

Turning to reproductive control, cultural constructions are often complex and contradictory. Engagement in sex during the first half of adolescence, and indeed in adolescence at all outside the confines of marriage, is not considerable acceptable in our society. Our views are quite different from those in most Western European nations, which seem to be more accepting of youthful sexuality, stressing the responsible management of fertility rather than abstinence (Jones et al., 1985; Jones, Forrest, Henshaw, Silverman, & Torres, 1988). Our cultural message clashes with reality, given that the majority of teenagers do have intercourse today, and that they see many of their elders engaging in nonmarital sexual relationships. Given the high rates of STDs and pregnancy during adolescence, questions are not being raised about the timing of the acquisition of various sexual behaviors and of information about and access to contraception (Brooks-Gunn, Boyer, & Hein, 1988; Brooks-Gunn & Furstenberg, 1989; Brooks-Gunn, Duke-Duncan, Ehrhardt, Hein, & Shafer, 1989).

Individual Factors

Biological Factors. The biological events of puberty might influence health behavior. With respect to dietary practices, as girls gain body fat and the rounded contours of a mature body, a large increase in concern about weight and caloric restriction occurs (Attie & Brooks-Gunn, in press; Sallis, in press). Increased hormonal levels are associated with sexual intercourse for boys and feelings of sexual arousal for boys and girls (Udry, Billy, Morris, Groff, & Raj, 1985; Udry, Talbert, & Morris, 1986). More general affective states may be associated with hormonal changes during puberty, such as depressive affect in girls, aggressive feelings in boys and girls, and mood lability in both sexes (Paikoff & Brooks-Gunn, 1990; Susman et al., 1987; Warren & Brooks-Gunn, 1989). Such emotional states may influence adherence in several health behavior domains, although little research has addressed this topic.

Emotional Factors. Changes in emotionality also might contribute to young adolescents' difficulty adhering to a health regime. Indeed, increases in negative affect, both depressive and aggressive emotions, have been documented for the first half of adolescence (Brooks-Gunn & Petersen, 1991; Rutter, Izard, & Read, 1986). These increases are due in part to the number of life events that occur during this period as well as to the biological changes associated with puberty (Brooks-Gunn, 1992; Brooks-Gunn & Warren, 1989; Simmons, Burgeson, & Reef, 1988). For example, the cumulative impact of simultaneous changes in the biological and social realm, rather than any one single event, is associated with depressive symptomatology. Links with health behaviors are typically not studied (see, as an exception, the work on depression and drug use by Kandel, Raveis, & Davies, 1991).

Social and Social-Cognitive Processes. Many cognitive and social-cognitive processes have been posited to influence adolescent adherence to health regimes. Processes discussed here are perceived costs and benefits of low adherence, perceived risks of certain health behaviors, understanding of future consequences, and decision-making skills. Others include the ability to delay gratification, an understanding of rule-governed behavior, a consideration of multiple perspectives on a problem, and refinement of interpersonal negotiation strategies. Self-efficacy could be considered still another relevant social-cognitive process (see Paikoff & Brooks-Gunn, in press).

Perceived Costs and Benefits. How do youth perceive the costs of low adherence, and do they see any offsetting benefits? And, do their perceptions differ from that of adults? Little research directly addresses these questions. However, in the nature of speculation, perceived benefits of low adherence are thought to influence youth's behavior. The obese teenager may rate going out to a fast food restaurant with friends as more beneficial than the long-term cost of high caloric content of a meal. With respect to sexuality, the immediate benefits of sexual arousal and perhaps peer acceptance and intimacy may outweigh the possible costs of pregnancy or a STD. Additionally, the cost of pregnancy itself, for some groups, may be seen as quite low. Boys are less likely to pay a price for getting a girl pregnant than are girls, or even boys 20 years ago: Over 90% of Black and over half of White teenage girls who bear children do so outside of marriage. For their partners, the cost of rearing a child is quite low (although recent state laws to ensure more child support will alter the actual cost of out-of-wedlock fatherhood; Garfinkel & McLanahan, 1990). And some girls may perceive the costs as relatively low if they believe that early parenthood will not reduce their prospects for eventual marriage or high school graduation.

Perceptions of Risk. Generally, health behavior is not changed unless the consequences are seen as severe (Janz & Becker, 1984). Therefore, for example, all other things being equal, a teenager would have to believe that she was very likely to become pregnant if engaging in unprotected intercourse, and that becoming pregnant would have serious negative consequences (i.e., becoming a mother earlier than anticipated, having to curtail educational and job aspirations, having to spend time caring for a baby rather than being in school or with friends, decreasing the likelihood of obtaining a good job or getting married). One of the major reasons given by teenagers for having unprotected intercourse is that they did not think they would conceive, suggesting that personal risk is minimized. Whether adolescents minimize personal risk more than adults is not known (Keating, 1990). Personal risk for an undesirable outcome tends to be underestimated by adults, and peers are believed to be at more risk than oneself (Weinstein, 1987).

Behavior defined as having a relatively high risk of negative consequences occurs in many behavioral domains more frequently in adolescence than at other ages (Irwin & Millstein, 1991). Possible mechanisms for low adherence in teenagers include: (a) cognitive difficulties in assessing personal risk, (b) lack of experience with the consequences of risk, (c) ignorance, and (d) denial.

Over the second decade of life, individuals are increasingly able to think about abstractions in more systematic, integrated, and internally consistent ways (Damon & Hart, 1982; Goldman & Goldman, 1982; Harter, 1983; Selman, 1980). Surprisingly few researchers, however, have attempted to document these processes with reference to sexual behavior. Age-related changes in understanding the process of conception occur from childhood to middle adolescence (Bernstein & Cowan, 1975; Goldman & Goldman, 1982). Many pregnant teenagers report that they took risks and procrastinated with respect to contraceptive use, suggesting that they have some awareness of pregnancy risk (Cobliner, 1974; Jones & Philliber, 1983; Rogel, Zuehlke, Petersen, Tobin-Richards, & Shelton, 1980; Zabin & Clark, 1981). Poor insight, lack of future orientation, or other high-level cognitive processes may explain in part such risk taking, but such notions have not been directly tested. At the same time, adolescents may have a hard time calculating precise probabilities about risk, despite the general recognition that "they took a chance." However, little research directly addresses this problem.

With respect to the effect of experience on risk estimation, if an event has not yet occurred, risk probabilities are usually underestimated by adults and probably by teenagers (Turner, Miller, & Moses, 1989). As an example, teenagers who become pregnant for the first time typically seem surprised (i.e., "it couldn't happen to me"; Brooks-Gunn & Furstenberg, 1989). Researchers have not yet investigated risk perception as a function of sexual experience, however.

Teenagers (as well as adults) are often misinformed about the time of the month when one is most likely to get pregnant and the effectiveness of various types of contraceptives. Unfortunately, little information exists about sexual knowledge and its association with sexual behavior. We do know that only one third of all teenagers are able to identify the cycle phase in which the risk of pregnancy is greatest (Dawson, 1986; Morrison, 1985; Zelnik & Kantner, 1977), with younger adolescents being less likely to be able to do so.

Denial is inferred from the fact that many teenagers probably do not accept themselves as sexual beings. Their sexual identity, having developed in a society that discourages expressions of teenage sexuality, is often characterized by ambivalence, secretiveness, and negativity. In such a scenario, taking personal responsibility for contraception or even assessing personal risk is probably difficult (Fisher, Byrne, & White, 1983; Winter, 1988). That pregnant teenagers report procrastinating or forgetting to use birth control is suggestive of denial of personal responsibility for their sexual behavior (Zabin & Clark, 1981). Whether and in what ways teenagers differ from adults and from each other with respect to these dimensions of risk assessment is not known (see Brooks-Gunn & Paikoff, in press, pp. 16–19; Paikoff & Brooks-Gunn, in press).

Understanding of Future Consequences. Understanding the future consequences of one's actions is a cornerstone of the theory of formal operations (Inhelder & Piaget, 1958). Current research suggests that adolescents become increasingly likely to consider the future consequences of decisions in hypothetical problem-solving situations from seventh to 12th grade (Lewis, 1981). Attitudes towards consequences of pregnancy may influence behavioral intentions regarding pregnancy resolution but appear not to influence contraceptive behavior (Paikoff, 1990; Paikoff & Brooks-Gunn, in press, p. 19).

Decision-Making Skills. Decision-making skills are believed to be important in the management of sexual behavior (Fischhoff, 1980; Furby & Beyth-Marom, in press; Gardner, in press). Adolescents in the second half of adolescence are quite similar in their decision processes (Furby & Beyth-Marom, in press; Gardner, in press), although little direct developmental comparative research has been conducted and not much is known about younger adolescents. Different-aged persons may, however, perceive the consequences of their decisions quite differently, as discussed earlier.

Environmental Factors

Peers and parents clearly influence adolescent adherence to a health regime.

Peers. One of the most accepted hallmarks of adolescence is the increased importance of peers, as seen in time spent with them, value of their opinions, beliefs that one's behavior is similar to one's peers, and conformity to one's perceptions of their opinions (Brown, 1990; Hartup, 1983). However, it is important to remember that some peer groups have values similar to those of parents and that great variation is seen in peer group beliefs and behavior, that parents still exert influence over their teenage offspring (Savin-Williams & Berndt, 1990). Most health behaviors are practiced with peers. How peers influence adherence to health regimes is not well studied. For example, sexuality, or at least its expression with others, is embedded in the peer network. However, we know little about how friends influence teenagers' sexual behavior (Brooks-Gunn & Furstenberg, 1989). At the very least, teenagers act on what they believe their friends are doing (leaving aside the question of whether their perceptions are accurate; Hofferth & Hayes, 1987; Newcomer, Gilbert, & Udry, 1980). Individual variation occurs: Blacks are less influenced by their peers than are Whites, boys less than girls, and older teens less than younger ones (Cvetkovich & Grote, 1980; Furstenberg, Moore, & Peterson, 1986; Smith & Udry, 1985). Perhaps peers are more salient when the behavior in question is less common or has acquired less "normative" status in a particular group (Brooks-Gunn & Paikoff, in press, p. 13).[3] Indeed, altering peer norms is one approach to changing adolescent health behavior.

---

[3]See Blyth, Simmons, and Zakin (1985), Gargiulo, Attie, Brooks-Gunn, and Warren (1987), and Magnusson, Stattin, and Allen (1985), for examples of this phenomenon for pubertal change.

Parents. Parents influence health behavior in a variety of ways. Parents provide direct training in certain aspects of health behavior (for example, diet). Parents clearly supervise their children's health behavior, as is illustrated by the parental role in the dispensing of medications to children and the monitoring of diet in obese and diabetic children (see Delamater, this volume). Social learning theory has highlighted parental influences as role models: Children and youth observe and imitate their parents' behaviors, including health behaviors. Indeed, parents' adherence to certain health regimes (diet and exercise) is modestly associated with child's adherence (see Epstein, this volume). Other parental influences are less direct, involving such factors as the parent–child relationship, the ability of parents to let children take more responsibility for their actions with age, and the familial context. The following discussion is speculative, given that links between such family factors and adherence have not been studied extensively; however, low parental conflict and high communication are predictive of some types of adherence (see Anderson, this volume; Delamater, this volume; Paikoff & Brooks-Gunn, in press).

It is believed that changes in the parent–child relationship occur during the transition to adolescence. Such changes may be associated with difficulties in adherence at this time. Do relationships undergo an alteration for young adolescents and, as the commonsense wisdom states, are they more conflictual? Generally, parent–child relationships are characterized as moving toward more individuation (Grotevant & Cooper, 1986) and more mutuality (Hartup, 1989). Parents of young adolescents seem to expect them to act in more mature ways, socially, emotionally, and cognitively (Block, 1978; Ruble, 1983; Simmons & Blyth, 1987). The changing body acts as a social stimulus for some of these expectations (Hill & Lynch, 1983). At the same time, pubertal children seem to expect to be granted more freedom in curfews, dress, and choice of friends (Simmons & Blyth, 1987), and they rate parental use of assertion less favorably (Paikoff, Collins, & Laursen, 1988). Actual behavior also undergoes a transformation. Time spent with parents, emotional closeness, and yielding to parents in decision making all decrease in the first half of adolescence (Csikszentmihalyi & Larson, 1984; Hill, 1988; Montemayor & Hanson, 1985; Steinberg, 1987; Youniss, 1985). And, a corresponding increase in parent–child conflict is seen (Montemayor, 1982; Paikoff & Brooks-Gunn, 1991a; Smetana, 1988). Such conflict, however, is *not* particularly intense, nor does it indicate a diminution of a strong bond between parent and child. However, both parties consider these conflicts as being significant. Interestingly, mother–daughter conflicts are more pronounced than conflicts in other parent–child combinations (Montemayor, 1982; Smetana, 1988).

In an elegant analysis of the social-cognitive processes underlying conflict during the adolescent transition, Smetana (1988) has queried 5th to 12th graders and their parents about the legitimacy of parental authority in a variety of social situations. Disagreements tend to occur for social convention and personal issues but not for morality issues. Adolescents tend to see more situations as personal jurisdiction than social convention issues, whereas parents have just the opposite interpretation. Interestingly, when asked to take the other's perspective, both parents and adolescents recognize each other's position. Thus, many adolescents understand but reject their parents' perspective for issues in which they believe personal jurisdiction is legitimate, whereas parents do just the same for issues in which they believe social conventions should take precedent. It is possible that such processes underlie some disagreements about adherence to a health regime: Youth may feel that their sexuality is subject to personal jurisdiction, whereas parents perceive sexual behavior as in the realm of social convention. A similar process could occur in obese youth: In this case, dietary intake has been under parental jurisdiction and the switch to personal jurisdiction is perceived as legitimate by parents only when youth follow the regime set up by the parents during childhood.

Less social-cognitive approaches to relationship changes might shed light on adolescent adherence problems. Youth must develop strategies to deal with parental control during the development of individuation. For example, in a study of mother–daughter conflict discussions, premenarcheal seventh graders were found to employ more aggressive, oppositional, and critical speech with their mothers than postmenarcheal seventh graders, whereas the latter group used more passive forms of resistance to maternal demands (Brooks-Gunn & Zahaykevich, 1989). In contrast, studies of boys suggest that they increase their use of assertive, aggressive opposition throughout the first half of adolescence (Steinberg & Hill, 1978). How such changes affect interaction patterns, maternal use of control, or possible gender differences in adherence is not well understood, but they may set the stage for struggles over adolescent behavior (see Anderson, this volume, for a discussion of relational conflict in families with a diabetic youth as well as the literature on parent–child conflict over eating in families with an eating-disordered daughter: Attie & Brooks-Gunn, 1989; Attie et al., 1990; Bruch, 1978; Minuchin, 1985).

Parental relationships probably influence health behavior more generally throughout adolescence, although research is sorely needed (Ooms, 1981). In the realm of teenage sexuality, close relationships with parents seem to be associated with later onset of intercourse (Inazu & Fox, 1980; Jessor & Jessor, 1977). However, few studies examine relationships prior to intercourse, different aspects of parent–child communication, or the context in which such discussions are embedded (Hofferth, 1987). Certain parental interaction styles are likely to promote ego development and autonomy, specifically those characterized as enabling, authoritative, and legitimizing (Baumrind, 1987; Brooks-Gunn & Zahaykevich, 1989; Grotevant & Cooper, 1986; Hauser, Powers, Noam, Jacobson, Weiss, & Follansbee 1984). Perhaps more autonomous youth make more well-informed health decisions. At the same time, the parental styles just mentioned could promote greater feelings of self-efficacy, which in turn could influence dietary practices and sexual behavior (Bandura, 1982). Such premises await further testing.

INTERVENTION APPROACHES TO ADHERENCE

Several different approaches have been used to promote adolescent health behaviors. Many of these rely on principles of behavioral change. Here, several approaches that have been used in pregnancy prevention programs are reviewed. These were chosen for their reliance on principles underlying health behavior change more generally (see Becker, 1985; Turner et al., 1989).

Education

Information Dissemination. Information dissemination is probably necessary but not sufficient for health behavior change. Dissemination programs have been conducted through the schools, on a community-wide basis, and in the media, both locally and nationally. School-based programs have been shown to be effective in increasing adolescent knowledge about sexuality (Hofferth & Miller, 1989; Kirby, 1984). However, sexual behavior is usually not affected (see, for exceptions, Dawson, 1986; Marsiglio & Mott, 1986). Because most sex education programs are not intensive or extensive (for example, only 20% of a sample of urban school districts surveyed in 1984 had sessions on contraceptives prior to the end of high school; Sonenstein & Pittman, 1984), adequate tests of the efficacy of information dissemination in sex education classes have not been conducted. Mass media campaigns are another approach to the dissemination of information about health behavior. They typically do not target teenagers specifically (although recent pregnancy prevention media campaigns are aimed at adolescents and young adults).

Fear Arousal. Fear arousal techniques, in and of themselves, have not been shown to be particularly effective agents of behavioral change (Turner et al., 1989). However, when they are coupled with information about specific behavior changes that will reduce risk and when they are presented in a manner as to arouse a high level of anxiety, fear arousal is effective in altering health behavior and is as effective as skill training programs (Becker, 1985; Job, 1988; Sutton, 1982).

Problem Solving and Skills Training Programs

Problem solving and skills training programs have been shown to influence contraceptive use. Several school programs train adolescents in specific skills relevant to postponement of initiation of sexual activity (see review by Donahue, 1987; Eisen & Zellman, 1987; Eisen, Zellman, & McAlister, 1985; Howard, 1988; Paikoff & Brooks-Gunn, in press-b). Programs are sometimes based on the Health Belief Model (Janz & Becker, 1984). In such interventions, students are taught about the role of others in influencing sexual behavior, supplied with specific social skills to resist peer pressure and have their misperceptions corrected (i.e., far fewer individuals engage in intercourse than many youth believe do so). Some programs are based conceptually on social learning theory (Bandura, 1977); peer leaders, social reinforcement, and role playing are likely to be employed.

In addition to direct motivational and social skills training techniques to promote adherence, training about situational constraints on behavior might prove helpful. If unprotected sex occurs most frequently in the context of drinking or drug use with peers, as it may given the possible disinhibitory effects of some substances (Stall, Coates, & Hoff, 1988), then programs could focus on skills to be used in such situations or on the avoidance of such situations.

Employment or Continuing Education Programs

Augmenting life options, specifically employment and education, is becoming an increasingly attractive program option for changes in fertility behavior (Hofferth & Miller, 1989). The assumption is that by providing the means to reach often unattainable goals (i.e., going to college when the family is unable to help or few students in the neighborhood or school attend), the desirability of delaying pregnancy and focusing on schooling will be enhanced (keeping in mind that teenagers with high educational aspirations and achievement are less likely to become pregnant and more likely to use contraception; Chilman, 1986; Furstenberg et al., 1987; Morrison, 1985; Paikoff & Brooks-Gunn, in press, p. 9).

Implications for Intervention

Several points need to be raised in light of this admittedly brief review of intervention strategies. First, and quite regrettably, intervention strategies are typically not discussed in terms of antecedent risk factors, such as those outlined earlier in this chapter. Intervention strategies need to be explicitly paired with, and developed, in the context of risk factors.

Second, strategies that are more "person focused" and "environmentally or contextually focused" need to be considered. The majority of current interventions focus on the individual, through information dissemination, fear arousal, and skill training. Another set focuses on the contexts in which health behaviors are expressed; these include peer training efforts, media campaigns, school- or community-wide interventions, and family-oriented programs. Because health behavior is determined by individual as well as contextual factors, intervention programs need to incorporate strategies to deal with both.

Third, intervention strategies vary widely with respect to the desired outcomes. Some have quite specific goals (i.e., delay of intercourse). These programs tend to overemphasize single risk factors, or a limited set, as contributing to a particular behavior (Felner & Felner, 1989). Other programs have more inclusive goals (i.e., including school success and avoidance of substance use as well as sexual behavioral change). These approaches are more likely to consider several risk factors. However, all programs would benefit from consideration of the multiple risk factors underlying the health behavior in question and inclusion of intervention components addressing as many risk factors as possible.

Fourth, very little work has been done on how difficult it is to sustain adolescent health behavior changes once they have been initiated. Nor is there research on whether behavior change is easier to sustain in adults than in adolescents, because so few programs target and compare both age groups. Applying the excellent work on relapse prevention in adults to younger groups is advisable. For example, factors associated with relapse or low adherence have been identified, typically via correlational analysis (Green, Wilson, & Lovato, 1986; Stall et al., 1988). Whether similar factors would be found for teenagers is not known. However, in the case of homosexual men and IV drug users, characteristics that have been shown to make the practice of safer sex more difficult might be more typical of adolescents than of adults (e.g., low personal efficacy, high sensation seeking, more suspectable to peer influences, low knowledge; Brooks-Gunn & Furstenberg, 1990; Des Jarlais & Friedman, 1988; Stall et al., 1988). If intensiveness of programs is associated with sustained behavior change, then the schools provide an excellent workshop. More intensive prevention programs could be offered, and booster sessions would be relatively easy to implement. If continued adherence is enhanced to a change in the social milieu, then school- or community-wide programs may have a greater chance of success than smaller scale programs.

BARRIERS TO STUDYING ADOLESCENTS

It may be more difficult to study adolescents then children or adults. Indeed, adolescent research, in particular that focusing on young adolescents, is believed to have languished because of difficulties in recruitment (Brooks-Gunn, 1989, 1990). When it comes to health-promoting behaviors, cultural and parental beliefs that youth do not (or should not) engage in particular behaviors impede research. Regardless of beliefs about the appropriateness of certain sexual behaviors, a relatively high percentage of teenagers 16 years of age and younger have had intercourse, with the majority using contraceptives sporadically or not all (Hofferth & Hayes, 1987; Jones et al., 1985).

Possible reasons for the relative paucity of research until recently include (a) societal prohibitions about teenage sexuality, (b) adult discomfort with puberty and sexuality, and (c) parental and youth reticence in study participation (Brooks-Gunn, 1990). First, societal prohibitions against sexuality make it difficult to query young adolescents about such behavior because they are not supposed to engage in them. Additionally, some individuals believe that asking or educating youth about sexuality is an implicit invitation to experiment; as an example, the main argument against sex education in the schools is that it may promote sexual activity (although evidence generally does not support this notion; see review by Paikoff & Brooks-Gunn, in press).

Second, what puberty means to most adults and how our society treats the onset of reproductive maturity structures the sexual discourse and, more generally, discourse about adolescence (see Brooks-Gunn, 1989; Brooks-Gunn & Reiter, 1990, for a discussion of more conceptual reasons for the "stepchild" status of pubertal and sexual research). Many adults are uncomfortable discussing the physical aspects of growth, probably because of cultural taboos about considering such topics and because the changes are associated with sexuality. Discomfort may lead to a denial of the importance of physical changes and sexual arousal for young adolescents.[4]

In addition, the pubertal experiences of many adults were not pleasant. For example, over 40% of women who are now over 60 were not prepared for menarche (Larsen, 1961). Being unprepared has been shown to be a particularly unsettling experience, influencing feelings about one's body and menstrual experiences into late adolescence and adulthood (Koff, Rierdan, & Sheingold, 1982; Ruble & Brooks-Gunn, 1982; Shainess, 1961). Men may be even less prepared for their own puberty, especially because ejaculation may be a more taboo subject than menarche, given the former's overt links with sexuality (Gaddis & Brooks-Gunn, 1985).

Finally, from a societal point of view, pubertal growth is not celebrated or even formally acknowledged today, as was the case in most world societies (Paige, 1983). Instead, it is not commented upon, or it is treated with secrecy, even within the family. For example, in the late 1970s in Central New Jersey, less than 20% of junior and senior high school girls told their father when they began to menstruate (although almost all told their mothers: Brooks-Gunn, 1987). In a small sample of boys from the same area, none told their mothers and one told his father that he had experienced an ejaculation (Gaddis & Brooks-Gunn, 1985). Consequently, family discourse about the body is rare, further reinforcing adult beliefs that body changes are not particularly salient to youth and adolescent beliefs that such topics are taboo.

---

[4]For example, in our research in 10 private schools, resistance to asking fifth graders about breast buds was initially encountered. School personnel were convinced that young girls either were not concerned about such changes or did not notice these changes in others (Brooks-Gunn, 1990).

Such a context makes it difficult to conduct research in schools on any health-promotion topics associated with reproduction or bodily changes (see Brooks-Gunn, 1990, for a more complete discussion of difficulties in and strategies for obtaining school permission). This is particularly true for studies of young adolescents; by late adolescence, it is acceptable to ask retrospectively about age of menarche and intercourse. However, it seems as though the spectra of AIDS is altering the research climate. Many school systems are implementing AIDS education curricula that by necessity deal with pubertal sexuality and drug use (Brooks-Gunn, Boyer, & Hein, 1988; Brooks-Gunn & Paikoff, in press; Hein, 1989). Virtually all adults are in favor of such programs. Will these changes make it easier to do research in these realms in the elementary and middle school? We do not know as of yet, but it seems highly likely.

Response rates for studies of puberty and sexuality range from 60% to 85% if positive rather than negative parental consent, as required by NIH, is obtained (Hill, 1982). It is often difficult to ascertain whether nonparticipation is due to parental worries, teenage reluctance, or some combination of both. However, in my longitudinal follow-up work, about half of refusals seem to be due to maternal reluctance and half to teenage demurring.

Are those teenagers and their families who participate in studies on such topics different from those who do not? In cases of original recruitment it is difficult to tell.[5] However, in longitudinal follow-ups, one may ascertain whether initial characteristics of those who stay in or leave a study are different. In most of my work on middle-class adolescent girls, few demographic or psychological differences emerge.

In my opinion, more barriers exist for the study of adolescents than for children or adults. Many health-associated behaviors are ones that society deems unacceptable for youth, that adults feel uncomfortable considering, that parents wish their offspring did not do, and that school personnel do not want to take responsibility for carrying out. Youth are sometimes reluctant because of concerns that parents or school personnel will find out what they are doing.

ASSESSING ADOLESCENT HEALTH BEHAVIORS

Three special measurement issues arise when considering adolescent health-promotion behaviors. These are sample selection, reliability of self-reports, and use of multiple respondents.

---

[5]In most studies the researcher does not have access, on an individual basis, to those who do not enter a study. However, schools will often provide basic demographic information on their student population, so that one may see in a general way how representative a sample is of the entire student body.

School, Clinic, and National Samples

Depending on the questions to be asked, a national survey (or, more likely, an extant data set), a school-based or community-based sample, or a clinic setting is used. Few community-based youth studies have been conducted, as the schools provide easy access to youth. About one-quarter to one-third of all teenagers do not complete high school, rendering the selection problem quite severe. School dropouts are more likely to have had sex early and to use contraception sporadically or not at all than those who manage to stay in school (Brunswick & Messeri, 1986; Elliott & Voss, 1974; Hofferth & Hayes, 1987; Kandel & Logan, 1984).

When studying adherence in obese or anorectic youth, clinic samples are typically used. It is difficult to estimate representativeness of such samples. For comparison purposes, matched samples from other clinic populations are often employed (however, other clinics often draw their clientele from different populations). Another approach is to select, randomly, several same-sex classmates from each obese or anorectic youth's school (keeping in mind that the school dropout selection problem exists from 10th grade on).

Self-Reports

How accurate are self-reports of behavior by adolescents, and are they less accurate than those of adults? The question is critical given that most studies rely on reports rather than observation, reports by others (i.e., parents, peers, teachers), or record reviews. Generally, adolescent reports of sexual and eating behavior seem to be quite accurate. Behaviors associated with eating are reported reliably by adolescents, in terms of height and weight, food records, and eating problems (Attie & Brooks-Gunn, 1989; Brooks-Gunn, Warren, Rosso, & Gargiulo, 1987; Frank et al., 1977; Garfinkel & Garner, 1982). Pubertal reports are reliable, even for Tanner stage classifications (Brooks-Gunn et al., 1987). Reports of onset of intercourse are accurate. Contraceptive use data may be subject to some bias; although youth who say that they use contraception regularly are less likely to be come pregnant, lending some face validity to such reports (Hofferth & Hayes, 1987). However, there are exceptions. We know that abortion is under-reported, and, by inference, those pregnancies that end in abortion. Whereas information on childbearing is accurate for women (and may be easily validated), fatherhood is believed to be under-reported (Furstenberg et al., 1987; Sonenstein, 1986).

Multiple Respondents

Another consideration is whether to rely on the target youth's reports, or to augment these by interviewing parents, teachers, or peers. Are youth more accurate reporters of their own behavior than others? The answer is a qualified yes. The incidence of sexual behavior and delinquency is higher from youth than parent reports (Furstenberg et al., 1987). And, parents do not know as much about their teenagers feelings as they think; correlations between daughters' and mothers' report of daughters' depressive feelings are low (Paikoff, Brooks-Gunn, & Warren, 1991; Weissman et al., 1987). Most developmentally oriented studies attempt to gather information from at least two people. However, few studies report on parent–youth divergence, nor on what such disagreements mean (Carlton-Ford, Paikoff, & Brooks-Gunn, 1991; Elliott & Ageton, 1980; Elliott, Huizinga, & Ageton, 1985; Elliott & Voss, 1974; McCord, 1990). However, perceptions not only may differ but may be differentially associated with health behavior. For example, maternal perceptions of the family environment, but not the daughters' ratings, were associated with daughters' eating problems in a sample of high school girls (Attie & Brooks-Gunn, 1989).

CONCLUSION

Promoting healthy behaviors is never an easy task. When it comes to adolescents, the problems may be even more daunting than they are with adults. Adolescents are in the midst of becoming adults, and all that this entails. In many cases, they have no prior experiences from which to construct the meanings of or to practice health-promoting behavior. Societal messages are often contradictory. Parents often are uncomfortable providing guidance or, in the eyes of adolescent, are unrealistic in their expectations (i.e., do not have sex). And, in the case of previous health regimes, parents are relinquishing control over their children's behavior during adolescence. Although peers provide support in the negotiation of adolescent tasks, they too are inventing meanings for the first time. Additionally, peers have their own agendas that may conflict with health promotion. If the costs of engaging in unhealthy behavior are perceived as low, if little societal support is given for behavior change, and if the context in which adolescents find themselves is not a target of intervention, then compliance with health-promoting behaviors will be sporadic at best.

Whereas young adolescents seem to have more difficulty adhering to health regimes than older adolescents or adults, surprisingly little information exists on this topic. Although possible mechanisms underlying lowered adherence in youth have been discussed in this chapter, virtually no comparative work on different-aged adolescents nor on youth and adults has been conducted. Whereas antecedent risk factors for low adherence have been identified, the relative strength of various biopsychosocial influences on health behavior has not.

As a final developmentally oriented note, different pathways to health promotion probably exist (Powers, Hauser, & Kilner, 1989). Subgroups of adolescents may be more likely to follow one pathway than another. For example, youth who are genetically at risk for obesity may need to use a combination of exercise and diet to control their weight and to maintain relatively constant surveillance over their dietary practices. Overweight youth with no familial history of obesity might successfully alter their weight via short-term dietary or exercise practices. Many adolescent athletes who are engaged in high-energy sports need not be concerned with caloric consumption during training but need to alter their practices during periods of inactivity due to injury or the end of the season (Brooks-Gunn, Burrow, & Warren, 1988; Warren, 1980). In contrast, athletes whose activities use less energy (such as dance) need to depend more on caloric intake to keep their weight at a certain level than do those whose activities burn more calories per hour of exercise (Brooks-Gunn et al., 1988). Similar examples have been given for sexual behavior (Brooks-Gunn & Paikoff, in press): Sexual well-being could be expressed by sexual abstinence, self-stimulating sexual behavior, or sexual intercourse with the practice of safe sex. Different subgroups of adolescents are likely to engage in different types of sexual behavior. Health promotion requires that these different pathways be identified, and the factors encouraging different types of healthy behavior be studied.

ACKNOWLEDGMENTS

This chapter was presented at a Workshop on "Developmental Aspects of Health Compliance Behavior," sponsored by the National Institute of Child Health and Human Development and the Bureau of Maternal and Child Health and Resources Development and held in Bethesda, July 1989. Support for the writing of this chapter was provided by the Russell Sage Foundation, when the author was a Visiting Scholar there. The research from which examples in the chapter were drawn was funded by NICHD, the W. T. Grant Foundation, the Ford Foundation, and the Robert Wood Johnson Foundation. Their generosity and continued support are greatly appreciated. I thank Norman Krasnegor for his thoughtful editorial comments.

REFERENCES

Attie, I., & Brooks-Gunn, J. (1987). Weight concerns as chronic stressors in women. In R. C. Barnett, L. Biener, & G. K. Naruch (Eds.), *Gender and stress* (pp. 218–254). New York: Free Press.

Attie, I., & Brooks-Gunn, J. (1989). The development of eating problems in adolescent girls: A longitudinal study. *Developmental Psychology, 25*(1), 70–79.

Attie, I., & Brooks-Gunn, J. (in press). Research strategies for studying the emergence of eating problems and disorders. In J. G. Crowther, S. E. Hobfoll, M. A. P. Stephens, & D. L. Tennenbaum (Eds.), *The etiology of bulimia: The individual and familial context*. Washington, DC: Hemisphere.

Attie, I., Brooks-Gunn, J., & Petersen, A. C. (1990). The emergence of eating problems: A developmental perspective. In M. Lewis & S. Miller (Eds.), *Handbook of developmental psychopathology* (pp. 409–420). New York: Grune & Stratton.

Bandura, A. (1977). Self-efficacy: Toward a unifying theory of behavioral change. *Psychological Review, 84*(2), 191–215.

Bandura, A. (1982). Self-efficacy mechanism in human agency. *American Psychologist, 37*, 122–147.

Baumrind, D. (1987). A developmental perspective on adolescent risk taking in contemporary America. *Adolescent Social Behavior and Health, 37*, 93–125.

Baydar, N., Brooks-Gunn, J., & Warren, M. P. (1991). *Determinants of depressive symptoms in adolescent girls: A four year longitudinal study.* Unpublished manuscript.

Becker, M. H. (1985). Patient adherence to prescribed therapies. *Medical Care, 23*(5), 539–555.

Bernstein, A. C., & Cowan, P. A. (1975). Children's concepts of how people get babies. *Child Development, 46*, 77–91.

Block, J. H. (1978). Another look at sex differentiation in the socialization behaviors of mothers and fathers. In J. Sherman & F. L. Denmark (Eds.), *The psychology of women: Future directions of research* (pp. 31–87). New York: Psychological Dimensions.

Blyth, D. A., Simmons, R. G., & Zakin, D. F. (1985). Satisfaction with body image for early adolescent females: The impact of pubertal timing within different school environments. *Journal of Youth and Adolescence, 14*(3), 207–225.

Brooks-Gunn, J. (1984). The psychological significance of different pubertal events to young girls. *Journal of Early Adolescence, 4*(4), 315–327.

Brooks-Gunn, J. (1987). Pubertal processes and girls' psychological adaptation. In R. Lerner & T. T. Foch (Eds.), *Biological–psychosocial interactions in early adolescence: A life-span perspective* (pp. 123–153). Hillsdale, NJ: Lawrence Erlbaum Associates.

Brooks-Gunn, J. (1988). Antecedents and consequences of variations in girls' maturational timing. *Journal of Adolescent Health Care, 9*(5), 365–373.

Brooks-Gunn, J. (1989). Pubertal processes and the early adolescent transition. In W. Damon (Ed.), *Child development today and tomorrow* (pp. 155–176). San Francisco: Jossey-Bass.

Brooks-Gunn, J. (1990). Barriers and impediments to conducting research with young adolescents. *Journal of Youth and Adolescence, 19*(5), 425–440.

Brooks-Gunn, J. (1992). Growing up female: Stressful events and the transition to adolescence. In T. Field, P. McCabe, & N. Schneiderman (Eds.), *Stress and coping in infancy and childhood* (pp. 119–145). Hillsdale, NJ: Lawrence Erlbaum Associates.

Brooks-Gunn, J., Boyer, C. B., & Hein, K. (1988). Preventing HIV infection and AIDS in children and adolescents: Behavioral research and intervention strategies. *American Psychologist, 43*(11), 958–964.

Brooks-Gunn, J., Burrow, C., & Warren, M. P. (1988). Attitudes toward eating and body weight in different groups of female adolescent athletes. *International Journal of Eating Disorders, 7*(6), 749–758.

Brooks-Gunn, J., Duke-Duncan, P., Ehrhardt, A., Hein, K., & Shafer, M. (1989). Adolescent HIV infection in Special Article: Nicholas, S. W., Sondheimer, D. L., Willoughby, A. D., Yaffe, S. J., & Katz, S. L., Human Immunodeficiency Virus infection in childhood, adolescence, & pregnancy: A status report and national research agenda. *Pediatrics, 83*, 299–301.

Brooks-Gunn, J., & Furstenberg, F. F., Jr. (1989). Adolescent sexual behavior. *American Psychologist, 44*(2), 249–257.

Brooks-Gunn, J., & Furstenberg, F. F., Jr. (1990). Coming of age in the era of AIDS: Sexual and contraceptive decisions. *Milbank Quarterly, 68*, 59–84.

Brooks-Gunn, J., & Paikoff, R. L. (in press). "Sex is a gamble, kissing is a game": Adolescent sexuality, contraception, and pregnancy. In S. P. Millstein, A. C. Petersen, & E. Nightingale (Eds.), *Promotion of health behavior in adolescence.* New York: Carnegie Corporation.

Brooks-Gunn, J., & Petersen, A. C. (Eds.). (1983). *Girls at puberty: Biological and psychosocial perspectives*. New York: Plenum Press.

Brooks-Gunn, J., & Petersen, A. C. (Eds.). (1991). Studying the emergence of depression and depressive symptoms during adolescence. *Journal of Youth and Adolescence, 20*(1).

Brooks-Gunn, J., Petersen, A. C., & Eichorn, D. (Eds.). (1985). Time of maturation and psychosocial functioning in adolescence. *Journal of Youth and Adolescence, 14* (Vol. 3 and 4).

Brooks-Gunn, J., & Reiter, E. O. (1990). The role of pubertal processes in the early adolescent transition. In S. Feldman & G. Elliott (Eds.), *At the threshold: The developing adolescent* (pp. 16–53). Cambridge, MA: Harvard University Press.

Brooks-Gunn, J., & Warren, M. P. (1989). Biological contributions to affective expression in young adolescent girls. *Child Development, 60*, 372–385.

Brooks-Gunn, J., Warren, M. P., Rosso, J., & Gargiulo, J. (1987). Validity of self-report measures of girls' pubertal status. *Child Development, 58*, 829–841.

Brooks-Gunn, J., & Zahaykevich, M. (1989). Parent–daughter relationships in early adolescence: A developmental perspective. In K. Kreppner & R. M. Lerner (Eds.), *Family systems and life-span development* (pp. 223–246). Hillsdale, NJ: Lawrence Erlbaum Associates.

Brown, B. B. (1990). Peer groups and peer cultures. In S. Feldman & G. Elliot (Eds.), *At the threshold: The developing adolescent* (pp. 171–196). Cambridge, MA: Harvard University Press.

Brownell, K. D., & Wadden, T. A. (1984). Confronting obesity in children: Behavioral and psychological factors. *Pediatric Annals, 13*(6), 473–480.

Bruch, H. (1978). *The golden cage*. Cambridge, MA: Harvard University Press.

Brunswich, A. F., & Messeri, P. (1986). Drugs, lifestyle, and health: A longitudinal study of urban black youth. *American Journal of Public Health, 76*, 52–57.

Carlton-Ford, S., Paikoff, R. L., & Brooks-Gunn, J. (1991). Methodological issues in the study of divergent views of the family. In R. L. Paikoff (Ed.), *New directions for child development: Shared views in the family during adolescence, 51*, (pp. 87–102). San Francisco: Jossey-Bass.

Chilman, C. S. (1986). Some psychosocial aspects of adolescent sexual and contraceptive behaviors in a changing American society. In J. B. Lancaster & B. A. Hamburg (Eds.), *School-age pregnancy and parenthood: Biosocial dimensions* (pp. 191–217). New York: Aldine De Gruyter.

Cobliner, W. G. (1974). Pregnancy in the single adolescent girl: The role of cognitive functions. *Journal of Youth and Adolescence, 3*(1), 17–29.

Csikszentmihalyi, M., & Larson, R. (1984). *Being adolescent: Conflict and growth in the teenage years*. New York: Basic Books.

Cvetkovich, G., & Grote, B. (1980). Psychological development and the social problem of teenage illegitimacy. In C. Chilman (Ed.), *Adolescent pregnancy and childbearing: Findings from research* (pp. 15–41). Washington, DC: U.S. Department of Health and Human Services.

Damon, W., & Hart, D. (1982). The development of self-understanding from infancy through adolescence. *Child Development, 53*, 841–864.

Dawson, D. A. (1986). The effects of sex education on adolescent behavior. *Family Planning Perspectives, 18*(4), 162–170.

Des Jarlais, D. C., & Friedman, S. R. (1988). The psychology of preventing AIDS among intravenous drug users: A social learning conceptualization. *American Psychologist, 43*(11), 865–870.

Donahue, M. J. (1987). *Human sexuality: Values and choices*. Technical report of the National Demonstration Project Field Test, Search Institute, Minneapolis, MN.

Eisen, M., & Zellman, G. L. (1987). Brief reports: Changes in incidence of sexual intercourse of unmarried teenagers following a community-based sex education program. *The Journal of Sex Research, 23*(4), 527–544.

Eisen, M., Zellman, G. L., & McAlister, A. (1985). A health brief model approach to adolescents' fertility control: Some pilot program findings. *Health Education Quarterly, 12*(2), 185–210.

Elliott, D. S., & Ageton, S. S. (1980). Reconciling race and class differences in self-reported and official estimates of delinquency. *American Sociological Review, 45,* 95–110.

Elliott, D. S., Huizinga, D., & Ageton, S. S. (1985). *Explaining delinquency and drug use.* Beverly Hills, CA: Sage.

Elliott, D. S., & Voss, H. L. (1974). *Delinquency and dropout.* Lexington, MA: Heath.

Ensminger, M. E. (1987). Adolescent sexual behavior as it relates to other transition behaviors in youth. In S. L. Hofferth & C. D. Hayes (Eds.), *Risking the future: Adolescent sexuality, pregnancy, and childbearing* (Vol. II, pp. 36–55). Washington, DC: National Academy Press.

Feldman, S. D., & Elliott, G. (Eds.). (1990). *At the threshold: The developing adolescent.* Cambridge, MA: Harvard University Press.

Felner, R. D., & Felner, T. Y. (1989). Primary prevention programs in the educational context: A transactional-ecological framework and analysis. In L. A. Bone & B. E. Compas (Eds.), *Primary prevention and promotion in the schools* (pp. 13–49). Newbury Park, CA: Sage.

Fischhoff, B. (1989). Making decisions about AIDS. In V. M. Mays, G. W. Albee, & S. F. Schneider (Eds.), *Primary prevention of AIDS* (pp. 168–205). Newbury Park, CA: Sage.

Fisher, W., Byrne, D., & White, L. (1983). In D. Byrne & W. Fisher (Eds.), *Adolescence, sex, and contraception* (pp. 207–239). Hillsdale, NJ: Lawrence Erlbaum Associates.

Frank, G. C., Berenson, G., Prentis, S., & Moore, M. C. (1977). Adopting the 24-hour recall for epidemiologic studies of school children. *Journal of American Dietetic Association, 71,* 26–31.

Furby, L., & Beyth-Marom, R. (in press). Risk taking in adolescence: A decision-making perspective. *Developmental Review.*

Furstenberg, F. F., Jr., Brooks-Gunn, J., & Morgan, S. P. (1987). *Adolescent mothers in later life.* New York: Cambridge University Press.

Furstenberg, F. F., Jr., Moore, K. A., & Peterson, J. L. (1986). Sex education and sexual experience among adolescents. *American Journal of Public Health, 75*(11), 1331–1332.

Gaddis, A., & Brooks-Gunn, J. (1985). The male experience of pubertal change. *Journal of Youth and Adolescence, 14*(1), 61–69.

Gardner, W. (in press). A life-span theory of risk-taking. In N. Bell (Ed.), *Adolescent and adult risk taking: The eighth Texas Tech Symposium on interfaces in psychology.*

Garfinkel, I., & McLanahan, S. (1990). The effects of the child support provisions of the Family Support Act of 1988 on child well-being. *Population Research and Policy Review, 9,* 205–234.

Garfinkel, P. E., & Garner, D. M. (1982). *Anorexia nervosa: A multidimensional perspective.* New York: Brunner/Mazel.

Gargiulo, J., Attie, I., Brooks-Gunn, J., & Warren, M. P. (1987). Girls' dating behavior as a function of social context and maturation. *Developmental Psychology, 23*(5), 730–737.

Garmezy, N., Masten, A. S., & Tellegen, A. (1984). The study of stress and competence in children: A building block for developmental psychopathology. *Child Development, 55,* 97–111.

Garmezy, N., & Rutter, M. (1988). *Stress, coping, and development in children.* Baltimore: Johns Hopkins Paperbacks.

Goldman, R. J., & Goldman, J. D. (1982). How children perceive the origin of babies and the roles of mothers and fathers in procreation: A cross-national study. *Child Development, 53,* 491–504.

Green, L. W., Wilson, A. L., & Lovato, C. Y. (1986). What changes can health promotion achieve and how long do these changes last? The trade-offs between expediency and durability. *Preventive Medicine, 15,* 508–521.

Grotevant, H. D., & Cooper, C. R. (1986). Individuation in family relationships. *Human Development, 29,* 82–100.

Gunnar, M. R., & Collins, W. A. (Eds.). (1988). *Transitions in adolescence: Minnesota Symposia on Child Psychology* (Vol. 21). Hillsdale, NJ: Lawrence Erlbaum Associates.

Harter, S. (1983). Developmental perspectives on the self-system. In E. M. Hetherington (Ed.), *Handbook of child psychology, Vol IV: Socialization, personality, and social development* (pp. 275–386). New York: Wiley.

Hartup, W. W. (1983). Peer relations. In E. M. Hetherington (Ed.), *Handbook of child psychology, Vol IV: Socialization, personality, and social development* (pp. 103–196). New York: Wiley.

Hartup, W. W. (1989). Social relationships and their developmental significance. *American Psychologist, 44*(2), 120–126.

Hauser, S., Powers, S. I., Noam, G. G., Jacobson, A. M., Weiss, B., & Follansbee, D. J. (1984). Familial contexts of adolescent ego development. *Child Development, 55*, 195–213.

Hayes, C. D. (Ed.). (1987). *Risking the future: Adolescent sexuality, pregnancy, and childbearing* (Vol. I). Washington, DC: National Academy of Sciences Press.

Hein, K. (1989). AIDS in adolescence. *Journal of Adolescent Health Care, 10*, 10–35.

Hill, J. P. (1982). Early adolescence (special issue). *Child Development, 53*(6), 1409–1412.

Hill, J. P. (1988). Adapting to menarche: Familial control and conflict. In M. R. Gunnar & W. A. Collins (Eds.), *Development during the transition to adolescence* (Vol. 21, pp. 43–77). Hillsdale, NJ: Lawrence Erlbaum Associates.

Hill, J. P., & Lynch, M. E. (1983). The intensification of gender-related role expectations during early adolescence. In J. Brooks-Gunn & A. C. Petersen (Eds.), *Girls at puberty: Biological and psychosocial perspectives* (pp. 201–228). New York: Plenum Press.

Hofferth, S. L. (1987). Factors affecting initiation of sexual intercourse. In S. L. Hofferth & C. D. Hayes (Eds.), *Risking the future: Adolescent sexuality, pregnancy, and childbearing* (Vol. II, pp. 7–35). Washington, DC: National Academy Press.

Hofferth, S. L., & Hayes, C. D. (Eds.). (1987). *Risking the future: Adolescent sexuality, pregnancy, and childbearing* (Vol. II). Washington, DC: National Academy of Sciences Press.

Hofferth, S. L., & Miller, B. C. (1989). An overview of adolescent pregnancy prevention programs and their evaluations. In J. J. Card (Ed.), *Evaluation program aimed at preventing teenage pregnancies* (pp. 25–40). Palo Alto, CA: Sociometrics Corporation.

Howard, M. (1988). Helping youth postpone sexual involvement. In D. Bennett & M. Williams (Eds.), *New universals: Adolescent health in a time of change*. Curtin, Australia: Brolga Press.

Inazu, J. K., & Fox, G. L. (1980). Maternal influence on the sexual behavior of teenage daughters. *Journal of Family Issues, 1*, 81–102.

Inhelder, B., & Piaget, J. (1958). *The growth of logical thinking from childhood to adolescence*. New York: Basic Books.

Irwin, C. E., & Millstein, S. G. (1991). Risk-taking behaviors during adolescence. In R. M. Lerner, A. C. Petersen, & J. Brooks-Gunn (Eds.), *Encyclopedia of adolescence* (pp. 935–943). New York: Garland Press.

Janz, N. K., & Becker, M. H. (1984). The health belief model: A decade later. *Health Education Quarterly, 11*(1), 1–47.

Jessor, R. (1992). Risk behavior in adolescence: A psychosocial framework for understanding and action. In D. E. Rogers & E. Ginzberg (Eds.), *Adolescents at risk: Medical and social perspectives* (pp. 19–34). Boulder, CO: Westview Press.

Jessor, R., & Jessor, S. L. (1977). *Problem behavior and psychosocial development*. New York: Academic Press.

Job, R. F. S. (1988). Effective and ineffective use of fear in health promoting campaigns. *American Journal of Public Health, 78*, 163–167.

Jones, E., Forrest, J., Goldman, N., Henshaw, S., Lincoln, R., Rosoff, J., Westoff, C., & Wulf, D. (1985). Teenage pregnancy in developed countries: Determinants and policy implications. *Family Planning Perspectives, 17*(2), 53–63.

Jones, E., Forrest, J. D., Henshaw, S. K., Silverman, J., & Torres, A. (1988). Unintended pregnancy, contraceptive practice and family planning services in developed countries. *Family Planning Perspectives, 20*(2), 53–67.

Jones, J. B., & Philliber, S. (1983). Sexually active but not pregnant: A comparison of teens who risk and teens who plan. *Journal of Youth and Adolescence, 12*(3), 235–251.

Kandel, D. B., & Logan, J. A. (1984). Patterns of drug use from adolescence to young adulthood: Periods of risk for initiation, continued use and discontinuation. *American Journal of Public Health, 74*(7), 660–666.

Kandel, D. B., Raveis, V. H., & Davies, M. (1991). Suicidal ideation in adolescence: Depression, substance use and other risk factors. *Journal of Youth and Adolescence, 20*(1).

Katchadourian, H. (1990). Sexuality. In S. S. Feldman & G. R. Elliott (Eds.), *At the threshold: The developing adolescent* (pp. 330–351). Cambridge, MA: Harvard University Press.

Keating, D. P. (1990). Adolescent thinking. In S. S. Feldman & G. R. Elliott (Eds.), *At the threshold: The developing adolescent* (pp. 54–90). Cambridge, MA: Harvard University Press.

Kirby, D. (1984). *Sexuality education: An evaluation of programs and their effects*. Santa Cruz, CA: Network Publications.

Koff, E., Rierdan, J., & Sheingold, K. (1982). Memories of menarche: Age, preparation, and prior knowledge as determinants of initial menstrual experience. *Journal of Youth and Adolescence, 11*, 1–9.

Lancelot, C., Brooks-Gunn, J., & Warren, M. P. (1991). A comparison of DSM–III and DSM–IIIR bulimia classifications. *International Journal of Eating Disorders, 10*(1), 57–66.

Larsen, V. L. (1961). Sources of menstrual information: A comparison of age groups. *Family Life Coordinator, 10*, 41–43.

Lerner, R. M. (1969). The development of stereotyped expectancies of body build behavior relations. *Child Development, 40*, 137–141.

Lerner, R. M. (1982). Children and adolescents as producers of their own development. *Developmental Review, 2*, 342–370.

Lerner, R. M., & Foch, T. T. (Eds.). (1987). *Biological–psychosocial interactions in early adolescence: A life-span perspective*. Hillsdale, NJ: Lawrence Erlbaum Associates.

Lewis, C. C. (1981). How adolescents approach decisions: Changes over grades seven to twelve and policy implications. *Child Development, 52*, 538–544.

Magnusson, D., Stattin, H., & Allen, V. L. (1985). Biological maturation and social development: A longitudinal study of some adjustment processes from mid-adolescence to adulthood. *Journal of Youth and Adolescence, 14*(4), 267–283.

Marsiglio, W., & Mott, F. (1986). The impact of sex education on sexual activity, contraception use and premarital pregnancy among American teenagers. *Family Planning Perspectives, 18*(4), 151–161.

McCord, J. (1990). Problem behaviors. In S. D. Feldman & G. Elliott (Eds.), *At the threshold: The developing adolescent* (pp. 414–430). Cambridge, MA: Harvard University Press.

Minuchin, P. (1985). Families and individual development: Provocations from the field of family therapy. *Child Development, 56*, 289–302.

Montemayor, R. (1982). The relationship between parent–adolescent conflict and the amount of time adolescents spend alone and with parents and peers. *Child Development, 53*, 1512–1519.

Montemayor, R., Adams, G. R., & Gullotta, T. P. (Eds.). (1990). *Advances in adolescent development, Vol. 2: From childhood to adolescence—a transitional period?* Newbury, CA: Sage.

Montemayor, R., & Hanson, E. A. (1985). A naturalistic view of conflict between adolescents and their parents and siblings. *Journal of Early Adolescence, 5*, 23–30.

Morrison, D. M. (1985). Adolescent contraceptive behavior: A review. *Psychological Bulletin, 98*(3), 538–568.

Newcomer, S. F., Gilbert, M., & Udry, J. R. (1980, September). *Perceived and actual same sex peer behavior as determined of adolescent sexual behavior*. Paper presented at the annual meeting of the American Psychological Association, Los Angeles.

Ooms, T. (Ed.). (1981). *Teenage pregnancy in a family context: Implications for policy*. Philadelphia: Temple University Press.

Paige, K. E. (1983). A bargaining theory of menarcheal responses in preindustrial cultures. In J.

Brooks-Gunn & A. C. Petersen (Eds.), *Girls at puberty: Biological and psychosocial perspectives* (pp. 301–322). New York: Plenum Press.

Paikoff, R. L. (1990). Attitudes toward consequences of pregnancy in young women attending a family planning clinic. *Journal of Adolescent Research, 5*(4), 467–484.

Paikoff, R. L., & Brooks-Gunn, J. (1990). Physiological processes: What role do they play during the transition to adolescence? In R. Montemayor, G. Adams, & T. Gullotta (Eds.), *Advances in adolescent development: Vol. 2, The transition from childhood to adolescence* (pp. 63–81). Newbury Park, CA: Sage.

Paikoff, R. L., & Brooks-Gunn, J. (1991). Do parent–child relationships change during puberty? *Psychological Bulletin, 110*(1), 47–66.

Paikoff, R. L., & Brooks-Gunn, J. (in press). Taking fewer chances: Teenage pregnancy prevention programs. *American Psychologist*.

Paikoff, R. L., Brooks-Gunn, J., & Warren, M. P. (1991). Effects of girls' hormonal status on affective expression over the course of one year. *Journal of Youth and Adolescence, 20*(1).

Paikoff, R. L., Collins, W. A., & Laursen, B. (1988). Perceptions of efficacy and legitimacy of parental influence techniques by children and early adolescents. *Journal of Early Adolescence, 8*(1), 37–52.

Powers, S., Hauser, S. T., & Kilner, L. (1989). Adolescent mental health. *American Psychologist, 44*(2), 200–208.

Rodin, J., Silberstein, L. R., & Striegel-Moore, R. (1984). Women and weight: A normative discontent. In T. B. Sonderegger (Ed.), *Nebraska Symposium on Motivation: No. 32, Psychology and gender* (pp. 267–307). Lincoln: University of Nebraska Press.

Rogel, M. J., Zuehlke, M. E., Petersen, A. C., Tobin-Richards, M., & Shelton, M. (1980). Contraceptive behavior in adolescence: A decision-making perspective. *Journal of Youth and Adolescence, 9*(6), 491–506.

Ruble, D. N. (1983). The development of social-comparison processes and their role in achievement-related self-socialization. In E. T. Higgins, D. N. Ruble, & W. W. Hartup (Eds.), *Social cognition and social development* (pp. 134–157). New York: Cambridge University Press.

Ruble, D. N., & Brooks-Gunn, J. (1982). The experience of menarche. *Child Development, 53*, 1557–1566.

Rutter, M., Izard, C. E., & Read, P. B. (Eds.). (1986). *Depression in young people: Developmental and clinical perspectives*. New York: The Guilford Press.

Sallis, J. F. (in press). Promoting healthful diet and physical activity. In S. G. Millstein, A. C. Petersen, & E. O. Nightingale (Eds.), *Promoting adolescent health: Rationale, goals and objectives*. Washington, DC: Carnegie Corporation.

Savin-Williams, R. C., & Berndt, T. J. (1990). Friendships and peer relations. In S. Feldman & G. Elliott (Eds.), *At the threshold: The developing adolescent* (pp. 277–307). Cambridge, MA: Harvard University Press.

Selman, R. L. (1980). *The growth of interpersonal understanding: Developmental and clinical analyses*. New York: Academic Press.

Shainess, N. (1961). A re-evaluation of some aspects of femininity through a study of menstruation: A preliminary report. *Comparative Psychiatry, 2*, 20–26.

Simmons, R. G., & Blyth, D. A. (1987). *Moving into adolescence: The impact of pubertal change and school context*. New York: Adline De Gruyter.

Simmons, R. G., Burgeson, R., & Reef, M. J. (1988). Cumulative change at entry to adolescence. In M. Gunnar & W. A. Collins (Eds.), *Development during transition to adolescence: Minnesota symposia on child psychology* (Vol. 21, pp. 123–150). Hillsdale, NJ: Lawrence Erlbaum Associates.

Smetana, J. G. (1988). Concepts of self and social convention: Adolescents' and parents' reasoning about hypothetical and actual family conflicts. In M. Gunnar & W. A. Collins (Eds.), *Develop-*

ment during transition to adolescence: Minnesota symposia on child psychology (Vol. 21, pp. 79–122). Hillsdale, NJ: Lawrence Erlbaum Associates.
Smith, E. A., & Udry, J. R. (1985). Coital and non-coital sexual behaviors of white and black adolescents. *American Journal of Public Health, 75,* 1200–1203.
Sonenstein, F. L. (1986). Risking paternity: Sex and contraception among adolescent males. In A. B. Elster & M. E. Lamb (Eds.), *Adolescent fatherhood* (pp. 31–54). Hillsdale, NJ: Lawrence Erlbaum Associates.
Sonenstein, F. L., & Pittman, K. J. (1984). The availability of sex education in large city school districts. *Family Planning Perspectives, 16,* 19–25.
Stall, R. D., Coates, T. J., & Hoff, C. (1988). Behavioral risk reduction for HIV infection among gay and bisexual men: A review of results from the United States. *American Psychologist, 43*(11), 878–885.
Stattin, H., & Magnusson, D. (1990). *Paths through life—Vol. 2: Pubertal maturation in female development.* Hillsdale, NJ: Lawrence Erlbaum Associates.
Steinberg, L. D. (1987). The impact of puberty on family relations: Effects of pubertal status and pubertal timing. *Developmental Psychology, 23,* 451–460.
Steinberg, L. D., & Hill, J. P. (1978). Patterns of family interaction as a function of age, the onset of puberty, and formal thinking. *Developmental Psychology, 14,* 683–684.
Stunkard, A. J., d'Aquili, E. E., Fox, S., & Filion, R. D. L. (1972). Influence of social class on obesity and thinness in children. *Journal of American Medical Association, 221,* 579–584.
Surgeon General. (1979). *Healthy people: The Surgeon General's report on health promotion and disease prevention.* Washington, DC: U.S. Department of Health, Education, & Welfare, Publication No. 79-55071, U.S. Government Printing Office.
Susman, E. J., Inoff-Germain, G., Nottelmann, E. D., Loriaux, D. L., Cutler, G. B., & Chrousos, G. P. (1987). Hormones, emotional dispositions, and aggressive attributes in young adolescents. *Child Development, 58,* 1114–1134.
Sutton, S. R. (1982). Fear-arousing communications: A critical examination of theory and research. In J. R. Eiser (Ed.), *Social psychology and behavioral medicine* (pp. 303–337). New York: Wiley.
Turner, C. F., Miller, H. G., & Moses, L. E. (Eds.). (1989). *AIDS: Sexual behavior and intravenous drug use.* Washington, DC: National Academy Press.
Udry, J. R. (1988). Biological predispositions and social control in adolescent sexual behavior. *American Sociological Review, 53,* 709–722.
Udry, J. R., Billy, J. O. G., Morris, N. M., Groff, T. R., & Raj, M. N. (1985). Serum androgenic hormones motive sexual behavior in adolescent boys. *Fertility and Sterility, 43*(1), 90–94.
Udry, J. R., Talbert, T., & Morris, N. M. (1986). Biosocial foundations for adolescent female sexuality. *Demography, 23*(2), 217–230.
Warren, M. P. (1980). The effects of exercise on pubertal progression and reproductive function in girls. *Journal of Clinical Endocrinology and Metabolism, 51*(5), 1150–1157.
Warren, M. P., & Brooks-Gunn, J. (1989). Mood and behavior at adolescence: Evidence for hormonal factors. *Journal of Clinical Endocrinology and Metabolism, 69*(1), 77–83.
Weinstein, N. D. (1987). Unrealistic optimism about susceptibility to health problems: Conclusions from a community-wide sample. *Journal of Behavioral Medicine, 10*(5), 481–500.
Weissman, M. M., et al. (1987). Assessing psychiatric disorders in children: Discrepancies between mothers' and children's reports. *Archives of General Psychiatry, 44*(8), 747–753.
Werner, E. E., & Smith, R. S. (1982). *Vulnerable but invincible: A longitudinal study of resilient children and youth.* New York: McGraw-Hill.
Winter, L. (1988). The role of sexual self-concept in the use of contraceptives. *Family Planning Perspectives, 20,* 123–127.
Youniss, J. (1985). *Adolescent relations with mothers, fathers and friends.* Chicago: University of Chicago Press.

Zabin, L. S., & Clark, S. D., Jr. (1981). Why they delay: A study of teenage family planning clinic patients. *Family Planning Perspectives, 13*(5), 205–217.

Zelnik, M., & Kantner, J. F. (1977). Sexual and contraceptive experience of young unmarried women in the United States, 1976 and 1971. *Family Planning Perspectives, 9*, 55–71.

Zelnik, M., & Kantner, J. F. (1978). Contraceptive practices and premarital pregnancy among women aged 15–19 in 1976. *Family Planning Perspectives, 10*(3), 135–142.

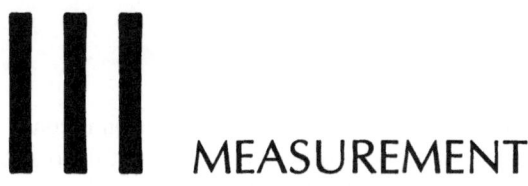

MEASUREMENT

Norman A. Krasnegor

The section on measurement contains two chapters. Both of these focus on how to assess the health compliance construct. The first chapter uses childhood diabetes as an example of a chronic disease in the context of which many compliance behaviors are required to avoid the deleterious consequences of the illness. The second chapter focuses mainly on measurement methodology associated with accurately characterizing whether or not compliance to medical regimes is occurring.

The chapter by Suzanne Bennett Johnson, "Chronic Diseases of Childhood: Assessing Compliance with Complex Medical Regimens," has as its focus the assessment of health compliance behavior to required medical regimens among children who are afflicted with chronic disease. The author employs insulin-dependent diabetes mellitus (IDDM) as the example of a chronic disease that involves compliance problems. Thus, the child or child/caregiver dyad are required to make complex measurements of body fluids (urine) to determine glucose levels and use this information to set the amount of insulin injected on a daily basis into the body of the diabetic child or change his or her daily diet.

Johnson addresses the issue whether compliance is a unitary or a multidimensional construct and comes down firmly on the side of it being multidimensional in nature. Her analysis of 13 diabetes compliance behaviors from a sample of IDDM children when subjected to a principle component analysis resulted in a five-factor solution that accounted for 70% of the variance. This conclusion is consonant with the theoretical characterization made by several of the contributors to this volume (see, e.g., Leventhal). The implication is that one should employ multiple measures to appropriately assess compliance behavior.

Johnson concurs with the observations of Iannotti and Bush, that cognitive development level interacts with capacity to comply with a complex regimen. She also agrees with Anderson and Coyne concerning the effects of miscommunication between health professionals and patient/caregiver on compliance efficacy. Johnson reports on studies that indicate that patients and/or parents of patients showed poor recall of recommendations made by providers. Johnson also points out the important observation concerning the confound between adherence and health status.

It is often assumed by health professionals that, in the case of IDDM, normal glucose levels represent excellent adherence. Whereas failure to comply to an adequate regime will usually affect health status, perfect compliance will not lead to good health if the regime itself is less than adequate. Johnson reviews a number of alternative strategies for assessing compliance. These are health status, physician ratings, self-reports, behavioral observations, permanent products (e.g., pill and bottle count; see Rudd, this section), and the 24-hour recall interview. In regard to this latter measure, Johnson reports that "when conducted with multiple informants on multiple occasions, [it] appears to provide the investigator with a reliable method of assessing a wide range of behaviors."

Finally, Johnson provides several guides for intervention. A cardinal principle for her is not to use "health status indicators, physician ratings, and general statements by the patient." She suggests that the 24-hour recall interview with multiple informants on multiple occasions should be employed first to assess compliance and follow this approach with behavioral techniques and permanent product measures for fine tuning.

The next chapter by Peter Rudd, "The Measurement of Compliance: Medication Taking," reviews the literature on medication taking of prescribed drugs. The work especially emphasizes measurement of compliance "despite constraints of patient cooperation." By and large, this chapter does not address the issue of how developmental factors affect compliance. Rather, the work takes a more generic perspective concerning the topic described. The examples provided are of adult populations; however, the methodology presented could apply to compliance of caretakers of pediatric populations or medication taking by adolescents.

Rudd provides an historic overview of some of the early compliance literature and identifies three major themes: (a) less than optimal medication taking by patients (epidemiological studies estimate that some patients take only 50% of their prescribed dosing regime), (b) a search for predictors and determinants of compliance (Rudd concludes as does Johnson that health status is not a good index of compliance), and (c) attempts to intervene in order to improve compliance (these interventions fall into the broad categories of educational, behavioral, and system-based).

Rudd gives an excellent overview on methods of measurement. He categorizes the alternatives into two groupings and provides a summary of the research findings that characterize the measures in terms of their effectiveness for measuring compliance. These are: (a) direct biological measures (e.g., assays of drug metabolites; markers); (b) indirect, nonbiological measures (e.g., self-report; pill counts; clinician's opinions). This latter grouping of measures is the one that Johnson pointed out were less than satisfactory for assessing compliance in chronically ill children.

A central theme of this chapter is that new technology can be employed to assess compliance. The particular device that Rudd focuses on is the *MEDICATION EVENT MONITORING SYSTEM (MEMS)*. This apparatus is a "modified plastic vial whose cap contains a microprocessor capable of recording the precise time and duration of each vial opening." Rudd describes research he and his colleagues have carried out with the device and its capacity to help measure compliance. Results of the studies suggest strongly that the technology will be quite useful to clinicians in assessing whether time/dose relationships are being handled adequately by patients, and whether the total dosing regime is being adhered to.

Rudd concludes his chapter by offering a series of guidelines to clinicians and investigators and recommendations concerning the needs for specific types of studies.

7 Chronic Diseases of Childhood: Assessing Compliance With Complex Medical Regimens

Suzanne Bennett Johnson
University of Florida Health Science Center

At the beginning of this century, the leading causes of death were influenza, pneumonia, diphtheria, tuberculosis, and gastrointestinal infections. Few of us know anyone who has died of such diseases today, pointing to the revolution in medicine that has occurred in the last century. This revolution was predicated on a theory, the germ theory of disease. As early as the 17th century, van Leeuwenhoek had discovered creatures too small to be seen by the naked eye. But it was two more centuries before Pasteur and Koch developed the germ theory of disease. This theory had profound implications for the care and treatment of the sick. Lister developed aseptic techniques, resulting in drastic reductions in fatalities from operations. Sanitation substantially reduced the spread of disease. Disease prevention became a reality through the development of effective vaccines. Previously life-threatening illness could be successfully treated with the advent of antibiotics and antiviral agents. Medicine's conquest of infectious disease has massively changed the health care challenges faced by our society. Chronic diseases and injuries from accidents, poisonings, and violence are our current health care problems. Behavioral factors, particularly habits such as smoking, dietary preferences, and alcohol use, play a major etiological role. In 1980, the Center for Disease Control of the U.S. Public Health Service estimated that 50% of mortality from the 10 leading causes of death in the United States can be traced to lifestyle behaviors (Miller, 1983).

With acute illness successfully controlled, chronic illness has become more evident. Improvements in the management of chronic conditions have further prolonged life, making chronic illness a large part of medical practice. Insulin, for example, was discovered in 1922. Before then, children with diabetes typically lived less than a year; now they have a life expectancy approximately 75%

of normal (Craig, 1981). Improvements in the management of childhood chronic illness continue. In 1967, the median length of survival was less than 2 years for children diagnosed with acute lymphoblastic leukemia. By 1983, 60%–65% of these children were surviving 5 years or longer (Miller & Miller, 1984). Similar progress has been made in the treatment of cystic fibrosis. Although still a fatal disease, 50% of youngsters are now surviving into their late teens or 20s (Matthews & Drotar, 1984). Any specific chronic illness in childhood is relatively rare. However, the total number of children suffering from any chronic condition is currently estimated at 10%–20% (Gortmaker & Sappenfield, 1984). Further, these children use a disproportionate amount of health care services. Smyth-Staruch, Breslau, Weitzman, and Gortmaker (1984) compared hospitalizations and the use of outpatient services during a 1-year period by 369 children with cystic fibrosis, cerebral palsy, myelodysplasia, or multiple physical handicaps. A random sample of 456 youngsters without congenital conditions served as controls. The average chronically ill or disabled child used 10 times more health care services than the average comparison child.

Childhood chronic conditions often require complex management regimens. Medicines may need to be ingested or injected on a daily basis. Often, there are dietary or activity demands or restrictions. The physician usually instructs the mother and child as to the appropriate treatment protocol, but it is the family that must carry out the protocol on a daily basis. The development of an effective medical treatment is simply not enough; the family must follow the treatment regimen as prescribed if the child is to benefit. However, the literature has consistently documented a link between regimen complexity and adherence; increased complexity is associated with poorer compliance (Haynes, Taylor, & Sackett, 1979).

Adherence is a behavioral and not a medical phenomenon. Consequently, adherence assessment and intervention strategies are not part of the usual medical armamentarium. Physicians have typically placed all responsibility for suboptimal adherence with the patient, failing to recognize their own roles in setting the context for adherence to occur. Fortunately, this situation is changing. There is recent but widespread recognition that patient behavior (in addition to physician prescriptions) is critical to patient health care, which has led to an increasing demand for psychological expertise. Hopefully, this will be followed by changes in medical education to include methods to encourage patient adherence, techniques to assess adherence, and intervention strategies to be used when suboptimal adherence occurs.

The purpose of this chapter is to provide the reader with an overview of methods and issues relevant to assessing compliance behaviors in children faced with complex medical regimens. Of primary interest are those regimens that require multiple adherence behaviors such as special diets, exercise, prescriptions/constraints, home-based medical testing or interventions, etc. Some of these regimens require pill taking, others do not. Pill taking per se is the focus of a separate chapter by Peter Rudd.

Throughout this chapter, insulin-dependent diabetes mellitus (IDDM) serves as an illustrative example. Adherence, of course, is disease specific; different adherence behaviors are required to treat different diseases. Consequently, the discussion of issues relevant to assessing adherence is eased by focusing on a particular disease. IDDM is one of the most common chronic diseases of childhood, affecting over 120,000 U.S. children (LaPorte & Tajima, 1985). The prevalence of IDDM is higher than for most other chronic diseases of childhood. It is equal to that of all childhood cancers combined and is much greater than that of other well-known diseases such as cystic fibrosis, muscular dystrophy, and rheumatoid arthritis (LaPorte & Cruikshanks, 1985). The disease demands an array of daily management behaviors, serving as an excellent example of medical regimen complexity.

The chapter is organized into several sections. First, a number of conceptual issues are addressed: defining adherence, characterizing adherence as a unitary versus a multidimensional concept, issues surrounding inadvertent noncompliance, and distinguishing between adherence and health status. Next, adherence assessment strategies are discussed with a particular focus on the use of the 24-hr recall interview. Finally, developmental issues are considered as well as guidelines for clinical practice and directions for future research.

DEFINING COMPLIANCE

Throughout this chapter, adherence and compliance are used as interchangeable terms. Some have argued that *adherence* is the preferred term because it places greater emphasis on the patient's role in choosing (or not) to adhere to a particular management regimen. In contrast, the term *compliance* implies patient subservience to a standard determined by some external authority (i.e., the physician).

Defining adherence (or compliance) to complex medical regimens is difficult for a number of reasons. Regimen complexity means that there are many different kinds of behaviors required, usually on a daily basis. Each of these behaviors must be clearly defined, if it is to be assessed. In IDDM, for example, adherence behaviors include insulin injections given once or twice a day that must be appropriately timed in relationship to meals. Small meals should be taken frequently, and certain foods, those high in concentrated sweets and fat, should be avoided. Regular exercise is considered beneficial because it improves insulin utilization and lowers blood glucose, but it must be carefully coordinated with food intake so as to avoid hypoglycemia (excessively low blood glucose). Because current treatment methods only crudely approximate normal pancreatic function, wide swings in blood glucose can and do occur. Consequently, patients are encouraged to test their blood glucose levels several times per day. These data are then used by the physician or patient to make changes in insulin dose, diet, or other aspects of the daily regimen in an effort to maintain blood glucose levels as close to normal as possible. This treatment regimen is complex not only because of the large number of behaviors required of the patient, but because of the relationships among regimen behaviors (e.g., insulin injections must be timed in relationship to meals, exercise and eating should be carefully coordinated).

Haynes (1979), one of the most cited authorities, defines compliance as follows: "the extent to which a person's behavior (in terms of taking medications, following diets, or executing lifestyle changes) coincides with medical or health advice" (pp. 2–3). This definition identifies the physician's medical advice as the standard to which the patient's behavior is compared. Unfortunately, for many aspects of complex treatment regimens, physicians' medical advice is nonexistent or so unclear that it cannot be successfully utilized as a standard. A review of patients' medical records highlights the very minimal nature of documented medical prescriptions. An insulin dose may be noted, but rarely are recommendations concerning diet, timing of insulin dose, glucose testing, and exercise provided. We do not know what the patient was told nor do we know how specific or general were the recommendations made. For example, although exercise is considered beneficial to patients with IDDM, not all patients are told to engage in regular exercise. Or, if exercise is mentioned, a very general prescription may be given (e.g., "get some exercise"). In such cases, it is extremely difficult to define adherence because a provider prescription is vaguely implied or stated in generalities. For this reason, Glasgow, Wilson, and McCaul (1985) have recommended that the term *levels of self-care behaviors* be utilized when there is no clear provider prescription available; they suggest that the terms *adherence* or *compliance* be reserved for those relatively rare regimen behaviors for which there exists a documented provider prescription. Glasgow et al. make an important point: Defining adherence requires some sense of an ideal standard, clearly documented by the physician or by the investigator. Ideal standards are necessarily disease specific, because different diseases demand different regimen behaviors.

Ideal standards can be ascertained in several different ways. Sometimes they can be gleaned from medical textbooks, statements from other "authorities" (e.g., the American Diabetes Association), or consensus statements of the medical community's standard practices. Such approaches assume that there are general standards that are applicable across most patients with a particular disease. When one or more components of a treatment are highly individualized (differing greatly across patients), patients' behavior must be compared to their own personalized standard. More difficult are those situations in which patients' behavior should vary in response to changing symptoms or conditions of the disease. For example, in IDDM populations, concentrated sweets are to be generally avoided.

However, during episodes of hypoglycemia (excessively low blood sugar), concentrated sweet ingestion would be defined as desirable and appropriate (or compliant) behavior. In this case, standards for adherence must be defined in terms of a conditional relationship between disease status and behavior.

COMPLIANCE AS A UNITARY VERSUS MULTIDIMENSIONAL CONCEPT

Physicians often describe patients as "compliant" or "noncompliant" as if adherence was a unitary trait or characteristic of the patient. Researchers have also treated adherence as a unitary construct, utilizing a clinician's rating, a composite score of patient self-ratings, or even a laboratory assay of health status, as a single index of adherence. Sometimes patients are dichotomized into "compliant" or "noncompliant" groups. Other times, compliance is measured using an interval scale. However, in all these examples, compliance is presumed to be an underlying unitary patient characteristic.

In IDDM populations there is increasing evidence that adherence behaviors are not strongly correlated with one another, and that a multidimensional conceptualization of adherence is more accurate and useful. We approached this problem by subjecting 13 diabetes adherence behaviors (1 glucose testing, 5 dietary, 4 injection, and 3 exercise behaviors, described in Table 7.1), quantified from a sample of 168 IDDM children and adolescents, to a principal component factor analysis (Johnson, Silverstein, Rosenbloom, Carter, & Cunningham, 1986). If diabetes adherence is a unitary construct, a single factor should have emerged. Instead, a five-factor solution resulted, accounting for over 70% of the variance. The five factors were rotated to simple structure using the varimax procedure to ease interpretation; the factors and their loadings are presented in Table 7.2. All three exercise measures loaded on the first factor and all four injection measures loaded on Factor 2. Dietary behaviors did not load on a single factor. The type of food consumed (Factor 3) was unrelated to the frequency of eating (Factor 4) and the amount of calories consumed (Factor 5). Glucose testing frequency was related to eating frequency (Factor 4); children who were careful to eat frequently also tested frequently. The amount of calories consumed was related to concentrated sweet consumption; children who ate excess calories also ate excess sweets (Factor 5). Confirmatory factor analysis was applied to the adherence data collected from a second sample of 162 IDDM children and adolescents (Johnson, Tomer, Cunningham, & Henretta, 1990). The first four factors were confirmed. Calories Consumed and Concentrated Sweets, which comprised Factor 5 in the initial exploratory factor analysis, exhibited a similar relationship to one another in both samples, but their relationships to the other adherence measures differed between samples. These data suggest that Calories Consumed and Concentrated Sweets are probably best treated as separate, single-indicator constructs.

TABLE 7.1
A Brief Description of 13 Adherence Measures Quantified from 24-Hour Recall Interview Data

Injection Behaviors

Injection Regularity: The degree to which injections are given at the same time every day.
Injection Interval: The degree to which the time between injections approaches ideal.
Injection-Meal Timing: The degree to which Injections are given 30-60 minutes before eating.
Regularity of Injection-Meal Timing: The degree to which the time between injection and eating is consistent across days.

Exercise Behaviors

Exercise Frequency: How often a youngster exercises on a daily basis.
Exercise Duration: How long a youngster exercises on any exercise occasion.
Exercise Type: The strenuousness of the youngster's exercise.

Dietary Behaviors

% Calories: Carbohydrate: Percentage of total calories consumed consisting of carbohydrates in relationship to the 60% ideal recommended by the American Diabetes Association (Nuttal & Brunzall, 1979).
% Calories: Fat: Percentage of total calories consumed consisting of fats in relationship to the 25% ideal recommended by the American Diabetes Association (Nuttal & Brunzall, 1979).
Calories Consumed: The youngster's ideal total number of daily calories (based on age, sex, and height) subtracted from the youngster's reported daily calorie comsumption.
Concentrated Sweets: The average number of concentrated sweet exchange units eaten on a daily basis (40 calories of any concentrated sweet equals one concentrated sweet exchange unit).
Eating Frequency: How often a youngster eats on a daily basis.

Glucose Testing

Testing Frequency: How often a youngster conducts a glucose test on a daily basis.

Note. For additional details concerning the definition and quantification of the 13 adherence measures, see Johnson et al. (1986)

Our factor analytic work and other investigators' correlational research with diabetic children (Glasgow, McCaul, & Schafer, 1987; Shafer, Glasgow, McCaul, & Dreher, 1983), diabetic adults (Orme & Binik, 1989), and children undergoing orthodontic treatments (Gross, Samson, Sanders, & Smith, 1988) support a multidimensional conceptualization of adherence. How the youngster and family manage a complex medical disease cannot be characterized by a unitary trait. Because different regimen behaviors are likely to be unrelated to one another, attempts to measure adherence using single-indicator assessment methods will inadequately capture this complexity; assessment methods that

TABLE 7.2
Factor Analysis of Adherence Measures: Factor Loadings
Johnson et al. (1986)

Adherence Measure	*Factor 1: Exercise	*Factor 2: Injection	*Factor 3: Diet Type	*Factor 4: Frequency	Factor 5: Diet Amount
Injection regularity	-.071	.736	.054	.018	-.077
Injection interval	.095	.852	.176	.005	.102
Injection-meal timing	.041	.724	.038	-.068	.003
Regularity of injection-meal timing	.007	.522	-.022	.361	.190
Calories consumed	-.090	.079	.262	-.408	.696
% Calories: fat	.006	.124	.965	.090	.070
% Calories: carbohydrates	.010	.108	.971	.028	.008
Concentrated sweets	-.011	.024	-.088	.216	.845
Eating frequency	-.048	-.075	.250	.740	-.116
Exercise duration	.959	.007	-.017	-.005	-.042
Exercise type	.941	-.086	.040	.028	-.007
Exercise frequency	.667	.109	-.010	.151	-.022
Glucose testing frequency	.239	.116	-.082	.656	.121
Percentage of variance accounted for	18.0	16.4	15.8	10.5	9.9

Note. High factor loadings are underscored, indicating the adherence measures belonging to each factor.
*Factors 1-4 were confirmed in a second study (Johnson et al., 1990).

focus on the multiple components of complex medical regimens are more appropriate.

INADVERTENT NONCOMPLIANCE

Assessing patient compliance behaviors is further complicated by well-documented patient knowledge and skill deficits as well as gaps in physician/patient communication. Patients may believe and report that they are highly compliant but, due to deficits in knowledge or skill, they may inadvertently behave in very noncompliant ways.

Studies of IDDM children injecting insulin or testing glucose have reported significant procedural errors in a substantial proportion of the children observed (Epstein, Coburn, Becker, Drash, & Siminerio, 1980; Johnson, Pollak, Silverstein, Rosenbloom, Spillar, McCallum, & Harkavy, 1982). Yet, these children believed that they were performing in a highly compliant manner. Skill deficits have been noted in other populations as well. Sergis-Deavenport and Varni (1983) monitored parents of hemophiliac boys as they demonstrated factor replacement techniques necessary for the home care of their children. Despite years of experience, these parents evidenced numerous errors of administration.

In children, skill and knowledge deficits are often associated with cognitive developmental level; younger children frequently perform more poorly than older children (Johnson et al., 1982). However, as the Sergis-Deavenport and Varni (1983) study illustrates, skill deficits are not limited to young children. Adults, who have sufficient cognitive capacity to fully understand and accurately conduct a disease-related task, often fail to do so.

In addition to skill deficits, there are frequent miscommunications between patient and provider. Although physicians typically instruct patients how to carry out a particular treatment protocol, there are surprisingly large discrepancies between what providers believe they have told their patients and what the patients actually recall. Page, Verstraete, Robb, & Etzwiler (1981) compared recommendations given by the health care providers in a childhood diabetes clinic with patients' and parents' recall of these recommendations. On the average, providers gave seven recommendations per patient. Patient (and parents of younger patients) recalled an average of two recommendations. However, 40% of the patient- or parent-recalled recommendations were not reported by the provider! Similar findings were reported by Falvo and Tippy (1988), who examined patient recall in a family practice clinic; only 50% of instructions given by the physician were recalled by the patients. When such large discrepancies exist between provider recommendations and patient recall, patients are likely to inadvertently behave in very noncompliant ways. The patient may believe and report that he or she is compliant with the treatment regimen but, due to mis-communication, the patient's behavior is highly inconsistent with the doctor's orders.

COMPLIANCE AND HEALTH STATUS:
CONCEPTUAL ISSUES

Chronic illnesses with complex management regimens place numerous daily demands on the patient and family. The physician serves as a consultant, making management prescriptions and suggestions, rather than providing direct daily care. The physician is dependent on the patient and family to operationalize medical advice. In diabetes, for example, the goal of treatment is to maintain blood glucose levels as close to normal as possible. The patient's and family's cooperation must be obtained if this goal is to be attained. The serious long-term complications of diabetes (i.e., blindness, renal disease, heart disease, leg amputations) are thought to be delayed, diminished, or even prevented by maintenance of blood glucose in or near the normal range. Consequently, there is great emphasis placed on patient adherence, because patient behavior on a daily basis is considered to be critical to the successful management of this disease.

Although adherence and health status are presumably linked, there have been surprisingly few empirical tests of this association. In fact, there exists a serious conceptual confounding of terms. In IDDM, compliance and diabetes control (i.e., how well the patient's blood glucose levels are maintained near the normal range) are often used interchangeably, as if they refer to the same construct or process. Many health providers simply assume that their healthy patients are compliant and those in poor health are noncompliant. The use of health status measures as indicators of compliance is often so ingrained that the provider and patient may be unaware of this confounding or its implications. Such confounding may be of little practical import if adherence behaviors were the sole determinants of patient health status. In fact, this is not the case. At the most basic level, a patient's health is determined by the adequacy of the treatment regimen. To be sure, an adequate treatment regimen will be rendered ineffective by patient failure to comply. At the same time, even perfect compliance will not render an inadequate treatment prescription effective. In IDDM, prescribed insulin doses that are too high or too low will negatively impact upon the child. Great care must be taken to select the appropriate insulin dose as well as the frequency and timing of its administration. Further, in IDDM and other chronic conditions of childhood, an adequate treatment prescription may become inadequate as a consequence of biological (e.g., increasing disease duration, puberty, onset of acute illnesses), environmental (e.g., increasing stress), or lifestyle (e.g., increased or decreased exercise) changes. Selecting an appropriate regimen prescription is not a static event; the health care provider must remain sensitive to the changing needs of the patient. This is particularly true for childhood populations who undergo marked biological, cognitive, and social-emotional change.

When compliance and health status are treated as interchangeable constructs, determinants of health status, other than compliance, may be ignored and remain unexplored. The patient may be subtly (or not so subtly) blamed for his or her condition. And, adherence/health status relationships remain untested. This is a serious problem that is not isolated to the IDDM literature (see Epstein & Cluss, 1982, for an excellent review). Whatever the illness, adherence and health status should be conceptualized, defined, and assessed as independent constructs.

COMPLIANCE ASSESSMENT STRATEGIES

Unfortunately, the most common compliance assessment strategies, health status indicators and physician ratings, confound compliance and health status. Self-reports of compliance are often employed but are fraught with their own methodological problems. Behavioral observations and permanent products have been used infrequently but offer useful information in limited circumstances. We have developed the 24-hour recall interview as a compliance assessment strategy; data relevant to this approach is described in the next section of this chapter.

Health Status Indicators

Psychologists and physicians often make the mistake of using a health status indicator as a measure of compliance. The extent of this problem is exemplified in a recent survey of U.S. pediatric diabetologists by Clarke, Snyder, and Nowacek (1985); over 89% of survey respondents reported using glycosylated hemoglobin levels (the most widely accepted measure of diabetes control) to assess compliance. These providers did not assess adherence behaviors directly. Rather, they inferred them from this single indicator of the patient's metabolic status. This approach not only confounds compliance and health status but offers no useful information about what the patient is (or is not) doing that is consistent (or inconsistent) with the prescribed treatment protocol.

Physician Ratings

Physician ratings of compliance also confound compliance and health status, but in a more subtle fashion. Physicians are usually aware of their patients' health status. Consequently, physician ratings of patient adherence could be and probably are influenced by this knowledge. Physician ratings of patient adherence may reflect physician beliefs about adherence/health status relationships rather than an accurate appraisal of patient adherence behaviors. Further, physicians are usually asked to make global ratings of their patients' adherence. Not only do these ratings confound compliance and health status but, like health status indicators, they tell us little about what each patient is or is not doing relevant to the treatment protocol.

Self-Reports

Health providers often simply ask the patient or parent about management of the child's illness. Unfortunately, what patients or parents say they do may bear little resemblance to their actual behavior. Certainly, the demand characteristics of the clinic setting are sufficient to entice at least some patients to tell the doctor what he or she wants to hear. Although there is some evidence that patient reports of noncompliance may be accurate (Epstein & Cluss, 1982), reports of highly compliant behavior remain suspect.

Some investigators use composite scores based on patient adherence ratings to specific regimen components (e.g., Hanson, Henggeler, & Burghen, 1987). Unfortunately, there is a paucity of psychometric evidence supporting the reliability and validity of composite scores. Also lacking is evidence relevant to composite scores' susceptibility to social desirability and other types of demand characteristics. Like physician ratings and health status indicators, composite scores also fail to reflect the underlying complexity of many medical regimen behaviors, providing insufficient information about what the patient is or is not doing relevant to the treatment protocol.

Self-recording of adherence behaviors on a daily basis in the form of diaries is a more labor-intensive approach used by several investigators (e.g., Glasgow, McCaul, & Schafer, 1987). In our own work, we have found daily written records to provide reliable estimates of adherence behaviors, if patients keep complete records. Unfortunately, in our particular patient sample, only half of those studied kept complete records, severely limiting the practical utility of this approach.

Behavioral Observations

Medical regimen behaviors, like all behaviors, can be scrutinized using behavioral observation techniques. Lowe and Lutzker (1979), for example, had a mother observe her diabetic daughter's foot care, glucose testing, and dietary behaviors. Reliability, intermittently assessed by the child's older sister and by the experimenters ranged from 81%–100% agreement. There is little doubt that good quality observational data can be obtained on an individual case basis. However, with complex medical regimens, the sheer number of behaviors required makes this approach impractical as a general assessment strategy. Behavioral observation procedures are probably must useful as a follow-up assessment technique in cases where problem behaviors are initially identified through a more general assessment screening. Observational methods are a particularly powerful means of documenting the effects of intervention programs designed to improve adherence to one or two components of a treatment regimen.

Permanent Products

Pill and bottle counts have long been used as an indirect method of assessing adherence in the adult, medical treatment literature. Peter Rudd's chapter in this volume deals extensively with the measurement issues relevant to medication taking per se. However, complex medical regimens require far more than pill ingestion, and some regimens, such as that associated with IDDM, require no pill ingestion at all. Counting permanent products is not a useful general assessment strategy because adherence behaviors are not always reliably associated with a permanent product that can be easily observed and measured. Nevertheless, sometimes permanent products associated with various aspects of the treatment regimen can be creatively used to corroborate self-reports or other types of adherence data. Gross (1983), for example, asked four 10- to 12-year-old boys to monitor their urine glucose four times per day. Because urine testing requires the use of test tablets, the boys' reports of the number of tests conducted could be verified by a weekly count of urine test tablets; the number of test tablets depleted on a weekly basis should have agreed with the boys' reports of the number of tests conducted. In this particular study, agreement between the boys' reports and the tablet count was 80%.

The recent development of meters for home blood glucose monitoring with large memory capacities offers a number of permanent products useful to patients, providers, and investigators interested in this particular aspect of diabetes care. These meters store in memory the date, time, as well as the result of each glucose test. The provider and patient can access the stored data to make treatment decisions. The interested investigator can also use the stored data to assess glucose-testing adherence or to evaluate the accuracy of patients' self-reports of glucose-testing behavior.

ASSESSMENT DISEASE MANAGEMENT USING 24-HOUR RECALL INTERVIEWS: CHILDHOOD DIABETES AS AN ILLUSTRATIVE EXAMPLE

The 24-hour recall interview has long been a standard dietary assessment technique and is considered the best of the available self-report methods (Marquis, Ware, & Relles, 1979). It seemed to us that, with modification, this approach might prove useful as a more general adherence assessment strategy. The available dietary literature suggested that it could provide an accurate reflection of dietary intake, even in children (e.g., Emmons & Hayes, 1973; Greger & Entyre, 1978; Samuelson, 1970; Stunkard & Waxman, 1981). The focus on specific behaviors during a recent time-limited period (i.e., the preceding 24 hours) seemed to offer a viable method of sampling adherence behaviors. Further, the method seemed more practical, and possibly less reactive, than diaries or other types of daily records.

However, modifications needed to be made if the 24-hour recall was to serve as a general adherence assessment strategy. First, all adherence behaviors needed to be recorded, not just those relevant to dietary intake. Second, we decided to conduct multiple 24-hour recall interviews in order to obtain a more representative sample of daily adherence behaviors. Third, serious consideration was given to the fact that all recall interviews are subject to errors of memory. We addressed this issue by emphasizing recall of recent behaviors (i.e., behaviors that occurred yesterday rather than behaviors that occurred last week or last month) and by interviewing both the child and the child's mother (or primary caretaker) independently, about the child's behavior during the preceding 24 hours. In this way, behaviors that were forgotten by the child might be remembered by the parent, and vice versa. Care was taken to conduct all interviews in temporal sequence, beginning with the time the child awoke in the morning and ending with the time he or she retired at night. The child was encouraged to report all of his experiences in chronological order, although only adherence behaviors related to the child's medical regimen were recorded. Interviewers were trained to prompt with questions in order to obtain sufficient detail concerning the types and amounts of foods eaten, duration and type of exercise, and so on.

We have conducted a series of studies using this assessment strategy with IDDM childhood populations. Thirteen different adherence behaviors are quantified based on the 24-hour recall interview data: 1 glucose testing, 4 injection, 3 exercise, and 5 dietary measures. Each is constructed so that a range of scores is possible, with higher scores indicating relative noncompliance and scores close to zero indicating relative compliance. A brief description of the 13 adherence measures is provided in Table 7.1. Originally, a 14th measure was included: the percentage of insulin injections prescribed that was actually taken. However, so few patients reported missing an insulin injection that this measure had to be dropped for lack of variability. The reader is referred to a previous manuscript for additional detail concerning the definition and quantification of the 13 adherence measures (Johnson, Silverstein, Rosenbloom, Carter, & Cunningham, 1986).

Estimates of parent/child agreement provide important psychometric information relevant to the reliability and validity of this procedure. Although perfect agreement cannot be expected because parents do not observe all their children's activities, statistically significant correlations between child and parent reports have been documented in three separate studies (Freund, Johnson, Silverstein, & Thomas, 1991; Johnson et al., 1986; Spevack, Johnson, & Riley, 1991; see Table 7.3); most are in the moderate to high range. The correlations depicted in Table 7.3 were based on data obtained from three 24-hour recall interviews conducted with each parent and with each child.

The Freund et al. (1991) study provided additional data relevant to interview frequency effects on estimates of parent/child agreement. These data are provided in Table 7.4. For eight of the 13 adherence measures, parent/child agree-

TABLE 7.3
Parent/Child Agreement for 13 Diabetes Management Behaviors

Adherence Measures	Johnson et al. (1986) (n = 168) r(p<)	Freund et al. (1991) (n = 78) r(p<)	Spevack et al. (1991) (n = 64) r(p<)
Injection Behaviors			
Injection regularity	.61 (.0001)	.62 (.0001)	.65 (.0001)
Injection interval	.77 (.0001)	.74 (.0001)	.75 (.0001)
Injection-meal timing	.67 (.0001)	.64 (.0001)	.54 (0001)
Regularity of injection-meal timing	.42 (.0001)	.33 (.005)	.09 (ns)
Exercise Behaviors			
Exercise frequency	.62 (.0001)	.75 (.0001)	.68 (.0001)
Exercise duration	.59 (.0001)	.72 (.0001)	.29 (.02)
Exercise type	.54 (.0001)	.76 (.0001)	.64 (.0001)
Dietary Behaviors			
Eating frequency	.45 (.0001)	.65 (.0001)	.72 (.0001)
Calories consumed	.77 (.0001)	.72 (.0001)	.73 (.0001)
% Calories: carbohydrate	.64 (.0001)	.76 (.0001)	.72 (.0001)
% Calories: fat	.64 (.0001)	.75 (.0001)	.78 (.0001)
Concentrated sweets	.62 (.0001)	.67 (.0001)	.63 (.0001)
Glucose Testing Behavior			
Testing frequency	.78 (.0001)	.94 (.0001)	.90 (.0001)

ment was significantly enhanced when nine, as compared to three, interviews were used to quantify the adherence measures. Because parent/child agreement was respectable for most measures based on three interviews, the increased reliability obtained with the use of nine interviews must be weighed against the additional costs of conducting more than three interviews.

In the Freund et al. (1991) investigation, nine interviews were conducted with the parent and with the child over a 3-month interval. This permitted an examination of the stability of adherence behaviors over the course of the investigation. Adherence measures quantified using the first three interviews collected during the first month of the study could be compared to the same measures quantified using interviews conducted during the second and third months of this investiga-

TABLE 7.4
Interview Frequency Effects on Parent/Child Agreement

Adherence Measure	3 Interviews r (p<)	9 Interviews r (p<)
Injection Behaviors		
*Injection regularity	.62 (.0001)	.81 (.0001)
Injection interval	.74 (.0001)	.72 (.0001)
*Injection-meal timing	.64 (.0001)	.85 (.0001)
*Regularity of injection-meal timing	.33 (.005)	.59 (.0001)
Exercise Behaviors		
Exercise frequency	.75 (.0001)	.76 (.0001)
*Exercise duration	.72 (.0001)	.90 (.0001)
Exercise type	.76 (.0001)	.76 (.0001)
Dietary Behaviors		
*Eating frequency	.65 (.0001)	.81 (.0001)
Calories consumed	.72 (.0001)	.77 (.0001)
*% Calories: carbohydrate	.76 (.0001)	.88 (.0001)
*% Calories: fat	.75 (.0001)	.88 (.0001)
*Concentrated sweets	.67 (.0001)	.82 (.0001)
Glucose Testing Behaviors		
Testing frequency	.94 (.0001)	.94 (.0001)

From Freund et al. (1991).
*Correlations significantly different.

tion. The relevant correlations are provided in Table 7.5. All correlations were statistically significant, with one exception, suggesting that diabetes regimen behaviors are quite stable over intervals as long as 3 months. There did appear to be some differences in the degree of stability exhibited by the different regimen behaviors. Glucose testing and dietary behaviors appeared to be the most stable, followed by exercise and injection behaviors. These data are consistent with that previously reported by Glasgow et al. (1987), who monitored adherence behaviors of adolescent and adult IDDM patients over 2-month and 6-month test–retest intervals. Although their method of assessing adherence varied from ours, the pattern of results obtained is quite similar. Glasgow et al. (1987) found glucose-testing behaviors to be the most stable, followed by dietary, insulin injection, and exercise behaviors. These authors' test–retest reliability estimates for the 6-month interval were generally lower than for the 2-month interval, suggesting that adherence behaviors may be quite stable over 2 or 3 months but significant variation may occur over longer intervals.

Although the available parent/child agreement and test–retest data support the

TABLE 7.5
Stability of Adherence Behaviors Over Three Months

Adherence Measure	Months 1 and 2 (n = 66 - 74) r(p<)	Months 2 and 3 (n = 65 - 72) r(p<)	Months 1 and 3 (n = 64 - 72) r(p<)
Injection			
Injection regularity	.24(.04)	.35(.004)	.06 (ns)
Injection interval	.49(.0001)	.43(.0003)	.38(.001)
Injection-meal timing	.71(.0001)	.58(.0001)	.65(.0001)
Regularity of injection-meal timing	.30(.01)	.31(.009)	.24(.05)
Exercise			
Exercise frequency	.40(.0005)	.63(.0001)	.47(.0001)
Exercise duration	.42(.0002)	.51(.0001)	.74(.0001)
Exercise type	.39(.0006)	.48(.0001)	.37(.001)
Diet			
Eating frequency	.74(.0001)	.77(.0001)	.63(.0001)
Calories consumed	.74(.0001)	.72(.0001)	.67(.0001)
% Calories: carbohydrate	.61(.0001)	.45(.0001)	.58(.0001)
% Calories: fat	.63(.0001)	.51(.0001)	.60(.0001)
Concentrated sweets	.53(.0001)	.51(.0001)	.53(.0001)
Glucose Testing			
Testing frequency	.76(.0001)	.75(.0001)	.72(.0001)

From Freund et al. (1991).

reliability of this method, they do not address the underestimation bias, due to errors of memory, that is frequently associated with recall data. Reynolds, Johnson, and Silverstein (1990) attempted to address this issue by comparing 24-hour recall interview data, obtained from 7- to 12-year-old children attending a diabetes summer camp, with actual observations of their behavior. There were only minor child/observer differences with regard to insulin injection and glucose-testing behaviors. However, underestimation was a problem for most of the dietary behaviors and for one of the exercise measures (see Table 7.6). The youngsters underestimated both the frequency of eating and the amount of food consumed. They also underestimated the strenuousness of their exercise but did not underestimate its frequency or duration. In this study, only relatively young children were interviewed and no parent report data were collected. Interviewing

TABLE 7.6
Observer Versus Child Report of Diabetes Management Behaviors

Adherence Measure	Mean Child Report	Mean Observer Report
Injection Behaviors		
*AM Injection time	7:28	7:41
PM Injection time	17:43	17:48
Exercise Behaviors		
Exercise frequency	3.0	3.6
Exercise duration (minutes)	47.2	45.7
*Exercise type (KCAL per min)	.0784	.0961
Dietary Behaviors		
Breakfast time	8:04	8:08
Dinner time	18:10	18:12
*Eating frequency	3.7	4.9
*Calories consumed	2336	2979
% Calories: carbohydrate	36.4	35.4
*Grams: carbohydrate	209	262
*% Calories: fat	47.4	50.0
*Grams: fat	125	166
*Concentrated sweets (exchange units)	2.2	3.4
Glucose Testing Behaviors		
Testing frequency	1.9	2.1
Test results (ranked data)	8.9	8.9

From Reynolds et al. (1990).
*Observer/Child reports significantly different, $p < .05$.

both parent and child and combining data from both respondents should help minimize the underestimation bias associated with single informant data.

A study by Spevack et al. (1991) provides additional validity data relevant to this procedure (see Table 7.7). Adherence was monitored before, during, and after a diabetes summer camp using the 24-hour recall assessment strategy. On nine of the 13 adherence measures, children exhibited significant change during camp as compared to pre or postcamp when the youngster was living at home. As expected, children were generally more adherent at camp, but these behavior changes were not maintained once the child returned home.

In summary, the 24-hour recall interview, when conducted with multiple informants on multiple occasions, appears to provide the investigator with a reliable method of assessing a wide range of adherence behaviors. Although this method has been primarily applied to IDDM populations, it could be readily modified for use with other chronic conditions of childhood.

TABLE 7.7
Adherence Behaviors Before, During, and After Diabetes Summer Camp

Adherence Measures[a]	2 Weeks Before Camp	During Camp	2 Weeks After Camp	6 Weeks After Camp	12 Weeks After Camp
Injection Behaviors					
[b]Injection regularity (minutes)	28.0	15.9	30.1	27.6	40.6
[b]Injection interval (minutes)	42.5	35.1	56.9	52.2	56.2
[b]Injection-meal timing (minutes before meal)	17.6	30.3	19.2	20.5	17.3
Regularity of injection-meal timing (minutes)	18.7	18.1	19.5	12.0	18.2
Exercise Behaviors					
[b]Exercise frequency (per day)	1.2	4.4	1.0	1.1	1.1
[b]Exercise duration (minutes)	20	42	14	15	14
Exercise type (kcal/min)	.03	.06	.02	.03	.03
Dietary Behaviors					
[b]Eating frequency (per day)	5.0	5.9	5.1	5.0	5.0
[b]Calories consumed (above or below ideal)	-72	382	-35	-65	59
% Calories: carbohydrate	35.7	36.7	34.6	35.2	36.7
% Calories: fat	48.7	47.0	49.5	48.9	47.7
Concentrated sweets (per day)	1.5	1.2	1.3	1.4	1.6
Glucose Testing Behaviors					
[b]Testing frequency (per day)	1.9	2.2	1.8	1.6	1.5

From Spevack et al. (1991).
[a] Presented are interpretations of the adherence measures using familiar measurement scales.
[b] Camp significantly different from before or after camp.

COMPLIANCE IN PEDIATRIC POPULATIONS: DEVELOPMENTAL ISSUES

Because our focus is on children, no discussion of adherence to complex medical regimens would be complete without some consideration of developmental issues. Age-related differences have been found in children's ability to acquire skills necessary for the management of their disease and to understand and communicate effectively with the health care provider. The reliability of adherence data reported by children differs depending on their age. Similarly, the actual level of adherence behaviors exhibited by children changes as they grow older.

Children's cognitive sophistication increases in age-related stages. Very young children rarely have the cognitive capability to carry out complex treatment tasks. Placing too much responsibility for disease management upon the child too early in his or her cognitive development may lead to numerous episodes of inadvertent noncompliance as a consequence of knowledge or skill deficits. Our research with childhood diabetic populations suggests that education programs addressing different adherence behaviors should be emphasized at different ages. For example, insulin injection seems best taught at about 9 years of age (Gilbert, Johnson, Spillar, McCallum, Silverstein, & Rosenbloom, 1982; Harkavy, Johnson, Silverstein, Spillar, McCallum, & Rosenbloom, 1983; Johnson et al., 1982). This does not preclude children from participating in these activities at a younger age than suggested. However, parental monitoring and supervision is necessary until the youngster shows competence.

Just as children vary developmentally in their ability to acquire knowledge and skills relevant to their disease, they vary in their ability to understand and communicate with the health care provider. Although investigators have not examined patient recall or provider instructions by patient age, they have examined the provider's ability to communicate with children of different cognitive developmental tasks. Perrin and Perrin (1983), for example, gave clinicians children's responses to five questions regarding illness mechanisms and asked them to estimate the children's ages on the basis of the quality of the responses. The health care providers participating in the study, who all worked regularly with children, consistently overestimated the age of the younger children's responses and underestimated the age of the older children's answers. In other words, they seemed to have difficulty detecting age-related differences in the youngsters' conceptual understanding of illness, treating youngsters of varying ages essentially the same. These findings suggest that patient adherence may be undermined by provider communications that are insensitive to the cognitive developmental capabilities of the child patient.

The reliability of children's reports about their own adherence behaviors has been examined, using the 24-hour recall approach, in IDDM children as young as 6 years of age. Compared to their older counterparts (e.g., 10- to 12-year-olds), younger children (6–9 years) show poorer parent/child agreement on adherence measures involving time (i.e., all four injection measures and the exercise duration measure). Relevant data from two separate studies are provided in Table 7.8. On simple frequency measures (e.g., eating, exercise, and testing frequency) and on more qualitative measures (e.g., type of exercise and type of foods consumed), young children demonstrate agreement with their parents that is comparable to the parent/child agreement exhibited by older youngsters. It is not surprising that 6- to 9-year olds have problems reliably reporting behaviors involving time because these require more complex mathematical concepts. However, data provided by Freund et al. (1991) suggest that, with practice, children as young as 6 years may become reliable reporters of all adherence behaviors, including those involving time. As was mentioned previously, parents and children in this study were interviewed on nine occasions across 3 months. This permitted an assessment of possible change in parent/child agreement across time. Although parent/child agreement exhibited marked stability for most adherence measures in all age groups, the youngest children studied

TABLE 7.8
Parent/Child Agreement for 6-9 and 10-12 Year Olds for 13 Diabetes Adherence Behaviors

	Johnson et al. (1986)		Freund et al. (1991)	
	6-9 Yrs	10-12 Yrs	6-9 Yrs	10-12 Yrs
	n = 26-31	n = 65-70	n = 8-12	n = 21-22
Adherence Measures	r (p<)	r (p<)	r (p<)	r (p<)
Injection Behaviors				
Injection regularity	.46 (.02)	.68 (.0001)	.16 (ns)	.82 (.0001)
Injection interval	.36 (.05)	.71 (.0001)	.31 (ns)	.64 (.002)
Injection-meal timing	.53 (.002)	.54 (.0001)	.18 (ns)	.61 (.0003)
Regularity of injection-meal timing	-.23 (.002)	.50 (.0001)	.18 (ns)	.20 (ns)
Exercise Behaviors				
Exercise frequency	.62 (.0001)	.72 (.0001)	.90 (.0001)	.49 (.02)
Exercise duration	.03 (ns)	.96 (.0001)	.20 (ns)	.38 (.08)
Exercise type	.74 (.0001)	.99 (.0001)	.86 (.0004)	.53 (.01)
Diet Behaviors				
Eating frequency	.67 (.0001)	.47 (.0001)	.83 (.0008)	.68 (.0006)
Calories consumed	.79 (.0001)	.80 (.0001)	.51 (ns)	.52 (.02)
% Calories: carbohydrate	.44 (.01)	.63 (.0001)	.90 (.0001)	.74 (.0002)
% Calories: fat	.50 (.005)	.63 (.0001)	.87 (.0002)	.72 (0004)
Concentrated sweets	.47 (.007)	.71 (.0001)	.80 (.002)	.83 (.0001)
Glucose Testing Behaviors				
Testing frequency	.81 (.0001)	.73 (.0001)	.92 (.0001)	.97 (.0001)

showed substantial improvement in parent/child agreement for the injection measures, all of which require an accurate report of the timing of injections and/or the timing of meals. As is depicted in Table 7.9, parent/child agreement for the 6- to 9-year olds markedly improved between interviews 1–3 and interviews 4–6. By interviews 4–6, these young children were exhibiting parent/child agreement comparable to the 10- to 12-year olds studied. Further, this improvement in parent/child agreement was maintained throughout the rest of the investigation. In summary, IDDM youngsters as young as 6 years of age appear to be reliable reporters concerning most adherence behaviors. Very young children do have some problems accurately reporting behaviors involving time. However, these problems appear to be overcome with practice.

Developmental differences also emerge when the actual level of adherence behaviors of different-aged children are examined. Adolescents are typically less adherent than their younger counterparts across a variety of disease conditions (Chacko, Wells, & Phillips, 1987; Dolgin, Katz, Doctors, & Siegel, 1986; Jacobson, Hauser, Wolfsdorf, Houlihan, Milley, Herskowitz, Wertlieb, & Watt, 1987; Tebbi, Cummings, Zevon, Smith, Richards, & Mallon, 1986). Relevant

TABLE 7.9
Parent/Child Agreement With Practice for 6-9 and 10-12 Year Olds for the Injection Adherence Measures

Adherence Measure	6-9 Years $N = 8\text{-}12$ $r\ (p<)$	10-12 Years $N = 19\text{-}22$ $r\ (p<)$
Injection Regularity		
Interviews 1-3	.16 (ns)	.82 (.0001)
Interviews 4-6	.88 (.002)	.50 (.02)
Interviews 7-9	.74 (.02)	.01 (.0001)
Injection Interval		
Interviews 1-3	.31 (ns)	.64 (.002)
Interviews 4-6	.89 (.003)	.87 (.0001)
Interviews 7-9	.76 (.02)	.89 (.0001)
Injection-Meal Timing		
Interviews 1-3	.18 (ns)	.61 (.003)
Interviews 4-6	.68 (.02)	.71 (.0004)
Interviews 7-9	.62 (.06)	.96 (.0001)
Regularity of Injection-Meal Timing		
Interviews 1-3	-.16 (ns)	.20 (ns)
Interviews 4-6	.67 (.07)	.49 (.03)
Interviews 7-9	.53 (ns)	.51 (.04)

From Freund et al. (1991).

data from two different studies, using the 24-hour recall interview method with IDDM youngsters, are presented in Table 7.10 (Johnson et al., 1986; Johnson, Freund, Silverstein, Hansen, & Malone, 1990). The cross-study consistency of significant age-related effects is noteworthy. In both studies, adolescents, when compared to younger patients, took their injections less regularly, exercised less frequently, ate less frequently, ate too few carbohydrates, ate too many fats, and glucose tested less often. Although the clinical literature has often remarked upon the disruptive influence of adolescence on adequate diabetes care (e.g., Tattersall & Lowe, 1981), there have been few empirical tests of this assertion.

TABLE 7.10
Age-Related Differences in Diabetes Adherence Behaviors
Johnson et al. (1986; 1990)

	Age Groups							
	6-9 Yrs.		10-12 Yrs.		13-15 Yrs.		16-19 Yrs.	
Adherence Measures* (N)	Study 1 (31-32)	Study 2 (12)	Study 1 (67-71)	Study 2 (21-22)	Study 1 (38-42)	Study 2 (26-28)	Study 1 (21-23)	Study 2 (16)
Injection Behaviors								
Injection regularity (min)[1,2]	29.4	41.4	36.0	37.7	52.2	43.0	64.8	59.9
Injection interval (min)[1]	38.4	56.1	48.0	53.2	72.0	54.1	99.6	83.4
Injection-meal timing[1] (minutes before meal)	25.8	17.0	18.6	24.8	9.6	13.9	1.8	23.5
Regularity of injection-meal timing (minutes)	23.5	28.2	18.8	18.6	23.9	23.1	42.6	33.1
Exercise Behaviors								
Exercise frequency[1,2] (per day)	1.9	2.1	2.0	1.9	1.7	1.7	1.3	1.3
Exercise duration (min)	20.6	20.3	23.0	15.8	19.4	17.8	20.2	17.9
Exercise type (kcal/min)	.029	.028	.032	.025	.026	.024	.021	.019
Dietary Behaviors								
Eating frequency[1,2] (per day)	5.4	5.3	5.3	5.3	5.2	4.8	4.8	4.5
Calories consumed[2] (above or below ideal)	9	533	44	538	-60	162	-233	-220
% Calories: carb.[1,2]	40.6	37.5	37.2	35.6	36.1	34.2	34.8	31.4
% Calories: fat[1,2]	44.4	46.6	47.2	49.0	48.4	49.8	50.0	53.0
Concentrated sweets (per day)	1.6	1.5	1.7	2.3	2.6	2.1	2.2	1.5
Glucose Testing Behaviors								
Testing frequency 1,2 (per day)	2.1	1.9	1.9	1.7	1.5	1.5	.9	.8

Study 1: Johnson et al. (1986).
Study 2: Johnson, Freund et al. (1990).
[1]Age-related significant differences for Study 1, $p < .05$.
[2]Age-related significant differences for Study 2, $p < .05$.
*Presented are interpretations of the adherence measures using familiar measurement scales.

The data presented in Table 7.10 suggest that the concerns frequently expressed by clinicians are quite justified; adolescents do appear to be remarkably nonadherent with the demands of their daily diabetes regimen. Similar, developmentally related differences in adherence have been documented in childhood cancer as well (Chacko et al., 1987; Dolgin et al., 1986).

GUIDELINES FOR CLINICAL PRACTICE AND DIRECTIONS FOR FUTURE RESEARCH

Physically ill patients are often referred to psychologists for health-related problems that are presumed to be behaviorally induced. If the patient is not doing well, the physician often assumes that the patient is not complying with the prescribed treatment regimen. Although this may be true, health status indicators tell us nothing about what the patient is or is not doing to manage a particular disease on a daily basis. In diabetes, for example, an elevated glycosylated hemoglobin level is an indication of poor diabetes control. It tells us that something is wrong but offers few clues as to the source of the problem. Physicians often assume that the patient is noncompliant, but other factors may be involved (e.g., an inappropriate insulin dose). Psychologists must take great care not to equate health status indicators with measures of adherence. Physicians often equate the two and pass on this conceptual confounding to the psychologist, along with the patient. Because of this conceptual confounding, physicians may blame patients whose health is deteriorating. Psychologists must avoid similar assumptions while conducting an objective assessment of the patient's medical regimen adherence behaviors. Only in this way can the psychologist ascertain if and how the patient's adherence behaviors are contributing to his or her health problems.

Assessing adherence behaviors is no easy task, particularly when complex medical regimens are involved. The psychologist must learn what the patient is supposed to do (or not do) on a daily basis to manage the disease. Usually multiple behaviors have to be defined. Further complexity is induced when multiple adherence behaviors are supposed to have a particular relationship to one another. Although physicians have often treated compliance as a unitary trait of the patient, psychologists would be wise to avoid such an overly simplistic conceptualization. If multiple behaviors are required of the patient to manage a particular illness, it is best to assess all relevant behaviors; assessing a single adherence behavior will probably not provide an accurate reflection of the vast array of compliance behaviors required of the patient.

The psychologist should carefully select an appropriate assessment strategy. To be avoided are health status indicators, physician ratings, and general statements by the patient. This type of information should not be totally ignored by the psychologist as it provides important insights as to the patient's current health, and the physician's and patient's perceptions of the problem. Patients who acknowledge failure to comply with the treatment regimen are probably truthful. However, much less confidence can be placed in patient reports of highly compliant behavior. Information of this type simply cannot provide an objective assessment of the patient's adherence behaviors because it is so easily colored by patient or provider beliefs about adherence/health status relationships or by the demand characteristics of the clinic setting. As a general assessment strategy, we have found the 24-hour recall interview, when conducted with multiple informants on multiple occasions, can provide a practical methodology for collecting reliable data on daily disease management behaviors in IDDM childhood populations. We believe it could be easily modified to serve as a useful general screening strategy for other illness populations as well. Behavioral observation techniques are good follow-up strategies once a limited number of problem behaviors have been identified. Permanent products can also be creatively used to corroborate self-reports or other types of adherence data.

Because this volume addresses assessment strategies relevant to children and families, developmental issues are of obvious import. When using 24-hour recall interviews to assess daily adherence behaviors, it is important to realize that young children (e.g., 6–8 years) may have difficulty accurately recalling time-related behaviors. They are not poor reporters in general as they are quite accurate when recalling what they did or how often they did it (but not when they did it or how long they did it). Further, it appears that with practice children as young as 6 years quickly learn to accurately recall all types of adherence behaviors, including those involving time. However, when the actual level of adherence behaviors is compared across childhood and adolescence, it appears that adolescents are far less adherent, at least among victims of diabetes and childhood cancer. Whether this is true for other chronic illnesses remains to be seen. But, given the adolescent's striving for independence, concerns with peer conformity, and increased experimentation, it would not be surprising if similar findings were reported for other childhood chronic conditions as well.

Clinicians should also be aware of behaviors that are rare but are of great significance. In IDDM populations, for example, skipping an insulin injection occurs infrequently. As an adherence measure, the percentage of insulin injections prescribed that are actually taken lacks sufficient variability to be useful for research purposes (also see Glasgow et al., 1987). Nevertheless, any individual child's failure to take insulin should be considered pathological from both a medical and psychological point of view; not only is insulin necessary for the child's survival, but the child's failure to take insulin marks him or her as clearly deviant from other youngsters with the same disease. The psychologist should know enough about the child's illness and its management to be able to detect unusual, but clinically significant, behaviors of this type.

The availability of a reliable and practical methodology for assessing medical regimen adherence behaviors enables the scientist–practitioner to address a number of important research questions. For many chronic conditions, the relationship between adherence behaviors and health status has not been well documented. The surprising paucity of research on this topic is probably the product of several factors. Compliance and health status have been so conceptually confounded that investigators have often failed to conceive of and assess each independently. Lack of psychometrically adequate measures of adherence has also contributed to the problem. There is little doubt that for some diseases there exists a powerful relationship between adherence behaviors and health outcomes, but for others the relationship is far more tenuous. In IDDM, for example, the relationship between adherence behaviors and metabolic status is not as strong or consistent as once was believed (Glasgow et al., 1987; Johnson, Freund et al., 1990). Only with adequate measurement strategies for assessing compliance can we successfully address these issues both within and across diseases.

Reliable and sensitive methods of measuring adherence also permit more effective study of factors that influence adherence. These factors are too numerous to name here, so only a few are highlighted. Physician–patient communication needs to be more carefully studied because the patient's understanding of what is or is not an adherent behavior is predicated on this relationship. Better ways to identify inadvertent noncompliance due to patient skill or knowledge deficits need to be identified. Family member responsibilities for the child's disease management is a topic of obvious importance but one that has received little empirical scrutiny. How much a parent supervises a child or how involved the parent is in the child's care may be powerful predictors of who is or is not adherent with a disease management protocol. We know that IDDM adolescents and adolescent victims of cancer are relatively nonadherent compared to younger children with the same disease. We need to assess this developmentally related phenomenon in other childhood chronic conditions. We also need to identify the factors that seem to be contributing to this problem during the adolescent years.

Intervention, of course, remains paramount. Physicians often refer patients to psychologists because they want the psychologist to intervene. When the patient referred is a chronically ill child, the usual hope is that the psychologist will help the patient and family more effectively manage the disease and, as a consequence, the child's health will improve or at least stabilize. A high-quality adherence assessment strategy permits the psychologist to identify which adherence behaviors need modification. The same adherence assessment strategy can be used to monitor the effects of intervention programs. Sometimes, a child may become more adherent, but no change in health status occurs (e.g., Epstein et al., 1981). If the psychologist has confidence in the validity of his or her adherence assessment data, the psychologist can enter into more meaningful discussions with the physician (and the patient) as to why the patient's changed behavior did not result in an expected change in health status. Perhaps a different behavior needs to be identified and changed or perhaps the physician needs to modify the child's disease management prescription. It is true that noncompliance will render an effective medical regimen ineffective. It is also true that even perfect adherence will not render an ineffective medical regimen effective. Physicians often assume that a patient's problem lies within the patient rather than in the physician's prescription. Sometimes, when a psychologist intervenes and improves a patient's adherence behaviors with no concomitant improvement in the patient's health status, the psychologist may assist the physician in redirecting his or her attention away from the patient's behavior and toward the disease management prescription. This is far easier to accomplish when the psychologist is confident in the reliability of the adherence data he or she has monitored and collected.

ACKNOWLEDGMENTS

This chapter was supported by grants #R01 HD13820 and K04 HD00686 from the National Institute of Child Health and Human Development.

REFERENCES

Chacko, M. R., Wells, R. D., & Phillips, S. A. (1987). Test of cure for gonorrhea in teenagers: Who complies and does continuity of care help? *Journal of Adolescent Health Care, 8*, 261–265.

Clarke, W. L., Snyder, A. L., & Nowacek, G. (1985). Outpatient pediatric diabetes-I. Current practices. *Journal of Chronic Diseases, 38*, 85–90.

Craig, O. (1981). *Childhood diabetes and its management* (2nd ed.). London: Buttersworth.

Dolgin, M. J., Katz, E. R., Doctors, S. R., & Siegel, S. E. (1986). Caregivers' perceptions of medical compliance in adolescents with cancer. *Journal of Adolescent Health Care, 7*, 22–27.

Emmons, L., & Hayes, M. (1973). Accuracy of 24-hour recalls of young children. *Journal of American Dietetic Association, 62*, 409–416.

Epstein, L. H., Beck, S., Figueroa, J., Farkas, G., Kazdin, A. E., Daneman, D., & Becker, D. (1981). The effects of targeting improvements in urine glucose on metabolic control in children with insulin dependent diabetes. *Journal of Applied Behavior Analysis, 14*(4), 365–375.

Epstein, L. H., & Cluss, P. A. (1982). A behavioral medicine perspective on adherence to long-term medical regimens. *Journal of Consulting and Clinical Psychology, 50*, 950–971.

Epstein, L. H., Coburn, P. C., Becker, D., Drash, A., & Siminerio, L. (1980). Measurement and modification of the accuracy of determinations of urine glucose concentration. *Diabetes Care, 3*, 535–536.

Falvo, D., & Tippy, P. (1988). Communicating information to patients: Patient satisfaction and adherence as associated with resident skill. *The Journal of Family Practice, 26*, 643–647.

Freund, A., Johnson, S. B., Silverstein, J., & Thomas, J. (1991). Assessing daily management of childhood diabetes using 24-hr recall interviews: Reliability and stability. *Health Psychology, 10*(3), 200–208.

Gilbert, B. O., Johnson, S. B., Spillar, R., McCallum, M., Silverstein, J., & Rosenbloom, A. (1982). The effects of a peer-modeling film on children learning to self-inject insulin. *Behavior Therapy, 13*, 186–193.

Glasgow, R. E., McCaul, K. D., & Schafer, L. C. (1987). Self-care behaviors and glycemic control in type I diabetes. *Journal of Chronic Disease, 40*(5), 399–417.

Glasgow, R. E., Wilson, W., & McCaul, K. D. (1985). Regimen adherence: A problematic construct in diabetes research. *Diabetes Care, 8*, 300–301.

Gortmaker, S. L., & Sappenfield, W. (1984). Chronic childhood disorders: Prevalence and impact. *Pediatric Clinics of North America, 31,* 3–18.

Greger, J. L., & Entyre, G. M. (1978). Validity of 24-hour dietary recalls by adolescent females. *American Journal of Public Health, 68,* 70–72.

Gross, A. M. (1983). Self-management training and medication compliance in children with diabetes. *Child and Family Behavior Therapy, 4,* 47–55.

Gross, A. M., Samson, G., Sanders, S., & Smith, C. (1988). Patient noncompliance: Are children consistent? *American Journal of Orthodontics and Dentofacial Orthopedics, 93,* 518–519.

Hanson, C. L., Henggeler, S. W., & Burghen, G. A. (1987). Race and sex differences in metabolic control of adolescents with IDDM: A function of psychosocial variables? *Diabetes Care, 10*(3), 313–318.

Harkavy, J., Johnson, S. B., Silverstein, J., Spillar, R., McCallum, M., & Rosenbloom, A. (1983). Who learns what at diabetes camp. *Journal of Pediatric Psychology, 8,* 143–153.

Haynes, R. B., Taylor, D. W., & Sackett, D. L. (Eds.). (1979). *Compliance in health care.* Baltimore: Johns Hopkins Press.

Jacobson, A. M., Hauser, S. T., Wolfsdorf, J. I., Houilhan, J., Milley, J. E., Herskowitz, R. D., Wertlieb, D., & Watt, E. (1987). Psychologic predictors of compliance in children with recent onset of diabetes mellitus. *Journal of Pediatrics, 110,* 805–811.

Johnson, S. B., Freund, A., Silverstein, J., Hansen, C. A., & Malone, J. (1990). Adherence/health status relationships in childhood diabetes. *Health Psychology, 9*(5), 606–631.

Johnson, S. B., Pollak, T., Silverstein, J. H., Rosenbloom, A. L., Spillar, R., McCallum, M., & Harkavy, J. (1982). Cognitive and behavioral knowledge about insulin dependent diabetes among children and parents. *Pediatrics, 69,* 708–713.

Johnson, S. B., Silverstein, J., Rosenbloom, A., Carter, R., & Cunningham, W. (1986). Assessing daily management in childhood diabetes. *Health Psychology, 5*(6), 545–564.

Johnson, S. B., Tomer, A., Cunningham, W. R., & Henretta, J. (1990). Adherence in childhood diabetes: Results of a confirmatory factor analysis. *Health Psychology, 9*(4), 493–501.

LaPorte, R. E., & Cruickshanks, K. J. (1985). Incidence and risk factors for insulin-dependent diabetes. In M. Harris & R. Hamman (Eds.), *Diabetes in America* (pp. II–1–III) (NIH Publication No. 85-1468). Bethesda, MD: U.S. Department of Health and Human Services/National Institutes of Health.

LaPorte, R. E., & Tajima, N. (1985). Prevalence of insulin-dependent diabetes. In M. Harris & R. Hamman (Eds.), *Diabetes in America* (pp. V–1–V–8) (NIH Publication No. 85-1468). Bethesda, MD: U.S. Department of Health and Human Services/National Institutes of Health.

Lowe, K., & Lutzker, J. F. (1979). Increasing compliance to a medical regimen with a juvenile diabetic. *Behavior Therapy, 10,* 57–64.

Marquis, K. H., Ware, J. E., Jr., & Relles, D. A. (1979). *Measures of diabetic patient knowledge, attitudes and behavior regarding self-care: Summary Report.* Atlanta: Center for Disease Control. (NTIS No. PB83-134528).

Matthews, L. W., & Drotar, D. (1984). Cystic fibrosis: A challenging long-term chronic disease. *Pediatric Clinics of North America, 31*(1), 133-154.

Miller, N. E. (1983). Behavioral medicine: Symbiosis between laboratory and clinic. *Annual Review of Psychology, 34,* 1–34.

Miller, L. P., & Miller, D. R. (1984). The pediatrician's role in caring for the child with cancer. *Pediatric Clinics of North America, 31*(1), 119-131.

Orme, C. M., & Binik, Y. M. (1989). Consistency of adherence across regimen demands. *Health Psychology, 8,* 27–43.

Page, P., Verstraete, D. G., Robb, J. R., & Etzwiler, D. D. (1981). Patient recall of self-care recommendations in diabetes. *Diabetes Care, 4,* 96–98.

Perrin, E. C., & Perrin, J. M. (1983). Clinician's assessments of children's understanding of illness. *American Journal Diseases of Children, 137,* 874–878.

Reynolds, L. A., Johnson, S. B., & Silverstein, J. (1990). Assessing daily diabetes management by 24-hr recall interview: The validity of children's reports. Manuscript submitted for publication. *Journal of Pediatric Psychology, 15*(4), 493–509.

Samuelson, G. (1970). An epidemiological study of child health and nutrition in a northern Swedish county. *Nutrition and Metabolism, 12*, 321–340.

Schafer, L. C., Glasgow, R. E., McCaul, K. D., & Dreher, M. (1983). Adherence to IDDM regimens: Relationship to psychosocial variables and metabolic control. *Diabetes Care, 6*(5), 493–498.

Sergis-Deavenport, E., & Varni, J. (1983). Behavioral assessment and management of adherence to factor replacement therapy in hemophilia. *Journal of Pediatric Psychology, 8*, 367–377.

Smyth-Staruch, K., Breslau, N., Weitzman, M., & Gortmaker, S. (1984). Use of health services by chronically ill and disabled children. *Medical Care, 22*, 310–328.

Spevack, M., Johnson, S. B., & Riley, W. (1991). The effect of diabetes summer camp on adherence behaviors and glycemic control. In J. Johnson & S. B. Johnson (Eds.), *Advances in child health psychology* (pp. 285–292). Gainesville: University of Florida Press.

Stunkard, A. J., & Waxman, M. (1981). Accuracy of self-reports of food intake. *Journal of the American Dietetic Association, 79*, 547–551.

Tattersall, R. B., & Lowe, J. (1981). Diabetes in adolescence. *Diabetologia, 20*, 517–523.

Tebbi, C. K., Cummings, K. M., Zevon, M. A., Smith, L., Richards, M., & Mallon, J. (1986). Compliance of pediatric and adolescent cancer patients. *Cancer, 58*, 1179–1184.

8 The Measurement of Compliance: Medication Taking

Peter Rudd
Stanford University Medical Center

This chapter reviews the special issue of medication taking with special emphasis on prescribed drugs and optimizing its measurement despite constraints of patient cooperation, evolving technology, and user effectiveness. The discussion addresses definitions and assumptions, historical developments, epidemiology, methods of measurement, linkage to therapeutics, and guidelines for clinicians and investigators.

INTRODUCTION

Definitions and Assumptions

Haynes (1979a) has defined compliance as the extent to which a person's behavior, in terms of taking medications, following diets, or making other lifestyle changes, coincides with medical advice. This broad definition further assumes a number of conditions (Feinstein, 1975; Sackett, 1977). It first assumes that the medical condition under consideration has been properly diagnosed. Second, the definition presupposes that effective treatment exists in a form shown to produce more good than harm. Third, it presumes that the clinician provides the recommendations in understandable and achievable form. For example, suboptimal compliance might result if the prescription were offered in ambiguous language or at a cost prohibitive for a particular patient.

These assumptions are hardly trivial. They underscore that compliance for medication taking is usually situation specific and subject to multiple positive and negative influences. It is of little value to measure or enhance adherence when the diagnosis is incorrect or the treatment proves generally harmful.

In most clinical settings, the clinician performs a therapeutic experiment at each return visit. Having previously prescribed treatment, the clinician then reviews the degree of achieving the therapeutic goal, assesses other possible consequences of the treatment, and determines the optimal follow-up. At each return visit, the clinician must decide whether the current treatment is appropriate, adequate, and advantageous compared to alternatives. This chapter reviews what is known about medication-taking behavior, recognizing that such knowledge is necessary but not sufficient for interpreting the therapeutic experiment.

Historical Evolution of the Compliance Literature

The early publications related to medication compliance fell into three broad categories. The first primarily documented the high prevalence of suboptimal medication taking. There may have been some risk of publication bias, which inadvertently favored selection of those submissions that offered the most extreme reports of deviant noncompliance. These early reports confirmed high prevalence rates of noncompliance among those in both acute (Bergman & Werner, 1963) and chronic (Neely & Patrick, 1968) regimens, both pediatric (Gordis, Markowitz, & Lilienfeld, 1969) and adult (Latiolais & Berry, 1969) populations, and both trivial (Porter, 1969) and potentially life-threatening illnesses (Johannsen, Hellmuth, & Sorauf, 1966).

A second major theme in the literature was the search for predictors or determinants. In rapid order, over 100 potential factors were identified and found to be associated with suboptimal compliance (Haynes, 1976a). These studies, however, were generally limited to relatively small samples and usually univariate in their analysis (Goldsmith, 1976). On few occasions were assessments made for potential interactions among the factors, and most were found to be only inconsistently associated when studies were pooled or compared (Haynes, 1976a).

Finally, the literature had a relatively small number of interventional studies, usually highly site specific (Haynes, 1976b). There was only limited documentation of the intervention's impact, especially over the long term. A reader of the early literature could understandably become both confused and discouraged by the lack of controlled trials with careful attention to confounding influences.

THE EPIDEMIOLOGY OF MEDICATION TAKING

The primitive measures of medication taking available in the past have limited our knowledge of the epidemiology of compliance in general and that of medication taking in particular. As a consequence, there should be caution in interpreting published reports about their incidence, prevalence, predictors, natural history, and interventional studies.

Incidence and Prevalence

Most of the studies on the frequency of suboptimal medication taking have distinguished acute from chronic conditions, symptomatic from asymptomatic diseases, and preventive maneuvers from curative treatments. With moderate variance, the trends for compliance with a variety of chronic conditions converge on approximately 50% of the prescribed regimen.

Several important epidemiological qualifications are relevant. The behavior of *inception cohorts*, those newly diagnosed and starting treatment for the first time, may differ markedly from that of *survivor cohorts*, those patients who stay under treatment and receive treatment for prolonged time. By self-selection, survivor cohorts are more likely to accept the value of therapy and therefore to adhere to the prescription. Kass et al. (1986b) used medication monitors to document that mean compliance in an inception cohort of 184 ambulatory glaucoma patients was significantly lower (65% vs. 76%; $p = 0.04$) than that among a survivor cohort.

Little is known about the natural history of medication taking among cohorts over time, especially as they pass through developmental stages. Sackett (1977) compared the medication-taking distributions of 134 ambulatory hypertensive steelworkers based on pill counts at 6 and 12 months after starting antihypertensive medications. The overall distribution of the compliance rates changed little over the second 6-month follow-up period. They observed a J-shaped distribution with 15%–30% taking none of the prescribed medications, 35%–50% taking 80% of their doses, and the remainder falling in the midzone. Rudd et al. (1989) used pill counts to track medication taking among a survivor cohort of stable hypertensives on complex regimens. Whereas mean compliance clustered near 100% for most subjects at most visits, individuals displayed marked variability from week to week, both within and between subjects. Suboptimal medication taking appeared to be a random rather than a systematic event in the population studied.

Determinants/Predictors of Suboptimal Medication Taking

Despite limited confidence in measures of compliance, many investigators have focused on determinants and predictors or subsequent suboptimal medication taking. Identifying a low-risk subpopulation at baseline would then allow clinicians' attention and effort to shift to the high-risk group to maximize impact. There has been a reluctance to accept as inevitable and irreducible what Charney

(1975) has called the "rough-and-ready natural law . . . [that] the physician will be expected to prescribe with only approximate accuracy and the patient will be expected to comply with only modest fidelity" (p. 1009).

Most early studies used univariate searches assessing the differential impact of single factors or gradations of single factors on outcome measures of medication taking. Few investigators quantified the relative contributions of multiple factors simultaneously or evaluated interactions among the factors. Not surprisingly, a huge number of possible determinants were identified (Haynes, Taylor, & Sackett, 1979). Unfortunately, few determinants passed muster as important predictors of subsequent medication-taking levels. Among sociodemographic features, only extremes of age and abject poverty consistently predict suboptimal adherence. Other characteristics, like gender, educational level, occupational status, marital status, income, ethnic background, and race offer little predictive value.

Somewhat more disappointing is the failure of clinical features, especially symptom level and objective signs of disease severity, to forecast the level of adherence. Greater levels of disability, however, are associated with higher adherence rates. Patients with frank psychiatric disease most consistently demonstrate poor adherence. In addition, patients' self-perception as socially isolated and the development of side effects from medication are associated with poor medication taking by self-report (Nelson, Stason, Neutra, & Solomon, 1980).

The regimen's specifics clearly affect compliance, particularly the dosing frequency and total number of regimen components (Haynes, Sackett, Taylor, Roberts, & Johnson, 1977). Whereas the number of different medications prescribed is inversely proportional to the compliance rate, the number of daily dosings has a less clear effect (Hulka, 1979). Patients unequivocally prefer once daily dosing for asymptomatic conditions. Yet direct comparison of once versus twice versus four times daily dosings shows only marginally superior results for once daily administration among outpatients (Cramer et al., 1989; Eisen et al., 1990; Taggart, Johnston, & McDevitt, 1981). Patients' apparent misinterpretation of prescription instructions may further adversely affect the results (Mazzullo, Lasagna, & Griner, 1974). Adherence rates fall as the prescribed duration of treatment increases (Hershey, Morton, Davis, & Reichgott, 1980). Use of child-resistant containers may also dramatically reduce medication-taking rates (Sherman, Warach, & Libow, 1979).

Patients' understanding of the regimen is obviously essential but not sufficient to ensure optimal medication-taking behavior (Greene, Weinberger, Jerin, & Mamlin, 1982). Their knowledge of the regimen is inversely proportional to the number of different medications prescribed (Brody, 1980). The level of understanding, in turn, may be linked in a complex manner with cognitive factors like memory and psychosocial factors like satisfaction with medical care provided

(Barsky, 1983; Ley, 1985). Many patients may be particularly misinformed about the best action if a dose of medication is missed (Ascione, Kirscht, & Shimp, 1986).

Medications' side effects may affect compliance (Cromer, Steinberg, Gardner, Thornton, & Shannon, 1989) and yet are cited as important obstacles to medication taking by less than 10% of respondents in most surveys of patients' perceptions (Haynes, 1979b). Nevertheless, up to 15% of participants receiving active antihypertensive medications in a 5-year primary prevention trial (Medical Research Council Working Party, 1985) withdrew because of intolerable side effects. Others have cited the negative impact of many medications on quality-of-life, thereby predisposing to suboptimal adherence (Williams, 1987).

Interventions to Enhance Medication Taking

The arena of interventions to enhance medication taking remains an important barometer of assumptions and prejudices about compliance itself. Interventions remained modest in scope as long as suboptimal adherence was viewed as the unique responsibility of the patient. Compliance traditionally held little interest for clinicians, who gave priority to proper diagnosis and prescription. Failure to adhere and therefore failure to respond to treatment was seen as a consequence of patients' choices. Slowly and perhaps reluctantly, the field has come to acknowledge the contributions that clinicians and investigators can make to inhibit or enhance medication-taking behavior. With the acknowledgment has come a growing sophistication about both the determinants of compliance and the focuses for selective interventions (Haynes, 1979c).

In broad categories, the interventions readily fall into three groups: educational, behavioral, and system-based subtypes. The educational interventions start with the assumption that inadequate information lies at the heart of the problem. If individuals better understood the potential seriousness of the condition, their susceptibility to negative consequences without treatment, the effectiveness of therapy, its relative safety and convenience, and the particulars of the regimen, then all would be well.

The investigational data from educational interventions only partially support this perspective. Knowledge of medical diagnosis and drug purpose does not correlate with self-reported medication-taking behavior (Klein, German, McPhee, Smith, & Levine, 1982). As a group, many patients seem well aware of the dangers of uncontrolled disease and their individual risk status. In fact, exaggeration or even reinforcement of such fear messages in isolation often prompts patients' denial or evasion (Leventhal, 1971). Similarly, emphasis on the effectiveness of the treatment seems necessary but not sufficient as an enabling factor. Usually combinations of interventions prove superior to single interventions (Levine et al., 1979). Others have found that combining written and oral instructions may create "information overload," especially when complex regimens are involved (Ascione & Shimp, 1984). Meta-analyses of 70 published evaluations of educational programs indicate that the largest impact occurs from one-to-one counseling, group education, or both in combination with audio-visual materials (Mullen, Green, & Persinger, 1985). Triaging among possible interventions may maximize impact and minimize cost for use of limited resources (Hatcher, Green, Levine, & Flagle, 1986).

The behavioral interventions begin from a different perspective. They acknowledge that many patients may not fully understand their medical conditions but that compliant behavior may be induced and maintained by reinforcing behaviors (Zifferblatt, 1975). Some efforts attempted contractual incentives by which the patient and clinician negotiate and sign contracts specifying the patient's behavior in exchange for the clinician's availability, punctuality, and thoughtful supervision of treatment (Steckel & Swain, 1977). Other forms of social support have included group therapy, patient-operated self-help groups, telephone counseling, and special worksite occupational nurses. Early efforts to employ special medication packaging yielded disappointing results (Crome, Akehurst, & Keet, 1980; Eshelman & Fitzloff, 1976), despite the ingenuity of some of the devices. Other efforts, especially when based on the concept of a drug calendar to remind patients to take the medications as prescribed, produced significant improvements in medication-taking behavior (Gabriel, Gagnon, & Bryan, 1977), including blister packaging rather than standard vials (Wong & Norman, 1987). As with the educational interventions, the behavioral maneuvers appeared most effective when applied serially and in combination rather than as single, poorly defined steps (Levy, 1985; Spector, McGrath, Uretsky, Newman, & Cohen, 1978).

Some of the most successful interventions have employed this very strategy in combining system-based maneuvers. These efforts assume that no single intervention component will succeed with all subjects, given the complex determinants of compliant behavior. By providing a battery of components that range from educational or behavioral through logistical and philosophical, these studies seek less to prove the unique value of any component than to affect change by any of a variety of simultaneous mechanisms. One of the early feasibility studies confirmed that a dedicated clinic pharmacist could produce dramatic improvement in medication taking and blood pressure control by soliciting drug-related side effects, adjusting the regimen in conjunction with prescribing physicians, and providing background information about the disease (McKenney, Slining, Henderson, Devins, & Barr, 1973). Mean compliance rates by pill count rose from 25% to 79% in the intervention group during the 5-month maneuver but returned promptly to baseline when the interventions were withheld. The study underscores pre-existing communication problems between clinicians and patients as well as the need for sustained reinforcement for improved medication taking to continue.

METHODS OF MEASUREMENT

Concepts and Qualifications

Issues of Measurement and Reactivity. As previously described, compliance refers to the extent of concordance between the prescription and the patient's behavior. Such a definition necessarily includes measuring both the prescription and the behavior. Unfortunately, there are inescapable trade-offs in gathering these different kinds of information. On the one hand, one may use a variety of intensive and sometimes invasive maneuvers to obtain objective and reproducible information, but the maneuvers themselves may affect the behavior under study. Individuals who know their behavior is closely monitored may behave in an entirely atypical manner and often in nonreproducible ways. The obvious and opposite extreme is to measure more naturalistic behavior but with far less control and confidence.

Forms of Improper Medication Taking. Beyond the absolute measure of medication taking, several additional aspects may require special measurement and yet provide important management clues. Using verbal self-report from 350 outpatients, Hulka et al. (Hulka, 1979; Hulka, Cassel, Kupper, & Burdette, 1976) identified three predominant types of medication errors: inadvertent errors of *commission, omission,* and *scheduling misconception.* Much less commonly, they found deliberate *scheduling noncompliance.* These distinctions have several obvious implications for management. For example, there is a substantial difference between (a) forgetting to take the pill despite knowing the proper regimen and (b) believing incorrectly that only two rather than three pills are needed daily. The causes and reinforcers of these four different behaviors are dissimilar. Whenever possible, therefore, the form(s) of medication-taking error should be specified in defining suboptimal compliance.

Medication Taking Versus Compliance. Conceptionally, medication-taking behavior carries several advantages over the more traditional idea of concordance with a specific prescription (i.e., compliance itself). By focusing on medication-taking behavior, the clinician or investigator acknowledges the importance of a specific time and place in which the medication dose is dispensed, consumed, and permitted to have its pharmacological effect. Despite its apparent simplicity, such behavior is dynamic rather than static. As such, the optimal measure would be applied close in time and space to the actual event and yet be able to confirm consumption of the medication and not merely dispensing. The optimal measure would further provide a distribution of behaviors, because they would unlikely be monotonic in frequency and degree. Even knowing the distribution itself would not eliminate the possibility that the biological or pharmacological effect may need to exceed a threshold for minimal effectiveness or fall below a threshold of danger to avoid toxicity.

Distortions of Averages. In this context, simple or composite averages for medication taking may be misleading. Rudd, Byyny, Zachary, LoVerde, Titus, Mitchell, and Marshall (1989) followed 120 ambulatory hypertensives for up to 12 months, using pill counts at 1- to 12-week intervals to determine intervisit compliance rates. Although the group's mean rate of medication taking varied little, weekly pill count data showed marked inter and intrasubject variability without discernible pattern. As the measurement interval lengthened, the apparent variability diminished, as under and overcompliance phases compensated for each other. Thus, the timeframe for assessing each regimen component should be specified to avoid misrepresentation.

Compliance by Component. Definitions of compliance should further specify and assess each of the regimen's components to be most meaningful. In particular, a multifaceted regimen may involve a separate learning curve for each of the components. The more numerous the prescribed behaviors are, the less likely that any one component will be followed. A patient may adhere rigidly to one ingredient and poorly to another, only to alter both patterns unexpectedly. Sometimes these changes may be linked to disruptive life events or other alterations in routine. Rudd and co-workers (1989) reported poor concordance for different drugs in the same regimen among ambulatory hypertensives over 1 month, once the regimen had been stabilized for efficacy. Thus, medication taking for one drug offered limited predictive value for any other component of the regimen.

Interactions. In addition, both simple and complex interactions among regimen components may occur to affect medication taking. This includes concomitant administration of other medications for the same condition, medications for other conditions, and nondrug components. To be comprehensive, definitions of compliance must acknowledge the possibility of dynamic and dramatic shifts among compliance levels by each component.

Continuous Versus Dichotomous. With such dynamic changes, medication-taking behavior should be described as a continuous rather than as a dichotomous variable. Few clinical situations correspond to simplistic models of patients exhibiting either "good" or "bad" compliance (Dirks & Kinsman, 1982). Such simplistic categories cover wide ranges in medication-taking behavior. Unfortunately, too many uncertainties usually prevail for dichotomous variables to suffice. For example, few clinicians are able to define precisely how much compliance is "enough." The relationship between delivered dosage and therapeutic effect is frequently vague or may display either a graded relationship or a discrete threshold for efficacy. Only continuous distributions of compliance allow a rational basis for studies to optimize therapeutics. In addition, simplistic categories of good versus bad compliance obscure any possible covariations between medication-taking behavior and the many possible factors that influence it.

The actual medication-taking distributions are rarely "normal" or bell-shaped. Consequently, measures of central tendency may inadequately summarize the distribution. Some instances of apparent overconsumption of medication may be an artifact of improper pill counts, whether by patient misrepresentation (e.g., by pill dumping prior to scheduled visits) or by staff error. Several investigators, however, have reported patient subgroups who systematically or periodically take more medication than they should, a practice with great potential dangers (Kass, Meltzer, Gordon, Cooper, & Goldberg, 1986b). This problem may be particularly ominous for those with important comorbidity that impairs drug metabolism. Practical but possible causes for such overcompliance may include forgetting that a dose has already been taken and then overcompensating for prior missed doses.

In summary, the best definition of compliance would seem to be the degree of dynamic correspondence between a clinical prescription for any regimen component and the patient's measured behavior in response to the prescription.

Interpreting the Therapeutic Experiment

Categories of Response. These several qualifications for defining compliance underscore the dilemma of interpreting the therapeutic experiment. The clinician needs to assign the clinical response to one of four categories, as illustrated by Fig. 8.1 (Sackett, Haynes, & Tugwell, 1985):

1. *high/good* (high medication compliance with achievement of the therapeutic goal) corresponding to the ideal situation or correct diagnosis, full patient cooperation, and complete pharmacological response.

2. *high/poor* (high compliance without the achievement of the therapeutic goal), suggesting an insufficiently vigorous regimen or perhaps pharmacological resistance.

3. *low/good* (low medication compliance but achieved therapeutic goal nonetheless), most consistent with an incorrect diagnosis or perhaps overzealous prescription for mild disease.

4. *low/poor* (low medication compliance without achievement of the therapeutic goal), corresponding to the classical noncomplier. The latter presumably does not need a more vigorous regimen, only the will and consistency to adhere to the existing prescription.

The clinician is frequently unable to classify the clinical response with certainty into one of these four categories. Sometimes, the clinician may fail to consider the possibility that suboptimal medication taking has caused the inability to achieve the therapeutic goal. Fearing the risks of poorly controlled disease, the clinician may escalate the regimen to larger doses or more potent medications. The patient then undergoes the alternative risks of treatment-related toxicity.

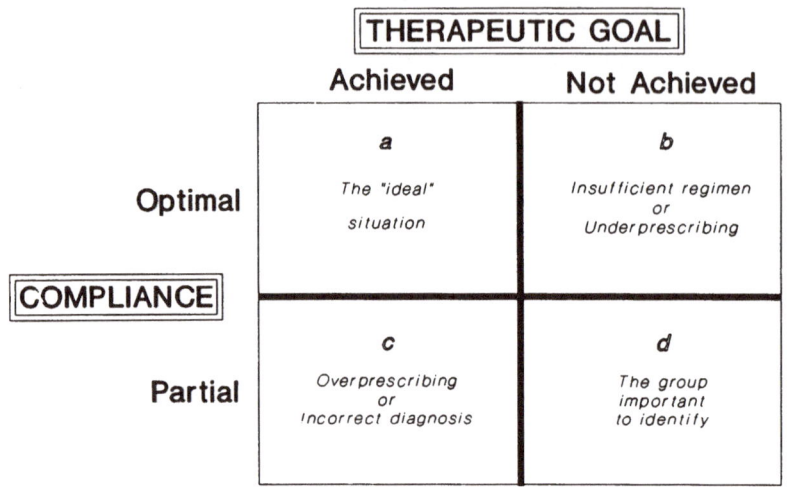

FIG. 8.1. Possible outcomes in the therapeutic experiment. Adapted from Sackett, Haynes, and Tugwell (1985). Reproduced by permission of Little, Brown.

Relative Frequency. There are only limited data to suggest the relative frequencies of misclassification. Taylor et al. (1978) reported the outcomes among 134 hypertensive steelworkers providing pill counts as the compliance measure with casual blood pressures during the home visit as a measure of therapeutic success. Using regression analysis, the investigators selected 80% compliance as the threshold for optimal medication taking, indicating that such a level was the minimal amount of medication taking associated with consistent reductions of blood pressure to the preselected goal level. They observed that only 23% of the group achieved goal blood pressure with high compliance. In contrast, 12% of the subjects achieved goal blood pressure despite suboptimal compliance, and 34% showed uncontrolled blood pressure despite high compliance. The remaining 31% exhibited both uncontrolled blood pressure and low compliance. Thus only 35% of the subjects achieved the goal blood pressure, and only 66% of these did so with near-optimal medication taking over the 12-month follow-up period.

Consequences of Misclassification. There are several consequences of misclassifying therapeutic outcomes. It is possible that up to two-thirds of patients might have their regimens adjusted incorrectly: (a) some incorrect adjustments due to clinicians' failing to consider the possibility of suboptimal medication taking as a cause of failure to achieve the therapeutic goal, and (b) other incorrect adjustments due to clinicians who ascribe all treatment failure to inadequate medication taking. In such cases, the clinicians might reinforce the existing but inadequate regimen, offering the patient incomplete protection despite full cooperation. Very similar findings in distribution of patients were found in other ambulatory treatment settings (Logan, Milne, Flanagan, & Haynes, 1983). Inui, Carter, Pecoraro, Pearlman, and Dohan, (1980) observed that 40% of their well-controlled hypertensives were "noncompliant" by pill count, suggesting overmedication or misdiagnosis. At least one report (Steiner et al., 1990) confirms that regimen reductions are sometimes possible without negative impact on clinical measures, suggesting that partial compliance with the prescription would be sufficient. The potential for misclassification, therefore, seems real and of considerable magnitude. Improving assessment of patients' medication-taking behavior remains pivotal to any progress.

Interpretive Dilemmas. The implications in some clinical settings will be more critical than in others. For individuals with conditions such as hypertension, diabetes mellitus, arthritis, or epilepsy, excessive prescription coupled with episodic full compliance carries the potential for suboptimal prophylaxis, intermittent drug toxicity, and potentially avoidable extra testing and/or hospitalization. Maronde et al. (1989) reported higher rates of rehospitalization among poorly compliant hypertensive outpatients compared to better complying counterparts. Perhaps even more dramatic, Psaty, Koepsell, Wagner, LoGerfo, and Inui (1990) demonstrated some lethal consequences of partial compliance. They observed nearly a five-fold increase in coronary heart disease events among a cohort of patients on β-blocker complying with less than 80% of the prescribed dose by refill rates compared to those complying close to 100%.

In clinical drug trials, several other interpretive dilemmas occur. Many trials select relatively stable, uncomplicated patients willing and able to comply with the demanding constraints and multiple return visits, frequent clinical and laboratory monitoring, and the uncertainties of receiving investigational drugs. Until recently, there were very few studies that even bothered to assess medication compliance. Soutter and Kennedy (1974) reported that only 19% of 768 trials reported in the *British Medical Journal* or *Lancet* in the period 1969–1972 included any measures of adherence. Gotzsche (1989) observed that compliance was measured in only 13% of 196 reports of nonsteroidal anti-inflammatory drug trials in the interval 1966–1985 and results explicitly reported in only 6%. Failure to include such assessment carries the risks of erroneously concluding (a) that true differences do not exist, when the lack of apparent difference may result from inadequate medication taking among those on the more effective treatment, or (b) that similar drugs have differing efficacy, when the differences really reflect only the medication-taking rates.

Several even more subtle issues emerge when special attention is paid to individuals exhibiting suboptimal compliance. Those with high versus low compliance may differ quantitatively in the extent to which they exhibit a therapeutic response. Haynes and Dantes (1987) reviewed several studies suggesting that a noncomplier, even to placebo treatment, may have other important differences, such as dying at nearly twice the rate as those who comply with placebo treatment in a coronary disease primary prevention trial. Intensive follow-up and careful reporting of noncompliance is therefore critical in the analysis of any trial.

Clinical Trial Constraints and Biases. Operationally, noncompliance may complicate achieving adequate sample size. By increasing within-group variance and diminishing observed treatment effect, noncompliance increases the minimal number of subjects to achieve statistical significance. The minimal sample size is directly proportional to the square of the standard deviation, itself an indication of the scatter around the mean. As mean compliance rates fall from 100% to 50%, the required sample size for each arm of a study may increase three- to four-fold (Goldsmith, 1979).

Several kinds of compliance bias may emerge as result of different ways of handling suboptimal compliance in the design and analysis of clinical trials. *Compliance bias* refers to several kinds of incorrect conclusions related to how subjects are selected, monitored, and/or analyzed (Feinstein, 1975, 1979; Goldsmith, 1979). A *compliance sample* may rise when patients' willingness to cooperate is one entry criterion for participation. As a result, the study subjects may be nonrepresentative of the patient population at large, limiting generalizability to other groups.

A second type of bias results from association between medication taking and other factors directly linked to one of the outcome variables. One example would be side effects from the principal drug (e.g., diuretic-induced impotence) that may prompt the patient to reduce the medication dosage. Once present, such a condition would produce different outcome rates among those subjects complying with the regimen than among those who did not, independent of the medication's therapeutic effects themselves. As a result, an ineffective regimen may appear beneficial or deleterious to those who adhered to it, when compared to those who did not comply. Alternatively, an effective regimen may seem useless if the compliance rate is sufficiently low.

Compliance bias may easily lead to erroneous results, although some mathematical compensation is possible (Palta & McHugh, 1980). Analysis by compliance subgroup, once compliance is defined as a continuous distribution, would permit defining a therapeutic gradient in which more adherence to a specified regimen may yield proportionally greater benefit.

Methods of Measurement

For compliance, as with most other aspects of science, measurement is the key. Measurement allows definition of the process, assessment of incidence and prevalence, exploration for predictors, and evaluation of interventions. Without proper measurement, none of these components is possible. As previously suggested, both the pattern and the rate of compliance are important.

Existing measures may be classified as either direct or indirect, biologic or nonbiologic. Several excellent reviews have recently described the array of traditional measures of compliance as well as their relative advantages and disadvantages (Caron, 1985; Dunbar, 1984; Norell, 1984; Roth, 1984; Rudd & Marshall, 1987).

Direct Biologic Measures. The direct measures, like *biologic assays* of active drug or metabolite, confirm actual drug ingestion. One may even take educated guesses about when drug ingestion last occurred if all the details of dosing, possible interfering substances, pharmacokinetics, and pharmacodynamics are all known. More realistically, clinicians and investigators rarely know all these details. Many of the analytical techniques are complex, expensive, and therefore impractical for most ambulatory settings (Nierenberg, 1987). Individual patients' metabolism offers complexities that further confound the effort. Perhaps, most importantly, biologic assays give little information about the consistency of medication taking, especially back farther than five half-lives for the index drug, the interval generally required for pharmacological equilibrium to be achieved. To interpret individual drug concentrations, one may need to establish threshold criteria corresponding to optimal medication taking. The criteria, in turn, will reflect arbitrary levels with trade-offs of sensitivity versus specificity (Beck et al., 1988). In sum, biological measures often raise as many questions as they answer.

Markers have become a tempting but frustrating alternative to direct biological assays. They consist of one of several biologically inert or subtherapeutic substances coupled in a predictable way with the ingestion of the active medication. Once ingested, the marker is monitored by direct assessment, free of the complexity surrounding the body's handling of the active drug. This approach retains several problems. Combining a marker like riboflavin or minute quantities of digoxin (Maenpaa et al., 1987a) or phenobarbital (Bignell, Mulcahy, Peaker, Pullar, & Feely, 1988) with another medication may result in a new "drug" according to FDA regulations. In addition, there may be marked patient-to-patient variability in excretion patterns, in inter and intraobserver variability in measuring urinary fluorescence, and in interference with other sources of the marker such as food supplements with riboflavin (Dubbert et al., 1985). Other approaches have used radioactive labeled markers such as chromium-51 or stable isotopes (Russell, 1984).

Indirect Nonbiological Measures. Indirect measures, in contrast, assess medication taking without confirming that the drug ingestion actually occurred. As a group, with the exception of medication monitors and self-monitoring diaries, these measures assess compliance in a process distant in time and space from the actual medication-taking event. As a consequence, several distortions may occur.

Patient self-report in all of its permutations tends to exaggerate the adequacy of compliance (Norell, 1981; Specter et al., 1986). Patients tend to report the specifics of interdose intervals more accurately than the issue of whether or not they omitted particular doses (Alfredsson & Norell, 1981). The longer the period of requested recall, the more likely the subject is to minimize deviation from the prescription. The outer limit of such accurate recall is probably less than 2 weeks. Beyond such an interval, self-report offers a simple estimate of average compliance, but little chance of an accurate, reproducible summary of specific doses taken versus missed (Strecher, Becker, Clark, & Prasada-Rao, 1989). Self-report may have the advantage of identifying individuals more likely to enhance their compliance when corrective interventions are applied (Sackett, 1977). In combination with a clinical measure like blood pressure and direct verbal inquiry, self-report may yield higher sensitivity than self-report alone for detecting suboptimal compliance in an ambulatory, hypertensive population (Inui, Carter, & Pecoraro, 1981).

Pill counts figure prominently in most ambulatory drug trials, both for screening prior to study entry during a placebo washout phase and for chronic monitoring of long-term medication taking. Subjects return the pill supply at each visit for surreptitious pill counts but quickly realize that their behavior is monitored in this fashion. Anecdotally, some subjects may appear to cooperate by returning near perfect or fully empty medication bottles whereas leaving many intact pills in clinic parking lots or waste containers. Pill counts then can give only a putative average compliance rate for a particular interval. As the interval lengthens, important deviations may be obscured by the average compliance rate.

Several logistical obstacles interfere with standard pill counts. These include subjects' forgetting to return pill vials, losing containers, sharing medication with other individuals, and storing medication in more than one place. Any patient's concern about being judged may also induce duplicitous behavior to simulate full adherence. The technique of pill counts, moreover, is very labor intensive, so that it is often impractical in nonresearch clinical settings (Fletcher, Pappius, & Harper, 1979).

Rudd et al. (1989) reported on 121 subjects followed prospectively with pill counts for ≤12 months in an antihypertensive drug trial. The compliance distribution for the entire but highly selected population of chronic hypertensives was unimodal but skewed, centered close to 100%. Nevertheless, fully 3% of the 1,052 intervisit pill counts exceeded 3 standard deviations above the group mean (i.e., greater than 135%). Such improbably high compliance rates likely represent a combination of partial dumping of unused or lost pill supplies (increasing the compliance rate numerator) combined with shorter than expected visit intervals (decreasing the denominator), because patients received 150% of the medication needed for the projected intervisit interval.

Prescription refills may serve as a less sensitizing alternative to the pill count but carry other shortcomings. The method monitors the prescribed dosing frequency and interval between prescription refills (Steiner, Koepsell, Fihn, & Inui, 1988). Patients may confound the technique by electing to obtain refills at more than one pharmacy or by sharing medications with others. Some settings, such as prepaid health plans and institutional programs, may use the approach because of centralized functions (Psaty, Koepsell, Wagner, LoGerfo, & Inui, 1990). There remains the possible confounding factor that in "free care" settings patients may lack the economic disincentives to purchase only those medications that they will actually consume.

Clinicians' opinions, when used, often prove a disappointing measure of compliance (Kass, Gordon, & Meltzer, 1986a; Norell, 1981). As a rule, clinicians' opinions are highly specific but relatively insensitive (Gilbert, Evans, Haynes, & Tugwell, 1980). More experienced clinicians did little better than more junior trainees (Caron & Roth, 1968). Brody (1980) has suggested that physicians may be both unaware of the importance of the relevant behavioral, psychological, and social aspects of care and have insufficient time, skills, or motivation to identify or manage these problems. *Therapeutic impact* is the measure perhaps most distant from the medication-taking event. Often a number of confounding factors like intercurrent stresses, comorbidity, concomitant medication, or other factors may interfere with consistent disease control or achievement of therapeutic goals. Thus, the degree of achieving the therapeutic goal does not always correspond to the compliance level.

Comparative Performance Among Measures. There have in fact been very few studies that directly compared simultaneous compliance measures for systematic distortion or concordance. Wandless, Mucklow, Smith, and Prudham (1979) assessed 81 elderly outpatients receiving a mean of 2.5 medications daily. They noted a correlation coefficient of 0.47 ($p < 0.001$) between self-report and prescription refill rates but only accounted for less than 25% of the variance. Only 58% of those reporting near-perfect compliance ($100 \pm 10\%$) by self-report exhibited equally desirable adherence rates by pill count. When patient self-report and prescription refill rates agreed, the investigators found confirmatory, near-optimal pill counts in 69% of patients. These data suggest that other objective measures must be integrated with patient self-report to enhance the overall predictive value. It remains unlikely that any single indirect measure of medication taking will be sufficient.

Fletcher et al. (1979) compared patient self-report, pill count, and serum drug concentration among 173 outpatients prescribed digoxin. Complete pill counts were possible in only 39% of subjects and were never available quickly enough to allow feedback during regular patient visits to clinic. Only 2% of pill counts among the 83% of subjects claiming perfect (100%) compliance confirmed perfect pill taking.

Haynes et al. (1980) evaluated 134 steelworkers during their first 6 months of antihypertensive treatment. The patients' self-reports showed high correlation ($r = 0.74$, $p < 0.001$) with compliance rates by pill count, but subjects overestimated their own compliance by an average of 17%. Interviews proved preferable in convenience and superior in correlation to pill counts, compared to qualitative urinary drug assays, drug-induced metabolic changes, or therapeutic outcome in blood pressure changes as alternative measures.

Maenpaa, Manninen, and Heinonen (1987b) employed a digoxin marker, capsule counting, and a compliance questionnaire among 1,739 subjects receiving gemfibrozil or placebo for a coronary artery disease primary prevention trial. The proportion of subjects exhibiting suboptimal compliance varied by the method: Of the 321 subjects (18.5% of cohort) exhibiting poor compliance by marker analysis, only 20% were detectable by questionnaire and only 44% by capsule count.

Rudd et al. (1989) examined several measures of medication taking among a stable survivor cohort of 121 chronic, ambulatory, hypertensive patients. To proceed beyond randomization, subjects had to exhibit sustained hypertension and pill count compliance rates of 75%–125% over a 3-week placebo washout phase. Thus, the cohort represented a group of individuals with stable asymptomatic disease and high compliance by traditional measures. The authors directly compared six measures: self-report by prospective global statement, 48-hour recall, pill counts, biologic assays of plasma drug concentrations, clinicians' opinions of average medication-taking rate, and therapeutic response in terms of change in blood pressure from baseline.

The study was hampered by the absence of a gold standard against which to compare the measures, and the authors observed only limited correlation and concordance among the measures. The lack of correlation may in part have been artifactual, due to the limited variability from preselecting individuals with relatively high compliance rates. Neither patients' self-reports nor the clinicians' estimates ever mentioned compliance levels greater than 100%, although pill counts frequently exceeded this level. Recall over 48 hours correlated better with pill count than did global self-report measures, especially at baseline. Although the biological assay confirmed that 29 of 30 eligible subjects consumed some of the study medication in the preceding day before clinical assessment, the consistency of compliance by bioassay class was poor. Only 41% of 17 subjects with "adequate" levels as defined by standardized criteria gave the same result 1 month later under identical conditions; 35% had lower values. Among the 7 subjects with initially "low" levels, 57% had satisfactory values in repeat testing.

Because most measures occurred far in time and space from any specific medication-taking event, the poor correlation and concordance among them may be disappointing but hardly surprising. All traditional measures of compliance prove imperfect. The advantages of cost, convenience, and acceptability have generally served as counterweights to accuracy, nonreactivity, and comprehensiveness. No single measure offers all virtues; trade-offs are inevitable.

EVOLUTION OF THE MEDICATION MONITOR

Concept of the Monitor

Several promising alternative measures of medication taking have emerged with technological advances. The basic concept is one of monitoring the actual dispensing of medication and recording the precise times at which the medication vial was opened with medication actually dispensed (Moulding, 1979; Rudd, 1979a; Rudd & Marshall, 1987). The monitors then provide a time tracing, which becomes the matrix on which the investigator places other observations, measurements, and potential predictors in search of associations. The monitors assess medication-taking events on a dynamic, hour-to-hour basis. It remains theoretically possible that a patient might systematically open and close the monitor and not actually take the medication, but such systematic deception over a prolonged period appears unlikely. Theoretically, such detailed temporal data on medication taking could provide a probe for factors that facilitate, cue, or inhibit specific occasions of dispensing and presumably consuming medication itself.

Early Development

Most of the early efforts used the model of antiglaucomatous eyedrops, employing microcircuitry and simple electronics to treatment for asymptomatic disease (Kass et al., 1986b; Norell, 1981). A number of other investigators (Eisen, Miller, Woodward, Spitznagel, Przybeck, 1990; Eisen, Woodward, Miller, Spitznagel, & Windham, 1987) developed electronic prototypes that struggled to overcome the mechanical–electronic interface to record the discrete dispensing of each pill. A number of relatively small, simple, and inexpensive electronic monitors have emerged recently that are suitable for both clinical trials and selective nonstudy situations.

Another promising approach has consisted of adapting bar code technology with both portable readers and computer-assisted instruction to assess suboptimal compliance and reduce its prevalence (Leirer, Morrow, Pariante, & Sheikh, 1988).

To date, several important observations have been made. Kass and co-workers (1986b) demonstrated great variability for interdose intervals among individuals taking antiglaucomatous eyedrops four times daily. Over 30% of the subjects exhibited intervals averaging more than 12 hours between dosings, allowing calculation of the proportion of time in which patients were "unprotected," given the known pharmacology of the drug. Among 720 hours-at-risk, 33% of the subjects had at least 23 (3%) of the hours uncovered. These data underscore the clinical superiority of pharmacological coverage rather than just dispensing the correct number of pills.

Several patterns of medication taking were described in this setting. Most common was *near-optimal pill taking* (49% of subjects), producing an average compliance rate of 90%–110% of prescribed doses. In decreasing frequency, the other patterns included *consistent underdosing* (40%) omitting 11%–70% of the prescribed doses; *drug holidays* (19%) with greater than or equal to 3 consecutive days without any dosing; *abrupt jumps* (17%) with major increases in dosing frequency from day to the next; *abrupt drops* (12%) involving major decreases in dosing frequency from one day to the next; and *consistent overdosing* (10%) dispensing 111%–147% of the prescribed dose. Only 1 patient in 91 displayed the desirable dosing pattern of "perfect" compliance using the medication monitor. Thus the monitor's precision in tracking medication taking over time represents its most impressive promise.

Medication Event Monitoring System

Overview. More recently, a different device has become available: the Medication Events Monitoring System (MEMS; Aprex Corp.; Fremont, CA). The device consists of a modified plastic vial whose cap contains a microprocessor capable of recording the precise time and duration of each vial opening. Internal circuitry permits the exclusion of multiple openings separated by less than 2 seconds. Early versions of the monitor contained sufficient memory reserve to record up to 350 consecutive opening events with excellent precision and reproducibility. More recent models permit recording more than 1,000 opening events over more than 6 months.

Nonconcordance with Pill Count. Rudd, Ahmed, Zachary, Barton, and Bonduelle (1990) applied the device in a short-term drug study comparing two antihypertensive agents (isradipine and enalapril) on a twice-daily basis among ambulatory subjects over 13 weeks. Subjects were given up to 150% of the pills required for the intervisit interval. By pill count, the two medications produced similar mean compliance rates for the entire study (91.5% vs. 98.7%; NS). For most subjects, the compliance rates by pill count for 1- to 2-week intervals clustered at 100 ± 20%, but the range extended from 0%–135%. Although there was modest correlation between pill counts and overall compliance measure by the electronic monitor ($r = 0.243$, $p < 0.02$), most outliers corresponded to low compliance by monitor despite near perfect compliance by pill count. The most deviant subject exhibited a mean compliance by pill count of 93% with eight return visits over 98 days, whereas his MEMS monitor confirmed only 21% appropriate openings for the intervals. In brief, major deviation in medication-taking behavior would have remained unsuspected without the monitor's data. As the criteria of compliance became more stringent, the mean values for medication-taking rates fell progressively below the optimal level of 100%. If one insisted that medications be dispensed at the prescribed interval of 12 ± 2 hours, less than half of all openings met this criterion. Even if one extended the acceptable range to 12 ± 6 hours, about 25% of openings failed even this criterion.

Nonconcordance with Self-Report. Most subjects appeared to increase their medication taking in the several days prior to scheduled visits, suggesting that the upcoming visit might have served as a reminder and/or incentive. Similar findings with the same technology were observed among outpatients on antiseizure medications (Cramer, Scheyer, & Mattson, 1990). The change in behavior, however, made it unlikely that all were at pharmacologic steady-state. In addition, subjects frequently underestimated the true interval between their last pill and the time of the clinical visit. Subjects claimed that the interval had been 0.5–10 hours, whereas MEMS opening showed a range of 0–26 hours for the same intervals ($r = 0.126$; NS).

Prescribed Versus Administered Dose. The monitor further allowed a comparison of the prescribed dose by the protocol versus the administered dose as measured by the MEMS monitor. In particular, the monitor allowed the assessment of both "under" and "overdosing" beyond the prescription.

Evaluating Possible Adverse Drug Reactions. A number of subjects reported symptoms potentially attributable to one or the other study medications. One subject reported approximately 1 week of vertigo at one follow-up visit. On the day preceding the presumptive dose-related symptom, the monitor indicated six openings rather than the customary one to three openings per day. Although the timing of the overdispensing in the day before the onset of symptoms might have been coincidental, it serves as a useful signal and probe for the investigator. In contrast, another subject reported 1 week of fatigue without temporal association to the vial openings by the monitor. Thus, the monitor provides one method to assess the temporal plausibility of reported adverse drug effects.

Assessment of Secondary Resistance. A similar approach may be useful in evaluating loss of responsiveness to treatment, both in clinical practice and during a clinical trial. Such secondary resistance may reflect the biology of the disease, the pharmacology of the medications, or the behavior of medication taking. Although indirect evidence from pill counts and self-reports are often sufficient to distinguish among these possible causes, sometimes only the medication monitor provides the critical distinction. "Secondary resistance" frequently becomes a matter of suboptimal medication-taking behavior, once precise data are available.

Interpreting the Therapeutic Experiment. Ultimately, the monitor offers value if it helps interpret the therapeutic experiment. Is the patient's lack of therapeutic response the result of an inadequate regimen, suboptimal medication taking, or both? Among 90 possible return visits among returning hypertensive outpatients, Rudd et al. (1990) reported both usable pill count and medication monitor data for 90%. Only 4 of the 81 visits (5%) were associated with suboptimal compliance by pill count, although goal blood pressure was often still achieved. Adding the monitor, however, uncovered previously undetected suboptimal medication-taking behavior. The desirable combination of achieving goal blood pressure and near-optimal compliance fell from 72% to 61%, a relative decline of 17%. Eight subjects at 15 visits exhibited inferior medication taking by monitor than by pill counts, whereas 3 subjects at 3 visits displayed the inverse. If one accepts the monitor as a de facto gold standard, pill counts misclassified subjects' responses in 18 of 81 occasions (22%). At 3 visits, the monitor confirmed that poor blood pressure control was associated with markedly prolonged intervals between dosings just before the visit. On only 1 of the 3 occasions was pill count similarly signaling low compliance; on 2 occasions, the pill count would have offered no insight into why the hypotensive effect was smaller than expected.

LINKAGE TO THERAPEUTICS

Clinical Trials

Sophisticated investigators usually succeed in controlling for most features that might impact on the outcome variables in clinical drug trials. Remaining hurdles, however, include whether or not ambulatory patients (a) come to scheduled visits and (b) take their medications as prescribed. Reducing ambiguity about medication compliance enhances the ability to interpret variability in the biology of the disease and the pharmacology of the drugs. It is particularly important to look at dose–response relationships to determine whether the initial regimen is appropriate, both in dose and frequency (Miller, Dalton, Vestal, Perkins, & Lyon, 1988). Pill counts and prescribed doses often fail to provide unambiguous dose–effect relationships, whereas medication monitors allow examination of some under and overdosing beyond the range of overlap. Even using pill counts, Joyce (1962) was able to demonstrate that oral medications for arthritis have differential therapeutic effects depending on whether or not the medication is actually taken.

Even more dramatically, the Lipid Research Council (1984a) illustrates the value of the compliance distribution for interpreting a clinical trial: oral cholestyramine versus placebo for hypercholesterolemia. About half the subjects in the LRC–CPPT took less than the full prescribed dose of cholestyramine, as measured by systematic packet counts upon return visits. The primary report (Lipid Research Council, 1984a) described an average reduction of 19% in nonfatal myocardial infarction and a 24% decline in definite coronary deaths among the cholestyramine-treated group, compared to controls. The companion piece (Lipid Research Council, 1984b), stratified the results by compliance level (0–6 packets per day by packet count). It reported a projected maximum of up to 49% reduction in coronary heart disease incidence, if all subjects had taken the full cholestyramine dosage of 24 gm/day rather than a wide distribution of doses (0–24 gm/day).

This powerful conclusion emerges from the compliance distribution itself. It might have remained buried by focus on the "average" effect and on the "intention-to-treat" classification of the subjects, rather than on the distribution of administered doses. By collecting information continuously, rather than just at scheduled visits, electronic monitors reduce the ambiguity from occult pill dumping. They allow assessment of a wider range of administered dosing patterns than is generally included by the prescriptions or protocol alone. Had such information been generated early in the product development of drugs like captopril, chlorthalidone, cimetidine, or ibuprofen, it is likely that a lower range of initial doses would have been marketed with less potential toxicity.

Possible Future Applications of Medication Monitors

The electronic monitoring of medication taking should permit several new kinds of studies at the interface of biology, pharmacology, and behavioral medicine. The monitors will allow focused exploitation of little experiments in nature. Patients can define their own dosing level in natural ways, detectable easily for the first time with devices like the MEMS. Cramer and co-workers (1989) recently described application of the MEMS monitor to ambulatory patients with seizure disorders. They observed that only 67% of 7,413 antiseizure doses were taken as prescribed, and that only 13% of patients with suboptimally low compliance were detected by pill count. Compliance rate was related to the prescribed dosing frequency (1 to 4 times per day; $p < 0.01$, ANOVA). Most impressively, 12 of 16 breakthrough seizures were associated with missed doses, as documented by the MEMS monitor among patients on chronic antiepileptic regimens. Optimal management might then focus on improving compliance rather than escalating the regimen.

In summary, the electronic monitor permits minimization of variance to maximize explanatory power. It allows more assessment in depth of smaller numbers of patients with more information generated, rather than blind insistence on larger trials with focus on only the average effect and on classification of subjects by "intention-to-treat." By using medication compliance as a covariable, investigators can stratify the outcome data to reveal new and important drug effects for both efficacy and safety. Subtle toxicities, resulting from or resolving with "drug holidays," may emerge for the first time. The growing field of "N-of-1" trials may employ such monitoring for confirming application of the intervention (Guyatt, Keller, Jaeschke, Rosenbloom, Adachi, & Newhouse, 1990). Essentially, the monitor transforms every regimen into a patient-initiated experiment in variable dosing. Clinical practice may then rethink the common pattern of frequent medication switching in favor of "fine tuning" with confirmed compliance.

GUIDELINES FOR CLINICIANS AND INVESTIGATORS

Despite uncertainty without better measures of compliance, these successful interventions suggest some initiatives that patients, clinicians, and investigators may pursue. *Patients' behaviors* include making the decision to control the disease, following the therapeutic regimen as prescribed, monitoring progress towards therapeutic goals, and resolving problems that block the therapeutic response. *Clinicians' behaviors* consist of supporting the patient in his/her behaviors, promoting adherence to the regimen, monitoring progress to the therapeutic goals, problem solving with the patient for all perceived obstacles, and working collaboratively with other health care providers (Coordinating Committee, 1984). Component actions may also include explaining events, reducing uncertainty, providing a basis for action, and strengthening the clinician–patient relationship (Coleman, 1985).

It is often particularly important to follow up selectively all those individuals who drop out of care or who fail to achieve the therapeutic goals after a reasonable interval of regimen adjustment. Inquiry about compliance should be a routine part of every visit, especially if asked in a nonjudgmental way about perceived obstacles to optimal compliance. Subsequently, negotiation may be necessary, directly addressing all perceived obstacles including subtle symptoms attributable to the medications. There should be specification of actions that the patient should take for any missed doses. The clinician is further responsible for providing lavish praise and simple rewards for success and for offering reassurance and constructive suggestions for failures to achieve the therapeutic goals.

For particularly high-risk subgroups, such as the very old, the confused, those on complex or changing regimens, and those failing to achieve the therapeutic goal, special efforts may be needed. These include simplifying the regimen whenever possible, trying to avoid mid-day dose administration, avoiding the introduction of many changes in the regimen all at once, providing both verbal and written reinforcement to ensure comprehension of the treatment plan, and linking medication-taking behavior to specific daily cues in the patient's usual routines. The clinician can further assist by adjusting treatment-setting policies to minimize waiting times, facilitate the patient's access for questions and concerns, enhance provider continuity, and encourage the patient's active participation in care. On occasion, it may be necessary to increase attention and supervision with more frequent outpatient visits and/or assistance from the patient's significant others or other health professionals like pharmacists or nurses. The use of more complex and expensive behavioral interventions, such as patient–provider contracts or special cuing pill dispensers, will be necessary only if simple efforts prove insufficient. The instructions should be legible and unambiguous, both on the prescription label and in supplementary written reinforcement.

These same guidelines are generally relevant to the setting of clinical investigation with the following additions: (a) defining the most important aspects of compliance for the particular trial and (b) designing and implementing multiple compliance measures in parallel based on the study population, research question, and logistical constraints. The outcome should be analyzed using compliance as both a continuous and dichotomous covariable. The data in support of clinicians and investigators embracing such guidelines and applying them to their patients is frankly disappointing. Much like patients who find a list of new behaviors somewhat daunting, clinicians and investigators may themselves drift along old patterns. More ambitious trials to enhance physicians' behaviors for improved medication taking by their patients have yielded inconsistent results (Cohen, Berner, & Duback, 1985; Inui, Yourtee, & Williamson, 1976; Maiman, Becker, Liptak, Nazarian, & Rounds, 1988).

CONCLUSIONS AND RECOMMENDATIONS

Despite troublesome measures of medication taking, suboptimal compliance appears to be frequent, complex, and multifactorial. Traditional measures have shown themselves to be relatively insensitive in terms of predictive value and sensitizing in terms of reactivity to the measurement process. Nevertheless, most of them are relatively specific, including therapists' opinions. A promising new group of measures in the form of electronic monitors will force re-examination of existing dogma and assumptions. These new measures should permit dynamic studies of ambulatory therapeutics with special reference to establishment of pharmacological steady state, evaluation of drug-associated toxicities, and appraisal for secondary resistance to treatment.

There remains a need for major prospective trials of simultaneous measures, using a gold standard in the form of a medication monitor or equivalent, especially in combination with some direct measure to confirm actual drug consumption. A further need exists for the development of more flexible monitor formats, less expensive models, more rapid feedback, and more clear linkage to remedial interventions. An exciting time is coming.

REFERENCES

Alfredsson, L. S., & Norell, S. E. (1981). Spacing between doses on a thrice-daily regimen. *British Medical Journal, 282,* 1036.

Ascione, F. J., Kirscht, J. P., & Shimp, L. A. (1986). An assessment of different components of patient medication knowledge. *Medical Care, 24,* 1018–1028.

Ascione, F. J., & Shimp, L. A. (1984). The effectiveness of four education strategies in the elderly. *Drug Intelligence and Clinical Pharmacology, 18,* 926–931.

Barsky, A. K. (1983). Nonpharmacologic aspects of medication. *Archives of Internal Medicine, 143,* 1544–1548.

Beck, N. C., Parker, J. C., Frank, R. G., Geden, E. A., Kay, D. R., Gamache, M., Shivvers, N., Smith, E., & Anderson, S. (1988). Patients with rheumatoid arthritis at high risk for noncompliance with salicylate treatment regimens. *Journal of Rheumatology, 15,* 1081–1084.

Bergman, A. B., & Werner, R. J. (1963). Failure of children to receive penicillin by mouth. *New England Journal of Medicine, 268,* 1334–1338.

Bignell, C. J., Mulcahy, F. M., Peaker, S., Pullar, T., & Feely, M. P. (1988). Measuring treatment compliance of men with non-gonococcal urethritis receiving oxytetracycline combined with low dose phenobarbitone. *Genitourinary Medicine, 64,* 312–315.

Brody, D. S. (1980). Physician recognition of behavioral, psychological, and social aspects of medical care. *Archives of Internal Medicine, 140,* 1286–1289.

Caron, H. S., & Roth, H. (1968). Patient cooperation with a medical regimen. *Journal of the American Medical Association, 203,* 922–926.

Caron, H. S. (1985). Compliance: The case for objective measurement. *Journal of Hypertension, 3,* (suppl. 1), 11–17.

Charney, E. (1975). Compliance and prescribance. *American Journal of Diseases of Children, 129,* 1009–1010.

Cohen, D., Berner, U., & Duback, U. C. (1985). Physician compliance in the management of hypertensive patients. *Journal of Hypertension, 3* (suppl. 1), 73–76.

Coleman, V. R. (1985). Physician behavior and compliance. *Journal of Hypertension, 3* (suppl. 1), 69–71.

Cramer, J. A., Mattson, R. H., Prevey, M. L., Scheyer, R. D., & Ouellette, V. L. (1989). How often is medication taken as prescribed: A novel assessment technique. *Journal of the American Medical Association, 261,* 3273–3277.

Cramer, J. A., Scheyer, R. D., & Mattson, R. H. (1990). Compliance declines between clinic visits. *Archives of Internal Medicine, 150,* 1509–1510.

Crome, P., Akehurst, M., & Keet, J. (1980). Drug compliance in elderly hospital in-patients; Trial of the Dosett box. *The Practitioner, 224,* 782–785.

Cromer, B. A., Steinberg, K., Gardner, L., Thornton, D., & Shannon, B. (1989). Psychosocial determinants of compliance in adolescents with iron deficiency. *American Journal of Diseases of Children, 143,* 55–58.

Dirks, J. F., & Kinsman, R. A. (1982). Nondichotomous patterns of medication usage: The yes–no fallacy. *Clinical Pharmacology and Therapeutics, 31,* 413–417.

Dubbert, P. M., King, A., Rapp, S. R., Brief, E., Martin, J. E., & Lake, M. (1985). Riboflavin as a tracer of medication compliance. *Journal of Behavioral Medicine, 8,* 287–299.

Dunbar, J. (1984). Adherence measures and their utility. *Controlled Clinical Trials, 5,* 515–521.

Eisen, S. A., Miller, D. K., Woodward, R. S., Spitznagel, E., & Przybeck, T. R. (1990). The effect of prescribed daily dose frequency on patient medication compliance. *Archives of Internal Medicine, 150,* 1881-1884.

Eisen, S. A., Woodward, R. S., Miller, G., Spitznagel, E., & Windham, C. A. (1987). The effect of medication compliance on the control of hypertension. *Journal of General Internal Medicine, 2,* 298-305.

Eshelman, F. N., & Fitzloff, J. (1976). Effect of packaging on patient compliance with an antihypertensive medication. *Current Therapeutic Research, 20,* 215-219.

Feinstein, A. R. (1975). Biostatistical problems in "compliance bias." *Clinical Pharmacology and Therapeutics, 16,* 846-857.

Feinstein, A. R. (1979). "Compliance bias" and the interpretation of therapeutic trials. In R. B. Haynes, D. W. Taylor, & D. L. Sackett (Eds.), *Compliance in health care,* (pp. 309-322). Baltimore: Johns Hopkins University Press.

Fletcher, S. W., Pappius, E. M., & Harper, S. J. (1979). Measurement of medication compliance in a clinical setting: Comparison of three methods in patients prescribed digoxin. *Archives of Internal Medicine, 139,* 635-638.

Gabriel, M., Gagnon, J. P., & Bryan, C. K. (1977). Improved patient compliance through use of a daily drug reminder chart. *American Journal of Public Health, 67,* 968-969.

Gilbert, J. R., Evans, E. E., Haynes, R. B., & Tugwell, P. (1980). Predicting compliance with a regimen of digoxin therapy in family practice. *Canadian Medical Association Journal, 123,* 119-123.

Goldsmith, C. H. (1976). Summaries of methodologic scores. In D. L. Sackett & R. B. Haynes (Eds.), *Compliance with therapeutic regimens* (pp. 276-279). Baltimore: Johns Hopkins University Press.

Goldsmith, C. H. (1979). The effect of compliance distributions on therapeutic trials. In R. B. Haynes, D. W. Taylor, & D. L. Sackett (Eds.), *Compliance in health care* (pp. 297-308). Baltimore: Johns Hopkins University Press.

Gordis, L., Markowitz, M., & Lilienfeld, A. M. (1969). Why patients don't follow medical advice: A study of children on long-term antistreptococcal prophylaxis. *Journal of Pediatrics, 75,* 957-68.

Gotzsche, P. C. (1989). Methodology and overt and hidden bias in reports of 196 double-blind trials of nonsteroidal antiinflammatory drugs in rheumatoid arthritis. *Controlled Clinical Trials, 10,* 31-56.

Greene, J. Y., Weinberger, M., Jerin, M. J., & Mamlin, J. J. (1982). Compliance with medication regimens among chronically ill, inner city patients. *Journal of Compliance in Health Care, 7,* 183-93.

Guyatt, G. H., Keller, J. L., Jaeschke, R., Rosenbloom, D., Adachi, J. D., & Newhouse, M. T. (1990). The n-of-1 randomized controlled trial: Clinical usefulness; Our three-year experience. *Annals of Internal Medicine, 112,* 293-299.

Hatcher, M. E., Green, L. W., Levine, D. M., & Flagle, C. E. (1986). Validation of a decision model for triaging hypertensive patients to alternate health education interventions. *Social Science and Medicine, 22,* 813-819.

Haynes, R. B. (1976a). A critical review of the "determinants" of patient compliance with therapeutic regimens. In D. L. Sackett & R. B. Haynes (Eds.), *Compliance with therapeutic regimens* (pp. 26-39). Baltimore: Johns Hopkins University Press.

Haynes, R. B. (1976b). Strategies for improving compliance: A methodologic analysis and review. In D. L. Sackett & R. B. Haynes (Eds.), *Compliance with therapeutic regimens* (pp. 69-82). Baltimore: Johns Hopkins University Press.

Haynes, R. B. (1979a). Introduction. In R. B. Haynes, D. W. Taylor, & D. L. Sackett (Eds.), *Compliance in health care* (pp. 1-7). Baltimore: Johns Hopkins University Press.

Haynes, R. B. (1979b). Determinants of compliance: The disease and the mechanics of treatment. In R. B. Haynes, D. W. Taylor, & D. L. Sackett (Eds.), *Compliance in health care* (pp. 49–62). Baltimore: Johns Hopkins University Press.

Haynes, R. B. (1979c). Strategies to improve compliance with referrals, appointments, and prescribed medical regimens. In R. B. Haynes, D. W. Taylor, & D. L. Sackett (Eds.), *Compliance in health care* (pp. 121–143). Baltimore: Johns Hopkins University Press.

Haynes, R. B., & Dantes, R. (1987). Patient compliance and the conduct and interpretation of therapeutic trials. *Controlled Clinical Trials, 8,* 12–19.

Haynes, R. B., Sackett, D. L., Taylor, D. W., Roberts, R. S., & Johnson, A. L. (1977). Manipulation of the therapeutic regimen to improve compliance: Conceptions and misconceptions. *Clinical Pharmacology and Therapeutics, 22,* 125–130.

Haynes, R. B., Taylor, D. W., & Sackett, D. L. (Eds.), (1979). *Compliance in health care.* Baltimore: Johns Hopkins University Press.

Haynes, R. B., Taylor, D. W., Sackett, D. L., Gibson, E. S., Bernholz, C. D., & Mukherjee, J. (1980). Can simple clinical measurements detect patient noncompliance? *Hypertension, 2,* 757–764.

Hershey, J. C., Morton, B. G., Davis, J. B., & Reichgott, M. J. (1980). Patient compliance with antihypertensive medication. *American Journal of Public Health, 70,* 1081–1089.

Hulka, B. S. (1979). Patient–clinician interactions and compliance. In R. B. Haynes, D. W. Taylor, & D. L. Sackett (Eds.), *Compliance in health care* (pp. 63–77). Baltimore: Johns Hopkins University Press.

Hulka, B. S., Cassel, J. C., Kupper, L. L., & Burdette, J. A. (1976). Communication, compliance, and concordance between physicians and patients with prescribed medications. *American Journal of Public Health, 66,* 847–853.

Inui, T. S., Carter, W. B., & Pecoraro, R. E. (1981). Screening for noncompliance among patients with hypertension: Is self-report the best available measure? *Medical Care, 19,* 1061–1064.

Inui, T. S., Carter, W. B., Pecoraro, R. E., Pearlman, R. A., & Dohan, J. J. (1980). Variations in patient compliance with common long-term drugs. *Medical Care, 18,* 986–993.

Inui, T. S., Yourtee, E. L., & Williamson, J. W. (1976). Improved outcomes in hypertension after physician tutorials; A controlled trial. *Annals of Internal Medicine, 84,* 646–651.

Johannsen, W. J., Hellmuth, G. A., & Sorauf, T. (1966). On accepting medical recommendations. *Archives of Environmental Health, 12,* 63–69.

Joyce, C. R. B. (1962). Patient co-operation and the sensitivity of clinical trials. *Journal of Chronic Diseases, 15,* 1025–1036.

Kass, M. A., Gordon, M., & Meltzer, D. W. (1986a). Can opthalmologists correctly identify patients defaulting from pilocarpine therapy? *American Journal of Ophthalmology, 101,* 524–530.

Kass, M. A., Meltzer, D. W., Gordon, M., Cooper, D., & Goldberg, J. (1986b). Compliance with topical pilocarpine treatment. *American Journal of Ophthalmology, 101,* 515–523.

Klein, L. E., German, P. S., McPhee, S. J., Smith, C. S., & Levine, D. M. (1982). Aging and its relationship to health knowledge and medication compliance. *Gerontology, 22,* 384–387.

Latiolais, C. J., & Berry, C. C. (1969). Misuse of prescription medications by out-patients. *Drug Intelligence and Clinical Pharmacy, 3,* 270–277.

Leirer, V. O., Morrow, D. G., Pariante, G. M., & Sheikh, J. I. (1988). Elders' nonadherence, its assessment, and computer assisted instruction for medication recall training. *Journal of the American Geriatrics Society, 36,* 877–884.

Leventhal, H. (1971). Fear appeals and persuasion: The differentiation of a motivational construct. *American Journal of Public Health, 61,* 1208–1224.

Levine, D. M., Green, L. W., Deeds, S. G., Chwalow, J., Russell, R. P., & Finlay, J. (1979). Health education for hypertensive patients. *Journal of the American Medical Association, 241,* 1700–1703.

Levy, R. L. (1985). Social support and compliance: Update. *Journal of Hypertension, 3* (suppl. 1), 45–49.
Ley, P. (1985). Doctor-patient communication: Some quantitative estimates of the role of cognitive factors in non-compliance. *Journal of Hypertension, 3* (Suppl.), S51–S55.
Lipid Research Clinics Program (1984a). The Lipid Research Clinics Coronary Primary Prevention Trial results: I. Reduction in incidence of coronary heart disease. *Journal of the American Medical Association, 251,* 351–364.
Lipid Research Clinics Program (1984b). The Lipid Research Clinics Coronary Primary Prevention Trial results: II. Relationship of reduction in incidence of coronary heart disease to cholesterol lowering. *Journal of the American Medical Association, 251,* 365–374.
Logan, A. G., Milne, B. J., Flanagan, P. T., & Haynes, R. B. (1983). Clinical effectiveness and cost-effectiveness of monitoring blood pressure of hypertensive employees at work. *Hypertension, 5,* 828–836.
Maenpaa, H., Javela, K., Pikkarainen, J., Malkonen, M., Heinonen, O. P., & Manninen, V. (1987a). Minimal doses of digoxin: A new marker for compliance to medication. *European Heart Journal, 8* (suppl. 1), 31–37.
Maenpaa, H., Manninen, V., & Heinonen, O. P. (1987b). Comparison of the digoxin marker with capsule counting and compliance questionnaire methods for measuring compliance to medication in a clinical trial. *European Heart Journal, 8* (suppl. 1), 39–43.
Maiman, L. A., Becker, M. H., Liptak, G. S., Nazarian, L. F., & Rounds, K. A. (1988). Improving pediatricians' compliance-enhancing practices: A randomized trial. *American Journal of Diseases of Children, 142,* 773–779.
Maronde, R. F., Chan, L. S., Larsen, F. J., Strandberg, L. R., Laventurier, M. F., & Sullivan, S. R. (1989). Underutilization of antihypertensive drugs and associated hospitalization. *Medical Care, 27,* 1159–1166.
Mazzullo, J. M., Lasagna, L., & Griner, P. F. (1974). Variations in interpretation of prescription instructions; The need for improved prescribing habits. *Journal of the American Medical Association, 227,* 929–931.
McKenney, J. M., Slining, J. D., Henderson, H. R., Devins, D., & Barr, M. (1973). The effect of clinical pharmacy services on patients with essential hypertension. *Circulation, 48,* 1104–1111.
Miller, L., Dalton, M., Vestal, R., Perkins, J. G., & Lyon, G. (1988). Delays in the drug approval process: Recent trends. *Journal of Clinical Research and Drug Development, 2,* 31–45.
Moulding, T. S. (1979). The unrealized potential of the medication monitor. *Clinical Pharmacology and Therapeutics, 25,* 131–136.
Mullen, P. D., Green, L. W., & Persinger, G. S. (1985). Clinical trials of patient education for chronic conditions: A comparative meta-analysis of intervention types. *Preventive Medicine, 14,* 753–781.
Neely, E., & Patrick, M. L. (1968). Problems of aged persons taking medications at home. *Nursing Research, 17,* 52–55.
Nelson, E. C., Stason, W. B., Neutra, R. R., & Solomon, H. S. (1980). Identification of the noncompliant hypertensive patient. *Preventive Medicine, 9,* 504–517.
Nierenberg, D. W. (1987). Measuring drug levels in the office: Rationale, possible advantages, and potential problems. *Medical Clinics of North America, 71,* 653–664.
Norell, S. E. (1981). Accuracy of patient interviews and estimates by clinical staff in determining medication compliance. *Social Science and Medicine, 15E,* 57–61.
Norell, S. E. (1984). Methods in assessing drug compliance. *Acta Medica Scandinavica,* Suppl. *683,* 35–40.
Palta, M., & McHugh, R. (1980). Planning the size of a cohort study in the presence of both losses to follow-up and non-compliance. *Journal of Chronic Diseases, 33,* 501–512.
Porter, A. M. W. (1969). Drug defaulting in a general practice. *British Medical Journal, 1,* 218–222.

Psaty, B. M., Koepsell, T. D., Wagner, E. D., LoGerfo, J. P., & Inui, T. S. (1990). The relative risk of incident coronary heart disease associated with recently stopping the use of beta-blockers. *Journal of the American Medical Association, 263,* 1653–1657.

Roth, H. P. (1984). Historical review: Comparison with other methods. *Controlled Clinical Trials, 5,* 476–480.

Rudd, P. (1979a). Medication packaging: Simple solutions to nonadherence problems? *Clinical Pharmacology and Therapeutics, 25,* 257–265.

Rudd, P., Ahmed, S., Zachary, V., Barton, C., & Bonduelle, D. (1990). Improved compliance measures: Applications in an ambulatory hypertensive drug trial. *Clinical Pharmacology and Therapeutics, 48,* 676–685.

Rudd, P., Byyny, R. L., Zachary, V., LoVerde, M. E., Titus, C., Mitchell, W. D., & Marshall, G. (1989). The natural history of medication compliance in a drug trial: Limitations of pill counts. *Clinical Pharmacology and Therapeutics, 46,* 169–176.

Rudd, P., & Marshall, G. (1987). Resolving problems of measuring compliance with medication monitors. *Journal of Compliance in Health Care, 2,* 23–35.

Russell, M. L. (1984). Behavioral aspects of the use of medical markers in clinical trials. *Controlled Clinical Trials, 5,* 526–534.

Sackett, D. L. (1977). Hypertension in the real world: Public reaction, physician response, and patient compliance. In J. Genest, E. Koiw, & O. Kuchel (Eds.), *Hypertension: Physiopathology and treatment* (pp. 1142–1149). New York: McGraw–Hill.

Sackett, D. L., Haynes, R. B., & Tugwell, P. (1985). *Clinical epidemiology: A basic science for clinical medicine* (pp. 199–222). Boston: Little, Brown.

Sherman, F. T., Warach, J. D., & Libow, L. S. (1979). Child-resistant containers for the elderly? *Journal of The American Medical Association, 241,* 1001–1002.

Soutter, B. R., & Kennedy, M. C. (1974). Patient compliance assessment in drug trials: Usage and methods. *Australia and New Zealand Journal of Medicine, 4,* 360–364.

Spector, R., McGrath, P., Uretsky, N., Newman, R., & Cohen, P. (1978). Does intervention by a nurse improve medication compliance? *Archives of Internal Medicine, 138,* 36–40.

Spector, S. L., Kinsman, R., Mawhinney, H., Siegel, S. C., Rachelsfsky, G. S., Katz, R. M., & Rohr, A. S. (1986). Compliance of patients with asthma with an experimental aerosolized medication: Implications for controlled clinical trials. *Journal of Allergy and Clinical Immunology, 77,* 65–70.

Steckel, S. B., & Swain, M. A. (1977). Contracting with patients to improve compliance. *Hospitals, Journal of The American Hospital Association, 51,* 81–84.

Steiner, J. F., Fihn, S. D., Koepsell, T. D., Blair, B., Kelleher, K., D'Alessandro, D., & Inui, T. S. (1990). Clinical predictors of treatment reduction in hypertensive patients. *Journal of General Internal Medicine, 5,* 203–210.

Steiner, J. F., Koepsell, T. D., Fihn, S. D., & Inui, T. S. (1988). A general method of compliance assessment using centralized pharmacy records: Description and validation. *Medical Care, 26,* 814–823.

Strecher, V. J., Becker, M. H., Clark, N. M., & Prasada-Rao, P. (1989). Using patients' descriptions of alcohol consumption, diet, medication compliance, and cigarette smoking; The validity of self-reports in research and practice. *Journal of General Internal Medicine, 4,* 160–166.

Taggart, A. J., Johnston, G. D., & McDevitt, D. G. (1981). Does the frequency of daily dosage influence compliance with digoxin therapy? *British Journal of Clinical Pharmacology, 1,* 31–34.

Taylor, D. W., Sackett, D. L., Haynes, R. B., Johnson, A. L., Gibson, E. S., & Roberts, R. S. (1978). Compliance with antihypertensive drug therapy. *Annals New York Academy of Science, 304,* 390–403.

Wandless, I., Mucklow, J. C., Smith, A., and Prudham, D. (1979). Compliance with prescribed medicines: A study of elderly patients in the community. *Journal of the Royal College of General Practitioners, 29,* 391–396.

Williams, G. H. (1987). Utility of behavioral science techniques in assessing adverse effects of antihypertensive agents. *American Journal of Kidney Diseases, 10* (suppl. 1), 61–65.

Wong, B. S. M., & Norman, D. C. (1987). Evaluation of a novel medication aid, the calendar blister-pak, and its effect on drug compliance in a geriatric outpatient clinic. *Journal of the American Geriatric Society, 35,* 21–26.

Zifferblatt, S. M. (1975). Increasing patient compliance through the applied analysis of behavior. *Preventive Medicine, 4,* 173–182.

IV PREVENTION

Norman A. Krasnegor

This section of the book contains three chapters. Each of the works deals with the topic of compliance in terms of behaviors that will be useful in preventing threats to health. The first chapter reviews approaches for preventing the risks to the health of children at both the public health level for the population as a whole and at the level of the individual family unit. The second chapter reviews longitudinal studies of childhood obesity and discusses the compliance mechanisms that were likely responsible for reducing weight and maintaining the loss over time. The third work presents a conceptual approach, the social action model, for elucidating the health compliance construct and points the way for formulating hypotheses to empirically study procedures for enhancing health compliance.

The first chapter in this section, "Improving Compliance in Childhood Injury Control" by Edward R. Christophersen, is concerned with issues that relate to parental compliance with injury control prevention. Unintentional injury is by far the leading cause of morbidity and mortality in pediatric populations. Unintentional injury is of major public health relevance because, in aggregate it causes health problems greater than the next six sources of childhood illnesses combined. Christophersen employs childhood injury as an example not only because of his familiarity with the topic but also for its heuristic value in demonstrating the varied ways that prevention approaches can be mounted to control incidence and prevalence. He provides an overview of the many tactics and strategies that can be used to reduce childhood injuries. The first approach discussed is that of legislation.

The author describes the varied laws that have been written (e.g., child-proof medicine bottles, window guards in tall apartment buildings to prevent falls, smoke detectors, seat belts, etc.) to create a safer environment and thereby reduce the chances for certain kinds of injuries. A second issue of relevance has to do with the type of strategy used to encourage safety and thereby reduce injury.

Christophersen differentiates between active and passive approaches. In the former, a person has to engage in certain behaviors (e.g., put a baby in a well-designed infant seat in a car and then strap the baby in). In the latter, no behavior is required for the safety device to be engaged (e.g., automatic safety belts; air bags). The main generalization from the literature on injury research is the less effort required, the more likely is the person to comply with the safety recommendation.

Christophersen reports on the utility of health education and concludes that when the message is given and in what context can dramatically influence parental compliance. For example, car seats given at the time of discharge from the hospital just after birth of a baby with encouraging comments by pediatricians and nurses at well child care visits led to an 85% rate of compliance for correctly using child restraint seats up to 1 year after discharge. Expectant parents were much more likely to reduce the temperature of their water heater to prevent scalding burns if the health message is delivered during parental education classes.

Christophersen outlines behavioral and group educational approaches. He provides examples of research findings that demonstrate the efficacy of rewards in motivating parents to comply with safety recommendations. Christophersen also describes studies that employ group health education to parents in the context of well baby visits to the pediatrician's office. Continuing education class approaches are also described. The main advantage of these latter strategies is that many parents can be serviced by a single provider and parents have more contact with the physician.

The next chapter, "Compliance and Long-Term Follow-Up for Childhood Obesity: Retrospective Analysis" by Leonard H. Epstein, has as its focus an overview of the author's pioneering longitudinal study of childhood obesity and the relationship between behavioral factors targeted for treatment and long-term outcome. Epstein reviews some of the variables necessary to modify eating, exercise, and treatment compliance patterns in children who were, at the start of the research, 8–12 years of age and 20%–100% above ideal weight for height, age, and sex. Regarding the compliance issue, the author describes findings that illuminate specific behaviors related to eating and exercise that influence long-term weight control and parental factors that influence these patterns of adherence.

Epstein describes the various behavioral intervention strategies employed with the groups of children and their families. Five years after commencing the study, follow-up data were collected from the families who had originally entered the study. Questionnaires were administered to assess the degree to which behavioral techniques learned during treatment were used by participants. The questions focused on changing eating and exercise habits and behaviors that were used to support such changes.

The results indicated that two variables were related to the percentage overweight change. These were the parent report of keeping within caloric range and parent report of the use of praise. Child weight was predicted by the percentage weight change in the first 6 months of treatment and the change in percentage over weight in the parents, over the 5 years. Epstein reports that three variables were correlated with weight change in the desired direction. These were: (a) general decrease in caloric intake; (b) compliance with the advice to decrease the intake of high-caloric, low-nutrient foods; and (c) compliance in association with the self-monitoring/self-regulation skill to plot weight. In addition to these three factors, the use of praise delivered reciprocally or conjointly by parents and their children was important for successes observed (in several of the conditions children and parents were treated together). Epstein concludes that mutual use of praise "may make a more supportive atmosphere more conducive to success than if the parent feels they are doing a lot of activities with little direct payoff from their child." Thus, a family-based approach, in which parents are treated along with their children, appears to be advantageous for long-term success. An interesting additional finding is that such parent–child treatment influences weight change in nontreated siblings. This result suggests that there is an additional benefit for using the parent–child dyad as the treatment target.

Epstein's work further suggests that parent–child reciprocal and conjoint reinforcement approaches may teach new ways of parenting and efficacious parent–child interaction patterns that allow both children and parents to exert influence that maintains mutually beneficial motivation to comply with health regimens.

The last chapter in this section, "Health Promotion and Disease Prevention: A Social Action Conception of Compliance Behavior" by Craig K. Ewart, provides a generic conceptualization of health promotion and disease prevention in the context of a social action model. Ewart differentiates between health ("an organism's capacity for self-protective action") and wellness ("the absence of disease"). He also points out that confusion has arisen about what compliance means. It can be viewed as: (a) the behavior(s) or action state that is the goal of intervention, (b) a process through which behaviors are changed, and (c) a behavioral product of the context in which behavioral change processes operate.

Ewart outlines a social action conception of compliance. According to Ewart, interventions designed to reduce or avoid health risk willy-nilly involve change of the individual. Compliance refers to the capacity of the individual to incorporate new goals and behaviors into an existing repertoire. Research on the topic then reduces to gaining an understanding of how such a process can or does occur.

Ewart articulates a *STATE* model of health protective action that assumes an equilibrium between behaviors that protect one's health and the effects that such behaviors generate. Essential to the model are three elements: (a) organized behaviors ("scripts"), (b) integrated behaviors (behaviors that can be run off without consciously attending to the pattern"), and (c) integrated behaviors that attain reinforcement value. He indicates that these three elements are contingent upon the effects that the action produces. Thus, the model implies a feedback loop that has built into it the idea of chaining, a concept derived from the experimental analysis of behavior. This idea implies that new behaviors, for example, should be initiated in close proximity to the goal because they (the behaviors) have a higher probability of being quickly reinforced by goal attainment. There is an interdependence between scripts of socially related individuals (e.g., family members); therefore, in order to best achieve change in the target individual, intervention should include such socially related individuals (the work of Epstein on weight control provides data on this point; i.e., sustained weight change was best for children who were treated along with parents).

Ewart contrasts the state model with a *PROCESS* model. Whereas the state model accounts for the features of health routines, it does not explicate how such routines originate. The process model indicates how new self-sustaining action systems are initiated and introduces the idea of "feedforward" processes that enable new goals, strategies, and environments. The process model also addresses the important topic of motivation and how it integrates with change in behavior.

Ewart points out that compliance behaviors are dependent on contextual factors. These include social settings (e.g., physical environment) and relationships (e.g., people) and biological contexts (e.g., developmental level; temperament). He also shows how the social action theory provides a useful framework for understanding compliance over the life-span. Ewart's ideas move one away from a parochial view of self-regulation toward a more social-contextual way of conceptualization. The suggestions contained in this chapter provide useful ways to frame hypotheses that should bear fruit in terms of more fully understanding the dynamic social processes that may govern the acquisition and maintenance of health compliance behaviors.

9 Improving Compliance in Childhood Injury Control

Edward R. Christophersen
Children's Mercy Hospital, Kansas City, Missouri

The hallmark of the field of pediatrics has long been assumed to be the prevention of maladies that affect our nation's young. Throughout much of medicine, particularly in pediatrics, prevention, rather than remediation, has been the preferred mode of practice. Numerous authors have identified injuries as a major etiological factor in brain damage and subsequent impaired cognitive functioning or mental retardation (Klauber, Barrett-Connor, Marshall, & Bowers, 1981). It is far easier to design transportation systems so that children are less likely to be injured than it is to design emergency transportation and hospitalization systems that can deal with brain damage after it has occurred. Historically, improvements in sanitation, pasteurization of milk, the ready availability of alternative sources of nutrition through commercially available infant formulas, immunization schedules, and the development of medications for many common childhood infectious diseases have substantially reduced the morbidity and mortality for children (Roberts & Brooks, 1987). Most of these advances have taken the form of more passive measures (measures that do not require much effort on the part of the recipient in order to realize a gain) as opposed to active measures (measures that do require effort on the part of the recipient). In fact, until these passive measures were in place, parents had to take active measures in the hope of preventing some of the problems associated with childhood. A review of the advances in the injury control literature, with suggestions for medicine in general, would be illustrative of the way that prevention strategies could be implemented. There have been several major areas in which pediatric health care has produced documented decreases in illnesses and deaths (Cataldo et al., 1986). This chapter reviews and discusses the published literature on improving parental compliance with injury control recommendations including legislative programs,

219

active versus passive strategies, health education approaches, behavioral approaches, and group health education approaches. Each approach has been effective in encouraging parents to implement injury control strategies. Combinations of these approaches have probably produced the largest effects.

LEGISLATION

Legislation has been used in a wide variety of different areas to reduce the harm that might otherwise befall our nation's children. Laws have been enacted and passed in an effort to reduce the number of children injured by ingestion of potentially harmful substances (by requiring childproof caps on medicine bottles and by limiting the number of tablets per bottle), by falls from tall apartment buildings (by installing window guards, Speigel & Lindaman, 1977), and suffocations (by requiring the use of magnet latches on refrigerator doors instead of the old latches that were virtually impossible to open from the inside). Present legislative efforts are being directed towards mandating the installation of air bags and/or automatic seat belts in all automobiles, smoke detectors in all residences, and the use of seat belts in all vehicles.

Legislation has already been used in a number of specific instances in the promotion of wellness. School districts require that children be immunized against certain diseases prior to being allowed to enroll for classes. Such legislation virtually forces parents to have their children immunized because the law also requires that children below a certain age must attend school. In general, such legislation does help to reduce the number of children at risk for contracting specific illnesses.

There has recently been much public discussion regarding the proposed requirement that adolescents remain enrolled in school if they want to be legally allowed to drive an automobile. This is a clear example of the use of legislation to reduce morbidity and mortality (available data demonstrate that higher driving ages are associated with lower accident and injury rates). There has also been legislation passed that prohibits individuals from smoking in public places such as hospitals, schools, and so on.

Innovative researchers might profitably concentrate their efforts at developing passive strategies, including legislation, to help reduce the likelihood of children developing hypertension, becoming obese, and initiating cigarette smoking. The literature on injury control suggests that such passive approaches have much greater likelihood of being successful than more active strategies. An example of such a passive procedure might be laws that minimize the amount of salt that can be in foods destined for consumption by infants and children (which would obviously be easier than asking each parent to monitor the salt intake of their children at every meal). The next section discusses active versus passive programs in greater detail.

Active Versus Passive Programs

Conceptually, most health education approaches can be placed on a continuum ranging from active programs to passive programs. Passive measures are those measures that require little or no effort on the part of the individual. Examples of passive measures are the pasteurization of milk and city sanitation systems that require no effort on the part of the individual. Active measures are those measures that require continuing effort on the part of the individual. Examples of active measures are child automobile restraint seats and monitoring of children for safety hazards. To put these same examples into perspective, one might ask how much progress would society have made towards reducing the number of children with problems related to unpasteurized milk if the only solution available was for parents to boil their own milk, each day, for their own children compared to dairies boiling all milk that is sold to the public. Historically, after the problems associated with unboiled milk were known, parents had to boil milk before they gave it to their children (an active procedure) until the time that pasteurization of milk was widespread (a passive procedure). Similarly, parents had to mix infant formulas, beginning with such products as dried milk (an active procedure), until infant formulas were widely available (a passive procedure). The widespread pasteurization of milk was brought about by legislation that was passed and enacted at the urging of public health professionals. If all injury control strategies could be placed on one continuum, according to the amount of effort that is required by the individual who is responsible for implementing the strategy, passive strategies would be those that required no effort on the individual's part. An example of a passive strategy is the automobile seat belt that automatically fits around the driver every time the car door is closed—thus, the label *passive*. An example of an active strategy is the traditional automobile seat belt that an individual must place around her or himself every time she or he enters an automobile—thus, the label *active*. There is a consensus in the injury control literature that active approaches are more difficult to implement and less effective than passive approaches (Williams, 1982). Table 9.1 provides examples of active and passive approaches to injury control.

As numerous researchers have already shown, although passive approaches are preferred, there are many instances when a passive approach is simply not possible. For example, although the government has mandated the administration of certain immunizations to children, it is still the responsibility of parents to get their children immunized and, under certain circumstances, to keep their children isolated when they are carrying an active and serious infectious disease.

Only in the last 10 years or so have automobile dashboards been designed so that a passenger hitting the dashboard is less likely to have their skull pierced by a protruding device such as a radio knob or a switch for one of the automobile functions. Similarly, passive seatbelts and airbags are now being installed in a substantial percentage of the automobiles built for sale in the United States for the current model year.

TABLE 9.1
Examples of Passive and Active Strategies

Passive			Active
Effort: None	Only Once	Occasional	Frequent
Automatic Seat Belts	Lower Hot Water Heater Setting	Check Smoke Detector	Seat Belts
Window Guards	Playground Covering		
Safety Caps			

The first body of literature related to medicine that has really consciously drawn upon the active/passive model of intervention is the area of injury control (which was previously referred to as accident prevention; Haddon, 1980). The injury control literature has shown quite dramatically that, the less effort that is required from the individual, the more likely the individual is to comply or adhere to a recommendation (Williams, 1982). That is the major reason that safety advocates have been so steadfast in their insistence on the installation of air bags in all new automobiles—airbags protect motor vehicle occupants from injuries sustained during vehicular collisions without requiring that the individual engage in any active behavior. With the understanding that legislation has proven to be very effective in reducing childhood injuries, and that passive procedures are generally preferable to active strategies, a discussion of the contributions made in the area of health education is in order.

Health Education

Most of the early efforts at reducing morbidity and mortality involved some form of health education (Pless, 1978). In their offices, health educators would inform their patients of the potential benefits and dangers of a particular behavior in which they were engaging. This advice included everything from discouraging smoking to recommending exercise to reduce hypertension. In the area of injury control, both Reisinger and his colleagues (Reisinger, Williams, Wells, et al., 1981) and Dershewitz (1979) tried brief (less than 2 minutes in duration) educational peptalks for restraint seat usage and smoke detector installation, respectively. Both studies reported some improvement in the parents' behavior related to injury control for their offspring. Dershewitz and Williamson (1977) reported on a study that compared the effectiveness of office-based health education strategies on two prevention strategies—the installation of small plastic covers for electrical wall outlets and the installation of plastic latches that would prevent toddlers from opening kitchen cabinets. Their data showed that parents would install the small plastic outlet covers but not the safety latches (the latches required a great deal more effort than the outlet covers). Later studies have shown that when a more comprehensive program was undertaken by the health-care provider for the health education message, more promising results emerged. Christophersen and his colleagues (Christophersen, Sosland-Edelman, & LeClaire, 1985) reported high rates of compliance with infant automobile restraint seat usage when a multidimensional program was used. Their program for automobile restraint seat usage included the passage of mandating state legislation, a hospital loaner program for provision of the restraint seats, nurses and physicians who encouraged and educated new parents about the need for restraint seat usage, and a community-wide educational program on the advantages of restraint seat usage (a combination of passive and active strategies). The parents in the study correctly used restraint seats more than 85% of the time at hospital discharge and at three 3-months, 6-months, and 12-months follow-up observations. In another study, Thomas and her colleagues (Thomas, Hassanein, & Christophersen, 1984) demonstrated the effectiveness of an alternative to the traditional one-on-one well-child visit—group well-child care, for encouraging parents of infants to turn down the hot water heaters in their homes. Other recent research (Williams, Barone, Hassanein, & Christophersen, 1989) showed that health education messages were more likely to result in a behavioral change if the messages were given to expectant parents, as a part of prenatal education, than if they were given to parents of toddlers. This study contrasted the results obtained using prenatal education groups and educational groups for parents of toddlers. The major educational message was that lowering hot water heater temperature settings can drastically reduce injuries from hot water scalds (the second leading cause of death in children). Families in the prenatal group that got the message had significantly lower hot water heater temperature settings than parents in the prenatal group that did not receive the message. There was no difference in the two groups from the toddler classes. When interviewed later, the expectant parents stated that they wanted to do anything they could to protect their children. The parents of toddlers made frequent comments to the effect that they hadn't turned down their hot water heater temperature settings before and their children had not received any scald burns. Parents may develop a false sense of security when they practice unsafe procedures in their home but do not experience any unpleasant effects from doing so. The authors suggest that expectant parents are more receptive to health education messages because they have a different history than the parents of toddlers. The time at which a health education message is delivered is obviously deserving of more study.

Another variation within the area of health education involves the use of the media (television, radio, and print media) for health education messages, which is an active approach in that the media message cannot usually be implemented without an active effort on the part of the recipient of the message. Kelly (1979) reported no effects in a carefully controlled study to measure the effectiveness of a television campaigns for health education. Using a cable television system that allowed the use of two different television inputs into different subscriber's homes, Kelly showed no differences between homes that received messages on the need to use automobile safety belts and homes that did not receive the messages. However, conclusions that it is impossible to use the media in an effective way for health education should not be based on this one study. Media messages have been used to explain the dangers of cigarette smoking with the results that many Americans are much better informed about these dangers. Whether such messages, alone, are sufficient is really not an issue, because virtually no recent campaign has relied exclusively on media messages for educating the public. The position taken in this chapter is that the combination of passive and active strategies is probably the most effective (Dershewitz & Christophersen, 1984). Some education strategies to injury control involve instructing parents in the use of behavioral approaches.

Behavioral Approaches

Whereas most health education approaches have probably been implemented through doctor's offices and hospitals, the vast majority of work in behavioral approaches has taken place through clinical research projects (Finney & Christophersen, 1984). The active/passive conceptualization can also be applied to what the health care provider must do as well as the patient and his or her family. Some programs for preventing problems with children require virtually no effort on the part of the parent or the health care provider. Some programs require little effort on the part of parents and health-care providers such as immunizations, which are administered only once (or at long intervals), and the installation of smoke detectors (that only need to be attended to episodically). Typically, behavioral approaches to changing health-related behaviors are active approaches for both the provider and for the patients/parents. A brief educational message, perhaps lasting 2 minutes (cf. Miller, Reisinger, Blatter, & Wucher, 1982), at first appears to require little effort on the provider's or the parent's part but in actuality may require a great deal of effort on the parent's part, and more effort on the provider's part than is immediately obvious.

Table 9.2 provides examples of passive versus active efforts that are made by health-care providers during their workday.

Thus, the procedures that require the most effort on the part of the patient, such as weight control, lifestyle changes related to the management of hypertension, and the management of behavior problems, also often require more effort on the part of the health-care provider. The attraction of educational efforts such as office video tapes and books or written handouts is that they take little effort on

TABLE 9.2
Examples of Passive Versus Active Efforts by Health-Care Providers

Active		Passive	
Large Effort	Periodic Effort	One Time Effort	No Effort
		Flouride	
			Pasturization
		Legislation Refrig. doors Passive restraints	
	Smoke detectors Immunizations Writing a Rx Educ. video tapes		
		Group well-child care Referral	
TX of obesity Tx of hypertension Counseling re: Injury control Behavior prolems			

the provider's part. Unfortunately, there hasn't been much support in the research literature for the use of video tapes and books or handouts for the reduction of problems such as obesity, hypertension, or behavior problems. Rather, what successful demonstrations that do exist typically take a significant effort on the part of the provider and the parent.

Among the active procedures, many standard behavioral procedures, including the use of tangible rewards and incentives, have been widely used in past research. Several researchers have applied these or similar procedures to injury control research. For example, Roberts and Turner (1986) used behavioral procedures for encouraging parents and children to use automobile safety belts or child restraint devices by rewarding parents for correctly using child restraint devices. Parents were rewarded with lottery tokens redeemable for prizes if their children were appropriately secured with an automobile seat belt when they arrived at their child's day care center. When the families began receiving rewards based upon their seat belt usage, there was a dramatic increase in their use of seat belts. After the rewards were removed, there was a gradual decline in seat belt usage. Sowers-Hoag, Thyer, and Bailey (1987) used behavioral practice, assertiveness training, and social and contrived reinforcers to establish and maintain automobile safety belt use in young children. Geller and his colleagues

(Geller, Bruff, & Nimmer, 1985) have also published clear demonstrations of the effectiveness of rewards on increasing the use of child safety devices. These studies demonstrate that such active procedures, initially developed in totally different settings, can have applicability when used in injury control research. The opposite point is probably also true—procedures developed in the injury control literature can be generalized to health-related problems.

One example of the use of behavioral procedures being applied to injury control is Mathews, Friman, Barone, Ross, and Christophersen (1987). They reported on a program for teaching mothers to use standard child management procedures (cf. Christophersen, 1988) to reduce the amount of dangerous behaviors in which their young children engaged. Mathews et al. (1987) showed that the use of procedures originally developed to reduce other inappropriate behaviors in young children were effective in reducing dangerous behaviors in young (less than 1-year-old) children. In this study, teenage mothers were taught, through modeling and demonstration, how to reward their children with brief physical contact (which is often used as a reward for children) for age-appropriate behaviors. They were also taught to punish dangerous behaviors by placing their child in their playpen for a brief disciplinary procedure (time-out). The children in the study engaged in potentially dangerous behaviors approximately 55% of the time prior to training. After the mothers were trained in the use of rewards and punishment, the children's potentially dangerous behaviors occurred less than 10% of the time. These results maintained for 6-month follow-up observations.

These types of studies contribute to our knowledge of how to encourage individuals to comply with active injury-control strategies. The field of injury control must also be in a position to identify more comprehensive programs that incorporate several different (active and passive) approaches. In the aggregate, these comprehensive approaches are complimentary and can produce an effect that could not be realized when one of the approaches (such as legislation or health education) is used in isolation. Gallagher, Hunter, and Guyer (1985) have reported very encouraging results from an evaluation of a Home Injury Prevention Program. The three strategies were regulatory (identification and abatement of violations of existing housing codes), educational (counseling on potential safety hazards in the home), and technological (installation and/or distribution of inexpensive safety devices at no cost to the family). Gallagher et al. (1985) showed that the homes in the intervention group had significant decreases in household hazards including both decreases in hazardous items in the house and decreases in hot water heater temperatures.

Counseling on home safety procedures as well as on behavior problems has been recommended by the American Academy of Pediatrics as a routine part of well-child care. However, the effectiveness of these approaches has been questioned given the limited amount of time available in the course of traditional well-child care. Thus, there is a need to evaluate alternative and augmentative strategies in the area of injury prevention.

Group Educational Approaches

Group well-child care refers to a recently developed alternative to the more traditional provider/patient, one-on-one interaction (cf. Osborn, 1985; Stein, 1978; Thomas, Hassanein, & Christophersen, 1984). Although the typical pediatric health care provider spends approximately 13 minutes on a well-child visit (Bergman, Dassel, & Wedgewood, 1966), less than 2 minutes of that time is spent on health education or anticipatory guidance (Reisinger & Bires, 1980). It is interesting to note that, when medical students are initially trained to perform physical examinations on patients, they are encouraged to perform the exam in exactly the same sequence each time (Leake, Barnard, & Christophersen, 1978), which, according to the behavioral literature, facilitates the learning of a response chain. Such a chain is easier to perform consistently. If health education is included in the office visit, regardless of the target behaviors of the health education efforts, a significant amount of time would be required on the part of the health-care provider. The effort required by the patient/parent if they intend to follow the provider's advice and recommendations is also increased. Several studies have reported only marginal results using these brief office interactions (Dershewitz & Williamson, 1977; Miller et al., 1982). One solution that has been proposed for dealing with the effort required in traditional well-child care is to conduct group well-child visits in which several parents are seen at the same time for a much longer office visit. Osborn (1985) reported seeing six mother/infant dyads together for a 45- to 60-minute office appointment. Thomas, Hassanein, and Christophersen (1984) reported seeing even more patients together (6 to 10 families together). Thomas, Hassanein, and Christophersen (1984) used a post-test-only control-group design to study the effects of burn-prevention counseling on 58 couples. Couples were randomly assigned to either an experimental group or a control group. In addition to the standard curriculum received by the control group, the experimental-group couples were provided with verbal and written information on checking the temperature of their hot water and the thermostat setting of their hot water heater. In subsequent home visits, 76% of the experimental group's homes had water temperatures measured at 130° or less, whereas only 23% of the couples in the control group showed hot water temperatures less than or equal to 130°. One of the main advantages of the group well-child format is that the provider can impart the same information to many families at one time, thereby reducing the amount of effort required of the provider. If the provider can explain the importance of checking and lowering hot water heater thermostat settings to 10 families at once, then he or she only needs to cover the same information one-tenth as many times. Parents report that the group well-child visits are more reassuring because they learn that other parents have almost exactly the same concerns and questions.

Christophersen, Barrish, Barrish, and Christophersen (1984) and Christophersen and Long (1987) reported on a Continuing Education for Parents program that can accommodate up to 40 families at one time. These parenting groups meet four times for 2 hours each for a total of 8 hours of instruction. These groups allow providers to see many patients at one time and allow for much more interaction between the provider and the families. In a recent study by the present author and his colleagues (Williams, Barone, Hassanein, & Christophersen, 1989), the effectiveness of the parent group model, for teaching parents injury control strategies, was examined. Seventy five women in their last trimester of pregnancy were randomly assigned, prospectively, to experimental (with accident-prevention information) and control (no accident-prevention information) groups. All participants were enrolled in a prenatal education class offered at an urban tertiary care hospital. The control group was provided with a 60-min presentation and discussion on what to expect during the first few months of life with a newborn infant, plus a presentation and written handouts about infant stimulation and feeding. The experimental group received a 60-min presentation and discussion about the first few months of life with an infant, plus specific injury control information on how to reduce the risk of tap water scalds, fire burns, and vehicular injury. On data collected during home visits, no differences were observed for smoke detector or infant restraint seat usage; however, differences were observed for hot water temperatures. Of the 40 experimental participants, 23 (58%) had the recommended hot water temperature of 130° Fahrenheit or less, whereas 11 of 35 (31%) of the control participants had temperatures of 130° Fahrenheit or less (hot water temperatures below approximately 130° Fahrenheit are generally considered to be safe. These results suggest that prenatal education classes may be an effective forum to introduce the topic of injury prevention. In this same study, a second experiment with parents with toddler-age children did not yield the same positive findings. Obviously, although educating parents in groups shows promise, a great deal of research must be done before the limitations of this model are known. Group education does, however, offer a feasible alternative to the traditional one-on-one office visit, and an alternative that requires substantially less time on the provider's part.

The main advantage of either group well-child care or parent groups is that one provider can see multiple families at the same time. The 1 hour spent with them is over four times as much as the total time spent during a routine well-child visit, as reported by Reisinger and Bires (1980). The greatly increased duration of the contact between the provider and the parents allows substantially more time for didactic presentations, discussion, questions and answers, demonstrations, and role modeling and rehearsing.

DISCUSSION

The commonsense notion that all a professional needs to do is to tell an individual what was healthy and what was unhealthy and they would forever engage in only the healthy behaviors, whereas enormously appealing, has never been proven to be true. The expectation that health-care recommendations will always be followed seems, at first glance, both simple and compelling. No one wants to be injured; when people know that a particular behavior could lead to injury, they should choose an alternative behavior. If so, health-care recommendations need only provide all the information required to avoid injury. Unfortunately, evidence indicates that this logic is too simple for many situations and reflects the fallacy that people take risks only because they lack information. Health-related behavior change (compliance) depends on the credibility of the presentation, the amount of effort required, its necessary frequency, its costs, the probability of injury if the recommendations are ignored, and whether the person is seeking information (Dershewitz & Christophersen, 1984; Janis, 1983; Miller, Reisinger, Blatter, & Wucher, 1982), as much as on the basic facts about risks.

In what is now almost a classic text, Haynes, Taylor, and Sackett (1979) reviewed most of the literature published up until that time and concluded that compliance with health-care recommendations was a major problem, one big enough to suggest that compliance is virtually a field of study in and of itself. Perhaps the greatest contribution of the Haynes et al. book was the focus on compliance and the magnitude of the problems that follow from noncompliance.

In general, research on the efficacy of health education continues to be inconclusive. Previous research in injury control has suggested some necessary components for effective health education. Compliance with health care recommendations may depend on the credibility of the presentation, the amount of effort required to initiate and maintain a safe environment, the costs associated with maintaining a safe environment, the likelihood of injury without change, and whether participants are receptive to the significance of the risk and to the suggested safer alternative (Becker & Maiman, 1975). Future research will be challenged by the task of identifying which methods to emphasize when educating toddler's parents about the risk of injury.

It is reasonable to assume that health education strategies have achieved some level of success in making us aware of risk factors. However, it is naive to assume that simply the awareness of risk will motivate safety-related behaviors. Future research on health education programs may show that the active/passive conceptualization from the injury control literature will be a productive model for other health education researchers to follow.

ACKNOWLEDGMENT

Preparation of this chapter was partially supported by a grant from the Centers for Disease Control.

REFERENCES

Bergman, A. B., Dassel, S. W., & Wedgewood, R. J. (1966). Time motion study of practicing pediatricians. *Pediatrics, 38*, 254.

Cataldo, M. F., Dershewitz, M. W., Christophersen, E. R., Finney, J. W., Fawcett, S. B., & Seekins, T. (1986). Childhood injury control. In N. A. Krasnegor, J. D. Arasteh, & M. F. Cataldo (Eds.), *Child health behavior: A behavioral pediatrics perspective* (pp. 217-253). New York: Wiley.

Christophersen, E. R. (1988). *Little people: Guidelines for commonsense child rearing.* Kansas City, MO: Westport Publishers.

Christophersen, E. R., Barrish, H. H., Barrish, I. J., & Christophersen, M. R. (1984). Continuing education for parents of infants and toddlers. In R. F. Dangel & R. A. Polster (Eds.), *Parent training: Foundations of research and practice* (pp. 127-143). New York: Guilford Press.

Christophersen, E. R., & Long, N. (1987). *Pediatric behavioral problems* (Monograph 103). Kansas City, MO: American Academy of Family Physicians.

Christophersen, E. R., Sosland-Edelman, D., & LeClaire, S. (1985). Evaluation of two comprehensive infant car seat loaner programs with 1-year follow-up. *Pediatrics, 76*(1), 36-42.

Dershewitz, R.A. (1979). Will mothers use free household safety devices? *American Journal of Diseases in Childhood, 133*, 61-64.

Dershewitz, R. A., & Christophersen, E. R. (1984). Childhood household safety: An overview. *American Journal of Diseases of Children, 138*, 85-88.

Dershewitz, R. A., & Williamson, J. W. (1977). Prevention of childhood household injuries: A controlled clinical trial. *American Journal of Public Health, 67*, 1148-1153.

Finney, J. W., & Christophersen, E. R. (1984). Behavioral pediatrics: Health education in pediatric primary care. In M. Hersen, R. M. Eisler, & P. M. Miller (Eds.), *Progress in behavior modification* (Vol. 16, pp. 185-229). New York: Academic Press.

Gallagher, S. S., Hunter, P., & Guyer, B. (1985). A home injury prevention program for children. *Pediatric Clinics of North America, 32*(1), 95-112.

Geller, E. S., Bruff, C. D., & Nimmer, J. G. (1985). "Flash for life": Community-based prompting for safety belt promotion. *Journal of Applied Behavior Analysis, 18*, 309-314.

Haddon, W. (1980). Advances in the epidemiology of injuries as a basis for public safety. *Public Health Report, 95*, 411.

Haynes, R. B., Taylor, D. W., & Sackett, D. R. (Eds.). (1979). *Compliance in health care.* Baltimore: Johns Hopkins University Press.

Janis, I. L. (1983). The role of social support in adherence to stressful decisions. *American Psychologist, 38*, 143-160.

Kelly, A. B. (1979). A media role for public health compliance? In R. B. Haynes, D. W. Taylor, & D. L. Sackett (Eds.), *Compliance in health care.* Baltimore: Johns Hopkins University Press.

Klauber, M. R., Barrett-Connor, E., Marshall, L. F., & Bowers, S. A. (1981). The epidemiology of head injury. A prospective study of an entire community—San Diego County, California, 1978. *American Journal of Epidemiology, 113*, 500-509.

Leake, H. C., Barnard, J. D., & Christophersen, E. R. (1978). Evaluation of pediatric resident's performance during the well-child visit. *Journal of Medical Education, 53*, 361-363.

Mathews, J. R., Friman, P. C., Barone, V. J., Ross, L. V., & Christophersen, E. R. (1987). Decreasing dangerous infant behaviors through parent instruction. *Journal of Applied Behavior Analysis, 20,* 165–169.

Miller, R. E., Reisinger, K. S., Blatter, M. M., & Wucher, F. (1982). Pediatric counseling and subsequent use of smoke detectors. *American Journal of Public Health, 72,* 392–393.

Osborn, L. M. (1985). Group well-child care. *Pediatric Clinics of North America, 12*(2), 355–366.

Pless, I. B. (1978). Accident prevention and health education: Back to the drawing board? *Pediatrics, 62*(3), 431–435.

Reisinger, K. S., & Bires, J. A. (1980). Anticipatory guidance in pediatric practice. *Pediatrics, 66*(6), 889–892.

Reisinger, K. S., Williams, A. F., Wells, J. F., John, E. C., Roberts, T. R., & Podgainy, H. J. (1981). Effect of pediatricians' counseling on infant restraint use. *Pediatrics, 67,* 201–206.

Roberts, M. C., & Brooks, P. H. (1987). Children's injuries: Issues in prevention and public policy. *Journal of Social Issues, 43*(2), 1–12.

Roberts, M. C., & Turner, D. S. (1986). Rewarding parents for their children's use of safety seats. *Journal of Pediatric Psychology, 11,* 25–36.

Sowers-Hoag, K. M., Thyer, B. A., & Bailey, J. S. (1987). Promoting automobile safety belt use by young children. *Journal of Applied Behavior Analysis, 20,* 133–138.

Speigel, C. N., & Lindaman, F. C. (1977). Children can't fly: A program to prevent childhood morbidity and mortality from window falls. *American Journal of Public Health, 67,* 1143–1147.

Stein, M. T. (1978). The providing of well-baby care with parent–infant groups. *Clinical Pediatrics, 17,* 825.

Thomas, K. A., Hassanein, R. S., & Christophersen, E. R. (1984). Evaluation of group well-child care for improving burn prevention practices in the home. *Pediatrics, 74*(5), 879–882.

Williams, A. F. (1982). Passive and active measures for controlling disease and injury. *Health Psychology, 1,* 399–409.

Williams, G. E., Barone, V. J., Hassanein, R., & Christophersen, E. R. (1989). *Parent compliance with health-care recommendations to decrease potential injuries to their children: An evaluation of group well-child care with parents of newborn infants and toddlers.* Unpublished manuscript.

10 Compliance and Long-Term Follow-Up for Childhood Obesity: Retrospective Analysis

Leonard H. Epstein
Alice Valoski
James McCurley
University of Pittsburgh School of Medicine

Obesity is a prevalent condition in childhood (Dietz, & Gortmaker, 1984; Stark, Atkins, Wolff, & Douglas, 1981), and obese children are more likely to become an obese adult than lean children (Abraham, Collins, & Nordsieck, 1971; Abraham & Nordsieck, 1960; Garn & LaVelle, 1985). Given the poor prognosis for obese adults (Brownell & Wadden, 1986), and the fact that obese children are likely to become obese adults, effective interventions for childhood obesity are needed to reduce the risk of obese children becoming obese adults.

The largest body of research on the treatment of childhood obesity has focused on behavioral treatments (Epstein & Wing, 1987). As we have previously discussed (Epstein & Wing, 1987), the treatment literature is sufficiently developed to warrant long-term evaluation. Behavioral treatments have shown superior weight losses to both no treatment control (Aragano, Cassady, & Drabman, 1979; Epstein, Wing, Koeske, & Valoski, 1984; Israel, Stolmaker, & Andrian, 1985; Israel, Stolmaker, Sharp, Silverman, & Simon, 1984; Kirschenbaum, Harris, & Tomarken, 1984; Senediak & Spence, 1985) and nonspecific attention placebo control treatments (Epstein, Wing, Steranchak, Dickson, & Michelson, 1980; Epstein, Wing, Woodall, Penner, & Kress, 1985; Graves, Meyers, & Clark, 1988).

Behavioral treatments for childhood obesity are designed to change eating and exercise habits of children by training parents and children in behavioral methods (Epstein & Wing, 1987). Basic behavioral skills taught in most programs include self-monitoring, calorie reduction, increasing exercise, modification of the environment (stimulus control), and the use of social and/or contractual reinforcement to support behavior change (Epstein & Wing, 1987). Controlled outcome research has begun to identify some variables that are important to modification of eating and exercise behavior and compliance to treatment recommendations. Research on compliance in childhood obesity has shown a relationship between compliance to both eating (Epstein, Wing, Koeske, Andrasik, & Ossip, 1981) and exercise (Epstein, Koeske, & Wing, 1984), and the following behavioral variables are related to positive short-term outcome: parental use of positive reinforcement versus negative reinforcement (Aragano et al., 1979), the inclusion of parents in treatment of their children (Epstein et al., 1981), parent training in behavioral principles (Israel et al., 1985), and family problem solving (Graves et al., 1988).

The focus of this chapter is the assessment of the relationship between behavioral factors targeted in behavioral family-based treatment and long-term outcome for obese children. Two aspects of compliance are analyzed. First, we attempt to identify the specific behaviors related to eating and exercise change that influence long-term weight control. Second, parental variables that influence the compliance to these eating and exercise changes are presented. These analyses are based on a database comprising four controlled outcome studies from our laboratories, which at the present time represent the only long-term follow-up of randomized, controlled studies of childhood obesity known to the investigators. The Childhood Obesity Research Program at the University of Pittsburgh has systematically been studying family-based treatment for childhood obesity for the last decade, and treatment development research has been completed on children from the ages of 2–5 (Epstein, Valoski, Koeske, & Wing, 1986), 5–8 (Epstein, Wing, Woodall, Penner, Kress, & Koeske, 1985) and 8–12 (Epstein & Wing, 1987).

This chapter is divided into five sections. In the first section, the methods for each of the four studies are reviewed. This is necessary to understand behavioral variables that may influence outcome. The second section presents the results of each study to document the effectiveness within each group of the major treatment procedures. Third, the methods for retrospective assessment and the analytic methods are reviewed. Fourth, analysis of behavioral factors across the four studies is presented. Finally, the results are discussed, and implications for future research are presented.

REVIEW OF RESEARCH METHODS AND DESIGNS

Five-year follow-up has been completed for four randomized, controlled outcome studies. There were several common characteristics across these studies. In each study obese preadolescent children and their parents were randomized to alternative treatments, with active treatments ranging from 8 to 12 weeks, and monthly meetings continuing to months 6 or 12. No booster sessions were used. Follow-up represented data collection and not additional treatment. The four studies have used somewhat different methods of implementing family-based intervention. The specifics of each intervention are described along with the major independent variables. Two of these studies have focused on family factors (Epstein, Wing, Koeske, & Valoski, 1987; Epstein, Wing, Valoski, & Gooding, 1987), and two on exercise (Epstein et al., 1984; Epstein, Wing, Koeske, & Valoski, 1985).

The initial study (Study 1) randomized families to groups that varied by which family members were targeted and reinforced for weight loss and habit change. All families received equal attention, measurement, and information, which included the stoplight diet (Epstein & Squires, 1988), and a flexible exercise program based on the Cooper point system (Cooper, 1977). The parent-plus-child group (1A) used a conjoint contingency system, in which both the obese child and parent were targeted, and the goals required both to show behavior change and weight loss in order to receive positive reinforcement. In the child-alone group (1B) the goal required only child behavior change and weight loss, independent of parent changes, and, in the nonspecific target control (1C), families were reinforced for attendance, independent of behavior change or weight loss. Results showed that over 5 years children in the parent-plus-child group had better long-term changes than children in the nonspecific target control group (Epstein et al., 1987). The nonspecific target control group served as the basis for subsequent comparisons of other family-based procedures in which both child and parent are targeted.

A second family study (Study 3) modified the initial family-based procedures in two ways. First, goals included only habit change, and not weight loss. Second, only the child was targeted and reinforced. The major independent variable was family history (at least one obese parent 3A/both parents lean 3B). All families were provided similar treatment programs, but obese children with a positive family history of obesity showed significantly less long-term weight control than obese children without a positive family history after 1 and 5 years (Epstein, Wing, Valoski, & Gooding, 1987).

The remaining studies (2 and 4) focused on exercise. They are based on a preliminary study that showed superior changes in percentage overweight over 6 and 17 months for children provided a lifestyle exercise program in comparison to a programmed aerobic exercise program (Epstein, Wing, Koeske, Ossip, & Beck, 1982). The first long-term exercise study (Study 2) used similar family-based procedures to those used in Study 3, including only setting goals based on behavior change and only reinforcing child behavior change. In this study families were randomized to diet-plus-lifestyle exercise (Group 2A) and diet-alone (Group 2B) groups (Epstein et al., 1984). No differences were shown for children or parents between these groups over 5 years.

The final long-term trial (Study 4) used a third variation of family-based treatments in which the goals remained based only on behavior change, but a reciprocal contracting system was used in which parents reinforced child behavior change and children independently reinforced parent change. The independent variables involved replicating the lifestyle (Group 4B) versus programmed aerobic exercise (Group 4A) comparison, with the addition of a calisthenics control group (4C). Children randomized to the lifestyle groups showed significantly greater weight change after 2 years compared to children in the programmed exercise and calisthenics groups (Epstein, Wing, Koeske, & Valoski, 1985), and preliminary analysis of these results showed significant differences at 5 years.

Methods

Subjects. Subjects were between 8–12 years of age, and 20%–100% over ideal weight for height, age, and sex (Jelliffe, 1966). Exclusion criteria for children include not being able to read, concurrent psychiatric diagnosis, unwillingness of at least one parent to attend all treatment meetings, and, for the exercise studies (Epstein, Wing, Koeske, & Valoski, 1984, 1985), no medical problem that contraindicates exercise. Children in all groups with the exception of the negative family history group (Epstein et al., 1987) had obese parents. These children are at greater risk of becoming obese adults than obese children with lean parents (Charney, Goodman, McBride, Lyon, & Pratt, 1976). The sample sizes, initial ages, baseline percentage overweight, and mean percentage overweight change over 5 years for children and their parents are presented in Tables 10.1 and 10.2, respectively.[1] The average SES (Hollingshead, 1975) for the total sample was 43.3, and the average family size 1.7 ± 1.4 siblings. In these four studies, 187 families were initially randomized, and data for 162 were available at 5 years, 86.6% of the total sample.

Treatment and Follow-up Procedures. At 5 years participants were contacted and follow-up data was collected in one of three ways. First, families who remained close to Pittsburgh were measured in our laboratories. Second, for families who had moved, or who were unable to attend the follow-up, physician or nurse reports were used. Third, a few families who were unable to comply with the previous methods self-reported heights and weights, which were adjusted to compensate for self-report bias using a database that compared measured and self-reported heights and weights based on 173 participants.[2] Families were paid for follow-up on a sliding scale, ranging from $100 for both parents

---

[1]The numbers presented in this table may be slightly different from data published in primary sources given differences in sample size and the use of a common computer-based system for calculating percentage overweight.

[2]The regression equations to estimate weight and height are as follows; Girls (Weight = 1.046 * self-reported weight in lbs), Boys (Weight = 1.017 * self-reported weight), Mothers (Weight = 1.019 * self-reported weight), Fathers (Weight = 1.011 * self-reported weight), Mothers & Daughters height (Height = .997 * self-reported height in cm.), Fathers & Sons (Height = .990 * self-reported height).

TABLE 10.1
Child Percentage Overweight Changes Over Five Years

Authors	Group	Number/Name	N	Age	0	0-60
Epstein, Wing, Koeske, & Valoski (1987)	1A	P + C	24	9.9	41.7 (15.3)	-12.6 (19.8)
	1B	Child	19		43.3 (15.0)	0.4 (18.6)
	1C	Non-spec Tar	19		46.2 (15.4)	7.8 (21.1)
Epstein, Wing, Koeske, & Valoski (1984)	2A	Diet + LS	12	10.5	45.1 (15.6)	-1.8 (22.0)
	2B	Diet	16		43.5 (10.7)	-6.8 (15.5)
Epstein, Wing, Valoski, & Gooding (1987)	3A	FH+	22	10.9	45.0 (16.1)	.1 (23.5)
	3B	FH-	16		39.9 (14.2)	-3.7 (17.3)
Epstein, Valoski, & Wing (1989)	4A	Diet + Aer	13	10.5	47.9 (16.1)	-6.2 (24.6)
	4B	Diet + LS	13		51.8 (16.4)	-12.0 (18.3)
	4C	Diet + Cal	8		47.7 (24.3)	6.5 (21.8)

and children coming to the laboratory for direct measurement, to $50 for nurse or physician reports, to $5 for self-reports.

Each family was asked to complete a questionnaire that assessed the extent to which participants used the behavioral treatment procedures that they were taught during treatment. These questions focused on three areas: changing eating habits, changing exercise habits, and behavior changes that support eating and exercise habit change. In addition, subjects were asked about their participation in other weight control programs, to ensure that effects of other programs they may have joined were not being attributed to our treatment program. The questionnaire, along with the means and standard deviations for children and parental responding, are presented in Table 10.3. Complete questionnaires were available for 125

TABLE 10.2
Parent Average Percentage Overweight Change Over Five Years

Authors	Group	Number/Name	N	Age	0	0-60
Epstein, Wing, Koeske, & Valoski (1987)	1A	P + C	24	40.8	33.0 (21.3)	0.3 (11.6)
	1B	Child	19	41.6	33.5 (19.3)	3.5 (13.3)
	1C	Non-spec Tar	19	38.7	36.9 (17.4)	7.6 (10.7)
Epstein, Wing, Koeske, & Valoski (1984)	2A	Diet + LS	11	38.5	31.7 (16.6)	-3.9 (10.1)
	2B	Diet	16	44.2	36.2 (18.6)	2.8 (10.9)
Epstein, Wing, Valoski, & Gooding (1987)	3A	FH+	22	40.2	32.9 (22.0)	4.3 (16.3)
	3B	FH-	16	37.8	8.8 (10.4)	5.0 (6.6)
Epstein, Valoski, & Wing (1989)	4A	Diet + Aer	13	39.0	54.7 (18.0)	-5.9 (15.3)
	4B	Diet + LS	13	41.3	52.5 (27.6)	-10.1 (26.2)
	4C	Diet + Cal	8	37.4	49.0 (11.1)	-1.0 (25.5)

TABLE 10.3
Means and Standard Deviations of Responses to Each Question. Children and Parents Filled out Separate Questionnaires

	Child		Parent	
	Mean	SD	Mean	SD

Rate the following questions using (1) completely satisfied - (5) completely dissatisfied

	Child Mean	Child SD	Parent Mean	Parent SD
satisfaction with your weight	3.9	1.1	4.2	1.1
satisfaction with child weight (parents only)			3.7	1.3

Rate how useful were the following techniques taught in the programs from (1) extremely helpful - (5) not at all helpful

Utility of

	Child Mean	Child SD	Parent Mean	Parent SD
treatment meetings	2.6	1.2	2.1	1.1
weighing yourself daily	2.4	1.2	2.2	1.2
goal setting	2.1	1.0	2.1	1.0
decreasing or eliminating red foods	2.0	1.0	1.7	1.0
selecting lower calorie foods	2.0	1.0	1.8	0.9
decreasing or eliminating snacks	2.2	1.1	1.9	0.9
controlling portion sizes	2.1	1.0	1.9	0.9
keeping within the calorie range	1.9	1.0	1.8	0.9
planning ahead for special occasions	2.7	1.2	2.4	1.1
other family members on the program	2.5	1.3	2.3	1.2
using praise	2.5	1.2	2.2	1.1
increasing activity	1.9	0.9	1.8	1.0

Indicate the frequency of the following behaviors: (1) daily, (2) every other day, (3) once a week, (4) once a month, (5) never

	Child Mean	Child SD	Parent Mean	Parent SD
weigh yourself	2.8	1.3	2.8	1.3
graph your weight	4.7	0.8	4.8	0.6
record your food intake	4.5	1.2	4.5	1.0

Reversed scoring on these items

	Child Mean	Child SD	Parent Mean	Parent SD
RED foods brought into the home	3.4	1.1	3.2	0.8
how often do you eat RED foods	3.7	1.1	3.8	0.9
how often do you serve family style	3.6	1.6	4.0	1.3

List any other weight control programs in which you participated during the past five years:

	Child Mean	Child SD	Parent Mean	Parent SD
number of other weight control programs joined	.8	1.07	0.7	0.7
months of participation	2.4	4.4	3.1	5.9
total pounds of weight lost	8.4	10.9	10.9	17.3

List any exercise programs in which you participated in the last five years:

	Child Mean	Child SD	Parent Mean	Parent SD
number of exercise programs joined	0.4	0.7	0.5	0.7
months of exercise participation	2.9	6.9	6.6	16.0
total pounds of exercise weight lost	2.1	6.4	1.7	4.3
total leisure metabolic units/year	6741	7415	2143	3065

How would you rate the childhood weight control program: (1) very positive - (5) very negative

	Child Mean	Child SD	Parent Mean	Parent SD
overall rating of program	2.0	.9	1.6	0.8

How successful do you feel the program was in helping you to make changes in your eating and exercise behaviors during the course of the program? (1) very helpful - (5) not very helpful

	Child Mean	Child SD	Parent Mean	Parent SD
habit change during program	2.4	1.1	2.2	1.2

(Continued)

(Table 10.3 Continued)

	Child		Parent	
	Mean	SD	Mean	SD
How successful do you feel the program was in helping you to make lasting changes in your eating and exercise habits? (1) very helpful -(5) not very helpful				
lasting habit change	3.1	1.1	3.2	1.1

Note. RED foods are high calorie/low nutrient density foods from the Stoplight Diet.

families, which represented 77% of the families for which 5-year data was available, and 69% of the families that were initially randomized.

In order to establish that no differences existed between families who provided retrospective questionnaires versus those who did not, t-tests were used to compare these groups at baseline in terms of differences in age, sex, initial child or parent percentage overweight, SES, and family size, as well as differences in percentage overweight change over 5 years. The means for these variables for both samples are shown in Table 10.4. No significant differences for any variables were shown, suggesting the sample assessed was representative of the larger sample that was treated.

Differences Between Treatments

The major focus of this chapter is to understand what behavior changes are related to long-term outcome. The statistical analysis of differences among the treatment groups is presented in a separate paper (Epstein, McCurley, Wing, & Valoski, 1990). To summarize these findings, significant differences were observed for treatment/control comparisons in two of the studies. The parent-plus-child target group (1A, −12.6) was significantly ($p < .005$) different from the control group (1C, +7.8) in Epstein, Wing, Koeske, and Valoski (1987), and the

TABLE 10.4
Comparisons for Subjects Who Completed Versus Did Not Complete the Retrospective Questionnaire

	Questionnaire	No Questionnaire
Child sex (0 = M, 1 = F)	.70 ± .46	.75 ± .43
Child age	10.6 ± 1.5	10.3 ± 1.5
Siblings	1.9 ± 1.3	1.7 ± 1.5
SES	44.7 ± 15.0	43.3 ± 13.0
% over child	45.9 ± 16.0	44.4 ± 15.4
% over parent	38.5 ± 22.2	34.5 ± 22.0
Child 0 - 5 change	-6.8 ± 20.7	-2.1 ± 20.8
Parent 0 - 5 change	-2.1 ± 19.1	2.1 ± 13.8

lifestyle exercise group (4B, −12.0) was significantly different ($p < .025$) from the calisthenics control (4C, +6.5) in Epstein et al. (1989). In addition, the lifestyle exercise group 4B was significantly different ($p < .01$) from the nontargeted control group 1C. In summary, each of the groups that showed long-term maintenance emphasized mutual reinforcement of parents and children, either using conjoint reinforcement (Epstein et al., 1987) or reciprocal reinforcement (Epstein et al., 1985).

Analysis of variance for parents showed a significant overall effect of treatment, but no within-study significant differences for parent changes. Three groups showed significantly greater percentage overweight changes than the nontargeted control group (1C) in Epstein et al. (1987). These were the diet-plus-lifestyle (4B) group ($p < .001$) and the diet-plus-programmed-aerobic exercise (4A) group ($p < .01$) from Epstein, Valoski, and Wing (1989) and the diet-plus-lifestyle (2A) group ($p < .025$) from Epstein, Wing, Koeske, and Valoski (1984).

Predictors of Long-Term Change

The analytic plan to understand how behavior change is related to long-term success involved first calculating the univariate relationships between retrospective questions and 5-year outcome for both child and parent percentage overweight change. Next, variables that were related to long-term success were entered into a multiple regression equation with change in percentage overweight over 5 years as the dependent variable. This was done in two steps for each equation, by first establishing the best predictors of child/parent outcome using only child or parent variables, and then combining the child and parent variables into the same equation. In addition to the retrospective variables, several other variables that had previously been shown to influence outcome were entered into the equations. These included initial changes in percentage overweight and changes in percentage overweight for the other participating family member.

Univariate Relationships to Long-Term Changes

The results for the univariate correlations for child and parent responses to the retrospective questionnaire in relationship to both child and parent changes in percentage overweight are shown in Table 10.5. Variables that were significant for either the children or parents were presented. Fifteen of the 25 variables were related to outcome for at least one of the percentage overweight changes. In order to compare the relationships among the variables, the probability levels for each correlation considered individually are presented. The subsequent multiple linear regression procedures will eliminate variables that share common variance with outcome. However, if any of these correlations are to be considered for univariate purposes, the overall significance level should be adjusted for the number of

TABLE 10.5
Variables That Were Significantly Related to Long-Term Success

| | Child Change | | | | Parent Change | | | |
| | Child | | Parent | | Child | | Parent | |
Respondee	r	p	r	p	r	p	r	p
utility of								
weighing yourself daily	.17	NS	.20	.05	.22	.05	.15	NS
goal setting	.08	NS	.24	.01	.11	NS	-.03	NS
decreasing or eliminating red foods	.13	NS	.22	.01	.13	NS	.02	NS
selecting lower calorie foods	.23	.05.	.21	.05	.19	.05	.10	NS
controlling portion sizes	.18	.05	.22	.01	.22	.01	-.05	NS
keeping within the calorie range	.13	NS	.28	.005	.20	.05	.04	NS
planning ahead for special occasions	.14	NS	.24	.008	.18	.05	-.09	NS
using praise	.14	NS	.29	.001	.05	NS	.03	NS
increasing activity	.08	NS	.27	.005	.08	NS	.03	NS
frequency of								
weigh yourself	.19	.05	.19	.05	.12	NS	.29	.001
graph your weight	.25	.005	.00	NS	.04	NS	.09	NS
reversed scoring on these items								
How often do you eat RED foods	.21	.02	.05	NS	.03	NS	.09	NS
number weight control programs joined	.10	NS	.00	NS	.08	NS	.21	.05
months of participation	.00	NS	.03	NS	.03	NS	.20	.05
total leisure metabolic units	-.20	.05	-.19	.05	-.11	NS	-.16	NS

correlations, and only correlations at the $p = .002$ should be considered to be significant.

Given these guidelines, two variables were related to child percentage overweight change in a univariate model, parent report of keeping within the calorie range ($p < .002$), and parent report of the use of praise ($p < .001$). When the adjusted correlations are considered for parent change, only the frequency of parental report of weighing was a significant predictor.

Ratings of satisfaction with the program suggest that both child change ($r = .43, p < .001$) and parent change ($r = .40, p < .001$) were related to satisfaction. Likewise, both child and parent ratings of program quality were related to outcome ($r = .21, p < .05; r = .19, p < .05$); child ratings of satisfaction were related to habit change during treatment ($r = .22, p < .05$), and child ratings of satisfaction with long-term change were also related to long-term outcome ($r = .47, p < .001$).

The univariate correlations between individual difference variables and initial and short-term treatment results are shown in Table 10.6. Child weight was predicted by two factors, initial percentage overweight change during the first 6 months of treatment ($p < .005$) and parent change in percentage overweight over 5 years ($p < .001$). When considering variables that relate to parent percentage

TABLE 10.6
Relationship Between Percentage Overweight Change Over Five Years and Baseline and Change Variables

Variable	Child		Parent	
	r	p	r	p
Age	-.14	NS	.01	NS
Sex	-.07	NS	-.03	NS
SES	.14	NS	-.02	NS
Siblings	-.01	NS	.04	NS
Percentage over 0	-.17	NS	-.25	<.05
Percentage over 0-6 mos	.24	<.005	.19	<.05
Weight 0	-.10	NS	-.21	<.05
Height 0	-.04	NS	-.04	NS
Height 0-5	.06	NS		
Baseline percentage over	-.02	NS	.07	NS
Parent or child 0-5 change	.28	,.001	.28	<.001

overweight change, adjusting correlations for multiple tests, then only one univariate correlation was significant, the relationship between child and parent long-term change ($p < .001$).

Multiple Regression Prediction of Long-Term Changes

The means for questionnaire responses and the univariate correlations were presented to provide investigators with an overview of the response patterns of subjects. However, given that multiple individual difference, treatment outcome, and retrospective report of behavioral variables were related to outcome, a multiple linear regression was used to better understand the role of individual variables in predicting outcome when other variables were considered in the prediction at the same time.

Child and parent percentage overweight changes were modeled separately using backward modeling procedures in which nonsignificant terms were sequentially removed. First, regression models were developed that began with only the (unadjusted) significant items from the retrospective questionnaire, and then (unadjusted) significant individual difference and outcome variables were added to the model. The final results for each model are shown in Table 10.7.

As shown in Table 10.7, four behavioral variables in addition to parent changes in percentage overweight were related to long-term outcome, child report of selecting low calorie meals, compliance to graphing weight, and compliance to eating fewer red foods, and one parent report variable, the use of parent praise. These variables, in combination with long-term parent change, had a multiple r of .51, accounting for 23% of the variance in long-term child percentage overweight change.

Changes in parent percentage overweight change were related to only one

TABLE 10.7
Multiple Linear Regression Models that Predict Child and Parent Changes in Percentage Overweight from 0-5 Years

Child Percent Overweight Change				
	Coefficient	SE	t	P
Constant	-59.8	11.81	-5.06	.000
(c) Selecting low-calorie meals	4.19	1.71	2.44	.016
(c) Graphing weight	5.58	2.06	2.71	.008
(c) Eating Red foods	3.32	1.51	2.20	.03
(p) Parent use of praise	4.51	1.48	3.04	.003
Parent 0-5	0.30	0.12	2.46	.015

Multiple $r = .51$; adjusted r squared $= .23$
$f(5,117) = 8.2, p < .001$

Parent Percent Overweight Change				
	Coefficient	SE	t	P
(p) weighing yourself	2.05	0.54	3.82	.000
Parent 0-6 change	0.33	0.11	2.99	.000
Child 0-5 change	0.13	0.06	2.14	.035

Multiple $r = .39$; adjusted r squared $= .14$
$f(5,117) = 9.92, p < .001$

behavioral variable, parent report of compliance to weighing themselves, along with two weight control variables, parent 0–6-month change, and child 0–5-year change. This model had a multiple $r = .39$, with an adjusted $r^2 = .14$.

DISCUSSION

The regression analyses assess contributions of individual-difference variables in combination with behavioral variables targeted during treatment to the long-term success of childhood obesity treatment programs. These analyses provide information that may be used to enhance future programs, as well as to provide insight into mechanisms that may be operating in groups that showed significant long-term success. The observation that initial treatment response was related to long-term outcome for both children and their parents is important because it suggests that compliance to initial treatment is relevant for understanding how initial treatment variables influence long-term outcome.

Before discussing the results, it is advisable to consider the limitations of retrospective questionnaires. A retrospective questionnaire that assesses the relationship between the utility of and compliance to behaviors that were taught 5 years previously to current weight control has several problems. First, there are problems in remembering the effectiveness of how specific behaviors may have influenced outcome. Second, post-hoc judgments about program effectiveness are likely to be influenced by current success or problems, which may cause inaccuracies in reporting on program-related activities. Third, the questionnaire did not focus on variability in outcomes that may occur over extended follow-up periods. When this research program began over 10 years ago, there was little discussion of mechanisms of relapse and relapse prevention (Brownell, Marlatt, Lichtenstein, & Wilson, 1986), and the treatment program did not focus on these variables and they were not assessed during follow-up. However, it is possible that the process of weight regulation does not involve learning skills that are always implemented, but rather that weight control behaviors and weight fluctuate on the basis of nonweight-related events, such as psychosocial stressors. Fourth, the influence of nonbehavioral variables such as metabolic rate (Epstein, Wing et al., 1989) that may influence weight or weight regulation were not assessed, which may have improved the prediction of success. Fifth, correlations do not indicate the direction of causality. A relationship between regular weight recording and weight control may represent the fact that recording and graphing does improve weight control, or that people who are able to regulate their weight like to record and graph their weight. Given these limitations, these data are still valuable because there are limited data available on long-term success of behavioral treatment programs (Brownell & Jeffery, 1987), and no other data are available on how behavioral factors may influence long-term success in children.

Two of the three behaviors noted by the children in predicting child change involved changes in eating behavior. Decreasing caloric intake represents the most important behavior changes for weight control and contributes more to weight loss than changes in activity (Wing & Jeffery, 1979). Thus, it is not surprising that selection of low calorie meals is related to outcome. Likewise, the stoplight diet for children (Epstein & Squires, 1988) focuses on reduction of high-calorie foods with low-nutrient density (RED foods), which we have previously shown is related to success in weight control (Epstein et al., 1981). It is interesting that both selection of low-calorie foods *and* compliance to reducing eating of RED foods independently are related to success. This may relate to the fact that people learn to make better choices of foods to eat within the YELLOW food category, which includes the staples of the diet. For example, whereas red meat, fish, or chicken represent alternative sources of high-quality protein, there are over twice as many calories in a 3-ounce serving of red meat than fish, and changes in these YELLOW foods may be related to long-term success.

The third variable reported by the child involved compliance to graphing weight, which is taught as a self-monitoring/self-regulation skill. It is interesting that parents report a similar behavior, weighing yourself, to be important in their efforts at weight regulation. Self-monitoring of weight is a simple behavior that provides regular feedback about the status of effects of daily behaviors designed to influence weight. The more children weigh themselves, the more feedback they will receive about the status of their behaviors, and thus the better they can regulate their weight. The present study provides no insight into the ideal frequencies for weight self-monitoring, but the more often children weigh themselves, the more feedback they will get to assist them in weight regulation.

Although the three variables just discussed are generic variables to all weight control programs, the other two variables that were related to outcome may be more interesting given the treatments that were studied and the focus of the research program on family-based interventions. The first variable, praise, is something that differentiates the treatment approaches in the two studies that showed long-term success. Praise is important because it may increase the probability that children will comply with the changes in eating and exercise behavior that are targeted. Whereas parent praise of child behavior was taught in all studies, in the two studies with positive outcomes the reinforcers used were either delivered conjointly (Epstein et al., 1981) or reciprocally (Epstein, Wing, Koeske, & Valoski, 1985). There are several ways in which these variables may influence outcome. For example, mutual reinforcement may support the use of behavioral techniques in both parents and children, such that parents may use techniques that influence compliance longer if the contingencies involve both parents and children than if parental behavior is never reinforced. Likewise, the emphasis on reinforcing both parent and child may make a more supportive atmosphere more conducive to success than if the parent feels he or she is doing a lot of activities with little compensation for themselves.

The relationship between parent and child success is important from the perspective of family-based treatment. As we have discussed previously (Epstein et al., 1990), one of the advantages of family-based treatment is that it can induce positive changes in both children and their parents. The fact that parent success is related to child success further supports this idea and suggests that family changes are in fact being made that influence multiple family members. Previous research on nontargeted family members has shown changes in siblings who were not targeted for treatment (Epstein, Nudelman, & Wing, 1987), suggesting variables were modified that can influence weight regulation across multiple family members.

It is interesting to consider factors that could produce similar changes in obese children and their parents over 5 years. First, parents could be serving as models for their children, which could influence child acquisition and maintenance of appropriate behavior (Harper & Sanders, 1975). For example, the fact that both parents and children rated self-monitoring of weight as very helpful in controlling weight suggests that children may imitate the parent who is doing this behavior. Second, parents may be modifying aspects of the environment that influence weight loss efforts of both parents and children separately. For example, if parents reduce the availability of high-fat, high-calorie foods in the house, then intake of both children and parents will be influenced, but independently. Third, the effects may be due to differences in motivation in parents who are successful than parents who are not successful. Successful parents may be more likely to emphasize continuation of behaviors in their children that are working than parents who are not as successful. Fourth, it may be easier to use parental praise and reinforcement if both parent and child are working on similar behaviors and both are successful.

It may be important that the same variables were not related to child and parent success. This may be due in part to differential treatment responsiveness in parents and children, with children doing somewhat better than their parents. On the other hand, the differences may be due to different variables influencing parents and their children. There are obvious developmental differences, as well as differences in peer influences and reasons for losing weight between parents and their children. If different variables do influence child and adult weight control efforts, it may be more important to emphasize common aspects of the environment that can influence parents and children independently than to focus on parent modeling and parent imitation as mechanisms for change.

Treatment and maintenance are often conceptualized as separate processes that depend on separate mechanisms (Stunkard & Penick, 1979). The present results show initial percentage overweight changes over 6 months and long-term success are related. This suggests that initial and long-term processes involved in family-based interventions are related, and skills learned during treatment may be important to long-term success. It is possible that the conjoint parent–child treatment program or the reciprocal reinforcement treatment program both teach new ways of parenting as well as changing parent–child interaction patterns to ones that work better than previous parenting behaviors and are maintained over time. Whereas child programs often focus on parental control of child behavior, there is a vast body of research showing children exert considerable control on parental behavior (Emery, Binkoff, Houts, & Carr, 1983).

Given the significant relationships between initial changes and/or behaviors taught during treatment and final outcome, long-term compliance to treatment recommendations and success can be improved by better outcomes during treatment (Brownell & Jeffery, 1987). Variations that are currently being used with adults that might be appropriate include increasing the duration of treatment (Brownell & Wadden, 1986; Perri, Nezu, Patti, & McCann, 1989), or the use of more aggressive dietary interventions such as the very low-calorie diet (Wadden, Stunkard, & Brownell, 1983), which also has been used with obese adolescents (Archibald, Harrison, & Pencharz, 1983; Dietz & Wolfe, 1985). Likewise, the addition of relapse prevention procedures (Brownell et al., 1986; Marlatt & Gordon, 1985; Perri, Shapiro, Ludwig, Twentyman, & McAdoo, 1984) may be useful in enhancing compliance to treatment recommendations and long-term success.

Whereas results based on retrospective reports must be confirmed using prospective designs, the present research provides guidelines for the types of program and compliance variables that can be considered in future studies. These prospective designs must include repeated objective assessment of compliance to eating and exercise behavior, as well as use of behavioral techniques. The current studies suggest that a variety of treatment variables are important to outcome, such as self-monitoring and changes in eating behaviors. In addition, family factors such as parent praise and changes in weight of other family members may be important in arranging an environment that promotes compliance to recommended changes. There are a variety of other factors that could influence outcome that should be evaluated, particularly in regard to behavioral factors that may be operative in family-based treatments. For example, child food and exercise perceptions (Epstein, Valoski, Wing, Perkins, Fernstrom, Marks, & McCurley, 1989), parent eating and exercise behavior patterns (Sallis, Patterson, McKenzie, & Nader, 1988), or parental perceptual biases (Wahler & Dumas, 1989) may be responsive to family-based treatment and compliance enhancing interventions and thus related to outcome.

ACKNOWLEDGMENTS

Appreciation is expressed to Rena R. Wing, Alice Valoski, and Joel Greenhouse for suggestions on design and analysis. The childhood obesity research presented was supported in part by grants HD MH 12520, HD 16411, HD 19532, and preparation of this chapter was supported by grant HD 20829, each of which was awarded to Dr. Epstein.

REFERENCES

Abraham, S., Collins, G., & Nordsieck, M. (1971). Relationship of childhood weight status to morbidity in adults. *Public Health Reports, 85,* 273–284.

Abraham, S., & Nordsieck, M. (1960). Relationship of excess weight in children and adults. *Public Health Reports, 75,* 263–273.

Aragano, J., Cassady, J., & Drabman, R. S. (1979). Treatment of overweight children through parental training and contingency contracting. *Journal of Applied Behavioral Analysis, 12,* 449–466.

Archibald, E. H., Harrison, J. E., & Pencharz, P. B. (1983). Effect of a weight-reducing high-protein diet on the body composition of obese adolescents. *American Journal of Diseases of Childhood, 137,* 658–662.

Brownell, K. D., & Jeffery, R. W. (1987). Improving long-term weight loss: Pushing the limits of treatment. *Behavior Therapy, 18,* 353–374.

Brownell, K. D., Marlatt, G. A., Lichtenstein, E., & Wilson, G. T. (1986). Understanding and preventing relapse. *American Psychologist, 41,* 756–782.

Brownell, K. D., & Wadden, T. A. (1986). Behavior therapy for obesity: Modern approaches and better results. In K. D. Brownell & J. P. Foreyt (Eds.), *Handbook of eating disorders* (pp. 180–197). New York: Basic Books.

Charney, E., Goodman, H. C., McBride, M., Lyon, B., & Pratt, R. (1976). Childhood antecedents of adult obesity. Do chubby infants become obese adults? *New England Journal of Medicine, 295*, 6-9.

Cooper, K. H. (1977). *The aerobics way*. New York: Evans.

Dietz, W. H., & Gortmaker, S. L. (1984). Factors within the physical environment associated with childhood obesity. *American Journal of Clinical Nutrition, 39*, 619-624.

Dietz, W. H., & Wolfe, R. R. (1985). Interrelationships of glucose and protein metabolism in obese adolescents during short-term hypocaloric dietary therapy. *American Journal of Clinical Nutrition, 42*, 380-390.

Emery, R. E., Binkoff, J. A., Houts, A. C., & Carr, E. G. (1983). Children as independent variables: Some clinical implications of child-effects. *Behavior Therapy, 14*, 398-412.

Epstein, L. H., Koeske, R., & Wing, R. R. (1984). Adherence to exercise in obese children. *Journal of Cardiac Rehabilitation, 4*, 185-195.

Epstein, L. H., McCurley, Wing, R. R., & Valoski, A. (1990). Five-year follow-up of family-based behavioral treatments for childhood obesity. *Journal of Consulting and Clinical Psychology, 58*, 661-664.

Epstein, L. H., Nudelman, S., & Wing, R. R. (1987). Long-term effects of family-based treatment for obesity on nontreated family members. *Behavior Therapy, 18*, 147-152.

Epstein, L. H., & Squires, S. (1988). *The stoplight diet for children*. Boston: Little/Brown.

Epstein, L. H., Valoski, A., Koeske, R., & Wing, R. R. (1986). Behavioral weight control in obese young children. *Journal of the American Dietetic Association, 86*, 91-95.

Epstein, L. H., Valoski, A., Wing, R. R. (1989). *Long-term follow-up comparing lifestyle exercise, aerobic exercise and calisthenics on weight loss in obese children*. Unpublished manuscript, University of Pittsburgh, Pittsburgh, PA.

Epstein, L. H., Valoski, A., Wing, R. R., Perkins, K. A., Fernstrom, M. H., Marks, B., & McCurley, J. (1989). Perception of eating and exercise in children as a function of child and parent weight status. *Appetite, 12*, 105-118.

Epstein, L. H., & Wing, R. R. (1987). Behavioral treatment of childhood obesity. *Psychological Bulletin, 101*, 91-95.

Epstein, L. H., Wing, R. R., Cluss, P., Fernstrom, M. H., Penner, B., Perkins, K. A., Nudelman, S., Marks, B., & Valoski, A. (1989). Resting metabolic rate in lean and obese children: Relationship to child and parent weight and percent-overweight change. *American Journal of Clinical Nutrition, 49*, 331-336.

Epstein, L. H., Wing, R. R., Koeske, R., Andrasik, F., & Ossip, D. J. (1981). Child and parent weight loss in family-based behavior modification programs. *Journal of Consulting and Clinical Psychology, 49*, 674-685.

Epstein, L. H., Wing, R. R., Koeske, R., Ossip, D. O., & Beck, S. (1982). A comparison of lifestyle change and programmed aerobic exercise on weight and fitness changes in obese children. *Behavior Therapy, 13*, 91-95.

Epstein, L. H., Wing, R. R., Koeske, R., & Valoski, A. (1984). The effects of diet plus exercise on weight change in parents and children. *Journal of Consulting and Clinical Psychology, 52*, 429-437.

Epstein, L. H., Wing, R. R., Koeske, R., & Valoski, A. (1985). A comparison of lifestyle exercise, aerobic exercise and calisthenics on weight loss in obese children. *Behavior Therapy, 16*, 345-356.

Epstein, L. H., Wing, R. R., Koeske, R., & Valoski, A. (1987). Long-term effects of family-based treatment of childhood obesity. *Journal of Consulting and Clinical Psychology, 55*, 91-95.

Epstein, L. H., Wing, R. R., Steranchak, L., Dickson, B., & Michelson, J. (1980). Comparison of family-based behavior modification and nutrition education for childhood obesity. *Journal of Pediatric Psychology, 5*, 25-36.

Epstein, L. H., Wing, R. R., Valoski, A., & Gooding, W. (1987). Long-term effects of parent weight on child weight loss. *Behavior Therapy, 18*, 219-226.

Epstein, L. H., Wing, R. R., Woodall, K., Penner, B. C., & Kress, M. J. (1985). The effect of diet and controlled exercise on weight loss in obese children. *Journal of Pediatrics, 107*, 358–361.

Epstein, L. H., Wing, R. R., Woodall, K., Penner, B. C., Kress, M. J., & Koeske, R. (1985). Effects of family based behavioral treatment on obese 5–8-year-old children. *Behavior Therapy, 16*, 205–212.

Garn, S. M., & Lavelle, M. (1985). Two-decade follow-up of fatness in early childhood. *American Journal of Diseases in Children, 139*, 181–185.

Graves, T., Meyers, A. W., & Clark, L. (1988). An evaluation of problem-solving training in the behavioral treatment of childhood obesity. *Journal of Consulting and Clinical Psychology, 56*, 246–250.

Harper, L. V., & Sanders, K. M. (1975). The effect of adults eating on young children's acceptance of unfamiliar foods. *Journal of Experimental Child Psychology, 20*, 206–214.

Hollingshead, A. B. (1975). *Four factor index of social status.* Unpublished manuscript, Yale University, New Haven, CT.

Israel, A. C., Stolmaker, L., & Andrian, C. A. G. (1985). The effects of training parents in general child management skills on a behavioral weight loss program for children. *Behavior Therapy, 16*, 169–180.

Israel, A. C., Stolmaker, L., Sharp, J. P., Silverman, W. K., & Simon, L. G. (1984). An evaluation of two methods of parental involvement in treating obese children. *Behavior Therapy, 15*, 266–272.

Jelliffe, D. B. (1966). *The assessment of the nutritional status of the community.* Geneva: World Health Organization Monograph No. 3.

Kirschenbaum, D. S., Harris, E. S., & Tomarken, A. J. (1984). Effects of parental involvement in behavioral weight loss therapy for preadolescents. *Behavior Therapy, 15*, 485–500.

Marlatt, G. A., & Gordon, J. R. (1985). *Relapse prevention: Maintenance strategies in addictive behavior change.* New York: Guilford.

Perri, M. G., Nezu, A. M., Patti, E. T., & McCann, K. L. (1989). Effect of length of treatment on weight loss. *Journal of Consulting and Clinical Psychology, 57*, 450–452.

Perri, M. G., Shapiro, R. M., Ludwig, W. W., Twentyman, C. T., & McAdoo, W. G. (1984). Maintenance strategies for the treatment of obesity: An evaluation of relapse prevention training and posttreatment contact by mail and telephone. *Journal of Consulting and Clinical Psychology, 52*, 404–413.

Sallis, J. F., Patterson, T. L., McKenzie, T. L., & Nader, P. R. (1988). Family variables and physical activity in preschool children. *Journal of Developmental and Behavioral Pediatrics, 9*, 57–61.

Senediak, C., & Spence, S. H. (1985). Rapid versus gradual scheduling of therapeutic contact in a family based behavioural weight control programme for children. *Behavioural Psychotherapy, 13*, 265–287.

Stark, O., Atkins, E., Wolff, O. H., & Douglas, J. W. B. (1981). Longitudinal study of obesity in the National Survey of Health and Development. *British Medical Journal, 283*, 13–17.

Stunkard, A. J., & Penick, S. B. (1979). Behavioral modification in the treatment of obesity: The problem of maintaining weight loss. *Archives of General Psychiatry, 36*, 801–806.

Wadden, T. A., Stunkard, A. J., & Brownell, K. D. (1983). Very-low-calorie diets: Their efficacy, safety, and future. *Annals of Internal Medicine, 99*, 55–79.

Wahler, R. G., & Dumas, J. E. (1989). Attentional problems in dysfunctional mother–child interactions: An interbehavioral model. *Psychological Bulletin, 105*, 116–130.

Wing, R. R., & Jeffery, R. J. (1979). Outpatient treatments of obesity: A comparison of methodology and results. *International Journal of Obesity, 3*, 261–279.

11   Health Promotion and Disease Prevention: A Social Action Conception of Compliance Behavior

Craig K. Ewart
Johns Hopkins University

Debates about *compliance*—what to call it and how to improve it—often manifest deeper contests between competing notions of health and illness. In this chapter I approach the question of behavioral compliance from a social action or problem-solving perspective in which *health,* defined as an organism's capacity for self-protective action, is distinguished from *wellness,* defined as the absence of disease. I maintain that compliance, properly understood, refers to a process through which people develop and enhance their capacity for self-protective activity. Confusion has arisen because compliance can—and must—be viewed simultaneously as a desired habit or *action state* that is the goal of behavioral intervention, a change *process* through which habits are altered, and a behavioral product of *contexts* in which habit-change processes operate. A tripartite view of compliance suggests new hypotheses and experiments to advance our understanding of health behavior change in children and generates guidelines for enhancing the long-term impact of health promotion efforts (Ewart, 1991).

In the first section of this chapter I present a social action conception of compliance behavior and show how it can help clarify the relationship between health promotion and disease prevention, as well as aid in reconciling conflicting views of the patient as an object of health care and its active consumer. I then describe the tripartite model, indicating ways in which action state, process, and contextual dimensions contribute to a more complete understanding of compliance behavior. Finally, by applying the model to the development of compliance capabilities, I outline some promising directions for early preventive intervention.

A SOCIAL ACTION CONCEPTION OF COMPLIANCE

Health Promotion Versus Disease Prevention

Health in the sense of self-protective or resistive potential, and wellness as the absence of disease or injury, are conceptually distinct phenomena that, together, determine one's level of physical and emotional well-being. Health and wellness also represent different strategies for relieving the burden of human misery imposed by injury and disease. Wellness, defined as absence of disease or injury, can be achieved by removing potential threats from the environment so that people never encounter them. A host of threats to children have disappeared in the wake of legislation requiring safer toys, fire-resistant bedding, and "child-resistant" packaging of medications and other hazardous substances.

These sanitary (wellness) strategies actively reshape human environments but are passive with respect to individuals, who do not even have to know that protective measures have been applied. Where sanitation is feasible, affordable, and effective, the problem of "noncompliance" simply does not exist; sanitary measures require no self-protective action on the part of persons they are meant to benefit. Preventive *sanitation* thus would seem to obviate concern about behavioral compliance and render the present volume superfluous. Yet in nations where public hygiene has vanquished yesterday's infectious epidemics, older threats have been replaced by cardiovascular diseases, cancer, and AIDS— multifaceted conditions whose varied genetic, behavioral, and environmental determinants are less susceptible to earlier models of sanitary control. Risk reduction requires personal action to alter health-endangering behaviors.[1]

Interventions on personal behavior attempt to enhance *health* by strengthening a person's ability to avoid, resist, or attenuate a disease or injury threat. Their goal is "health promotion" as distinct from "disease prevention"—the objective of environmental strategies promoting wellness.[2] Health promotion and disease prevention represent complementary approaches whose relative roles are determined by their comparative feasibility, efficacy, and cost in the face of specific

---

[1]This continues to be true in large regions of the world where poverty, malnutrition, and political conflict, by creating insurmountable barriers to water and sewage treatment, have made infectious diarrheal illnesses of children the world's leading cause of death. Parents must be trained to administer electrolyte solutions that prevent fatal dehydration.

[2]There is a tendency to call a health intervention an "environmental" strategy if it is achieved via legislation or policy directives, and to describe it as "health promotion" if it involves educational messages or clinic programs delivered face to face. In fact, many so-called environmental strategies are really aimed at fostering health-promoting activities in the face of threats that are not amenable to environmental control. For example, threatening to fine parents for failing to secure their children in protective car seats is an individually oriented strategy designed to influence a personal health decision by modifying its anticipated consequences. Instead of removing the danger (as passive air bag systems are designed to do), these legislative interventions attempt to manipulate peoples' environments in ways that will encourage them to modify their behavior.

health threats. When used together, health promotion and disease prevention tactics may even have a synergistic effect (Jeffery, 1989).

Confusion between notions of health and wellness has arisen from the practice of applying a "wellness" label to health enhancement programs aimed at disease-free individuals who might not be inclined to enroll in "health" classes. In this context, wellness more accurately describes the market segment at whom health promotion is targeted (i.e., a program for "well" people) than the intervention itself, which typically is designed to strengthen one's ability to resist or avoid disease, that is, to enhance personal health.

Health as Capacity for Self-Protective Action

Interventions to improve one's capacity to avoid, resist, or reduce health threats involve modifying the individual in some way—health promotion is active with respect to persons. An important public health achievement has been the development of innoculation techniques that alter the way an individual's immune system "behaves" when challenged by a pathogenic agent. The health of a living system can be defined in terms of its capacity for self-regulation, that is, its ability to establish and maintain feedback functions that allow the system to achieve a state of dynamic equilibrium (Seeman, 1989). In this view, innoculation—and many other medical treatments—can be said to operate by enhancing or repairing the self-regulatory behavior of specific physiologic subsystems.

To regulate its functions, a system requires a criterion of effective functioning, feedback concerning the degree to which states of the system approximate this criterion or goal, and the ability to engage in compensating activities to reduce perceived discrepancies. Events that disrupt such functions tend to "disregulate" the system leading to conditions we label *disease* (Schwartz, 1983). On the other hand, "health" is the ability to resist disregulation by maintaining goal orientation, feedback, and compensatory processes under stress. An index of this capability—and hence of health—is the amount or variety of disruptive elements a system can accommodate without becoming disregulated. For example, resistance to infection is indexed by the type and quantity of invading microorganisms that one's immune system can identify and destroy.

Health and "Compliance"

How does a systems view of health and illness affect the way we view "compliance?" Indeed, some writers would banish this term altogether, on grounds that it suggests passive subservience to a physician's advice. Compliance has more than one meaning, however. In a *systems* context, compliance refers to a system's stress-resistive potential, as when one speaks of a physical structure's ability to accommodate the burden imposed by increasing loads. In a systems view, compliance denotes *functional flexibility* rather than obedience; to speak of a biological, cognitive, or social system's compliance is to describe its resilient strength.

At the level of personal health behavior, compliance as assimilative flexibility refers to a person's ability to incorporate new and potentially discrepant goals, information, performance skills, or action patterns into established behavioral repetoires and routines. The task of compliance research is to investigate processes by which new goals, skills, or information are assimilated. Instead of equating noncompliance with "disobedience," the present social action definition suggests that a patient's "failure" to comply is better understood as signifying a breakdown of goal setting, feedback, or compensatory functions under conditions of inappropriate demand.

Debates about semantics can obscure more serious conceptual problems. The complaint that compliance connotes subservience reflects the fundamental inadequacy of a sanitary model of medical care. In a sanitary view, physicians "make people well" by discovering and removing illness threats from their bodies. After initial consent, a patient passively "undergoes" treatment. Surgical interventions to remove malignant neoplasms or dangerously infected tissues exemplify the sanitary paradigm, but it is doubtful if this wellness metaphor adequately describes most health care situations. Certainly it does not apply to contexts where the patient is expected to incorporate new behavior patterns related to medication use, exercise, dietary change, or other self-protective activities. Even surgery is not considered highly successful when it fails to restore self-regulating capabilities of endangered systems, an objective that usually requires rehabilitative behavioral intervention. Fostering health (self-regulation) requires active collaboration of caregiver and patient in a process of defining, negotiating, improvising, and problem solving (Leventhal, Zimmerman, & Gutman, 1984).

TRIPARTITE MODEL OF HEALTH BEHAVIOR CHANGE

Conflicting views of compliance reflect the fact that the task of developing and sustaining effective health protective action is a process that must be approached from multiple perspectives; existing views have tended to focus on one aspect of the problem while ignoring other essential aspects (Leventhal et al., 1984). The framework developed here defines compliance from three points of view, each of which is essential to fostering effective health protective activity (Ewart, 1991). First, it is helpful to view compliance as an action *state,* or an idealized condition of equillibrium between health-enhancing activities and their varied consequences. A state model of health protective action constitutes the goal or reference criterion for effective functioning within a systems perspective. Without such a model, it is difficult to establish self-regulatory objectives or to determine when health intervention goals are being met.

A state perspective has important limitations, however. For one thing, it fails to specify how a desired state is to be achieved. Equally important is the fact that once established the equilibrium envisioned in the state model frequently is punctuated by disruptions. Thus one needs a *process* dimension that tells how new action systems are established. Leventhal has noted that well-known health belief and decision theory models proposed by researchers have not been widely adopted by developers of health behavior change interventions (Leventhal et al., 1984). Although these models predict health actions with varying degrees of success, they leave a large amount of behavioral variance unexplained. Moreover, it has not been easy to relate these predictors to behavioral processes that interventionists can modify to encourage change. Much needed is a model to integrate change mechanisms that can be activated via well-established and empirically tested methods.

Process models can be difficult to develop, however, because a model that fits one patient group or care setting may not apply to others, and, even within the same individual, different causal processes may predominate in different times or settings. Thus some writers have advocated developmental models that divide the change process into discrete stages, distinguishing for example between initial compliance, early adherence, and later "maintenance" phases (DiClemente et al., 1991; Kristeller & Rodin, 1984; Prochaska & DiClemente, 1983). In the present social-contextual view, however, stages of change are not a function of time but rather of *generalization* processes in which self-change skills and problem-solving strategies developed in one context are activated in new and different contexts (Stokes & Baer, 1977; Stokes & Osnes, 1989). Time is important only to the extent that changing action *contexts* demand and support different action strategies.

For example, over a period of several months, an ill child may have to learn to cope with pain within a hospital environment, then with convalescence at home, and later with a return to school. Successive time periods are behaviorally important if they correspond to changes in physical, social, or biologic contexts that differentially activate or constrain the various action mechanisms specified in the process model.

A *contextual* model of health protective action integrates self-change processes with biological and macrosocial factors that affect an individual's self-regulatory capabilities. Physical environments, social models, activity structures created by work or leisure pursuits, one's biologic condition, current mood, or level of maturational development may significantly limit or augment capacity for change. A *contextual* analysis makes it possible to determine which action processes or mechanisms are likely to govern self-regulatory capabilities under particular life circumstances or developmental phases.

Action state, process, and contextual dimensions of the tripartite model provide an integrative framework for applying known facts and mechanisms of social, cognitive, and behavioral psychologies to the task of promoting widescale health-protective activity. In the remainder of this chapter, I examine how these perspectives enhance our ability to promote heart-healthy behavior in children and their families.

STATE MODEL OF HEALTH PROTECTIVE ACTION

A state model of self-protective action is depicted in Fig. 11.1. The model defines the goal of health promotion as the creation of a self-sustaining equilibrium between health protective behaviors and the effects they generate. The model provides a goal, or criterion, for effective self-regulation. It presents an idealized view of a system that is continually changing in response to external and internal demands. Such a view is valuable, nonetheless, because it specifies the critical or defining features of sustained self-protective action. These include diet and exercise behaviors, for example, their experienced effects, and microsocial influences moderating connections between these behaviors and their outcomes.

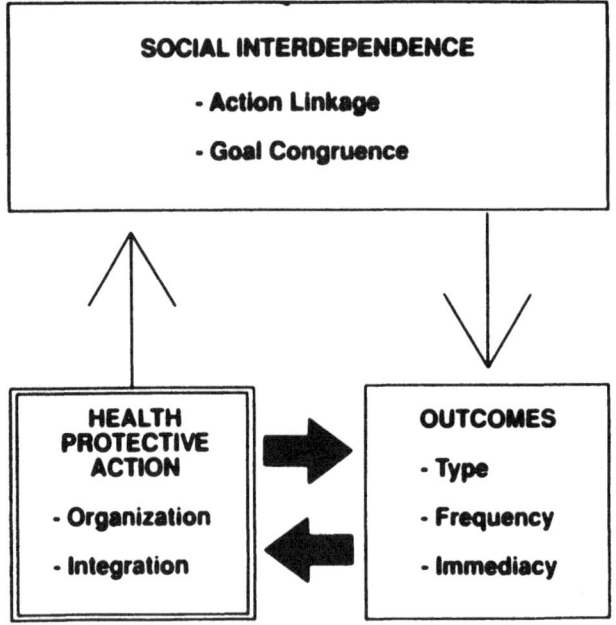

FIG. 11.1. *Action State* model of self-protective behavior. Habitual routines entail negative feedback loops that are extensively interconnected with the routines of intimate others. From Ewart (1991). Social action theory for a public health psychology. *American Psychologist, 46,* 931–946. Copyright (1991) by the American Psychological Association. Reprinted by permission.

Health Protective Action

Actions that are frequent or sustained tend to exhibit a high level of *organization,* that is, they are comprised of predictable action sequences, behavior chains, or "scripts," in which successive events in an action sequence reinforce preceding events while guiding or prompting subsequent action (Kazdin, 1984). Disruption of a highly established action sequence is frustrating and prompts vigorous effort to complete the action that was blocked. Indeed, the amount of effort one will expend to complete a disrupted action sequence, including how much one ruminates about sequences that cannot be completed (Klinger, 1975), indicates the extent to which the activity in question has become established as a persisting component of one's behavioral repertoire. Well-established behavioral routines also tend to co-occur with other behaviors in predictable "clusters." Such patterns tend to be idiosyncratic but highly stable within individuals (Baer, 1981; Kazdin, 1982). For example, as families take up exercising, their social and work activities may come to be organized around exercise routines, and a hierarchy of pursuits may be developed for occasions when preferred activities cannot be performed.

Integration is a second characteristic of actions that are performed frequently: One can do them without consciously attending to the component actions that comprise the larger pattern. As action sequences become better organized with frequent practice, attention shifts to their consequences rather than to features of the act itself (Abelson, 1981). The ability to engage in exercise or food preparation activities "unconsciously," while attending to other matters, indexes the degree to which that activity has become a well-developed component of one's usual routine. Behaviors that have become well established also acquire *reinforcement value,* that is, the opportunity to perform the behavior can become an inducement to engage in less well-established activities (Timberlake & Allison, 1974).

The preceding action characteristics provide concrete goals for interventions to promote self-protective activities: Programs must help parents and children construct smoothly flowing, well-rehearsed action scripts appropriate to the variety of situations and settings in which they function daily. These scripts must be organized within the larger structure of one's activities, and a hierarchy of alternative action sequences should be created for occasions when preferred scripts cannot be performed.

Consequences

An action's organization, integration, and reinforcement value are *contingent* upon effects the action generates. First, an act must produce consequences that are valued by the actor. The *type* of outcome that makes a behavior worth performing can vary greatly from person to person and does not necessarily correspond to the changes in health or risk status that are targeted by intervention programs. People may engage in health protective activities to obtain material outcomes, social status or support, favorable self-appraisals, or because they feel good. The Action State model says that behaviors are more likely to be maintained if they generate outcomes that are strongly desired, occur soon after the behavior is performed, and are frequently experienced. Arrows between the Action and Consequences boxes in Fig. 11.1 indicate that actions and their outcomes constitute a negative feedback loop; the experienced or threatened loss of an outcome causes increased effort to obtain that outcome.

This feedback function suggests that the starting place for developing intervention goals is with an analysis of the relationship between desired action sequences and their potential consequences. Such analysis often reveals behavior chains comprising an orderly temporal sequence in which component behavioral events are causally linked. Terminal components frequently are valued goals or reinforcers for earlier events in the sequence, suggesting that later behaviors in the action chain are harder to change because they are temporally closer to reinforcement (Kazdin, 1984). Thus, if one wants to disrupt an undesired action sequence, one should try to prevent the earlier events from occurring as they are weakly reinforced and hence easier to disrupt. It is easier to disrupt an action sequence leading to ice cream consumption by deleting ice cream from the weekly shopping list than by purchasing it and trying not to take it out of the refrigerator when tempted.

On the other hand, if one wants to encourage a new action sequence, it is best to start by encouraging behaviors close to the terminal goal because they will be more quickly reinforced by goal attainment. For example, if an objective is to help families reduce dietary fat consumption, it is best to invite them first to enjoy a delicious low-fat meal, then involve them in meal preparation, followed by lessons on how to shop for needed ingredients, and, finally, how to develop convenient meal plans for the months ahead (Ewart, 1989a).

Social Interdependence

An individual's frequently performed action sequences tend to become interconnected with, and altered by, the actions of others. Observational studies of family interactions disclose patterns of reciprocal interpersonal influence and interdependence that can shape people's actions in ways of which they may be unaware (Gottman & Levenson, 1986; Patterson, 1982). The Action State model suggests how these influences may be incorporated into the analysis of individual health protective actions.

Family members experience satisfaction or distress in the degree to which they are able to establish highly routinized action sequences leading to valued outcomes or goals related to work, recreation, leisure, and self-care (Berscheid, 1983; Berscheid, Snyder, & Omoto, 1989). Important action scripts frequently serve several goals; for example, in preparing dinner together, a husband and wife may achieve the goal of satisfying their hunger while also attaining goals relating to their need for companionship, information, or problem solving. The very act of sharing household tasks may satisfy the goal of being assured that other family members are committed to family life. Disruption of valued routines may cause frustration and dysphoria if valued goals cannot be attained via other means (Mandler, 1975), especially if the disruption occurs at a point in the action sequence that is temporally close to the terminal goal. If the disruption is perceived to be unjustified or preventable, the disruption may cause anger (Averill, 1982; Shaver, Schwartz, Kirson, & O'Connor, 1987).

In families, action sequences leading to important goals often become interconnected such that one person's ability to complete a highly practiced routine depends on the actions of other family members. Thus, shared meal preparation may require both partners to arrive home by a specified time, a contingency that renders each individual's action sequence vulnerable to disruption by the other partner. This vulnerability to disrupted action, and attendant emotion, can be said to define "interdependence," or the degree of "closeness" in social relationships (Berscheid, 1983). The birth of children often fosters greater interdependence within a marriage because parents must cooperate in child care if each is to attain valued goals. A parent's routines also become interlinked with those of the child, and siblings tend to develop numerous linked action sequences, especially if they are close in age. The degree of interdependence within a family is a function of the number and importance of shared routines, which in turn will vary with family members' outside involvment in work and social activities, and the number, age, and spacing of children.

As members of a family or other social unit become more interdependent, their ability to regulate their actions and achieve valued goals is more easily threatened by changes in another family member's activities. Modification of diet or exercise patterns by one family member has the potential to affect other family members' happiness, making it difficult for otherwise well-meaning family members to provide needed assistance and emotional support. Note that the disruptiveness of participating in health behavior change is predicted by family members' degree of *action linkage,* or interdependence, and not by the affection they feel for each other or for the family unit. Action linkage and degree of satisfaction with marital or family relationships are separate constructs; interdependence pertains to the number of activities family members depend on each other to perform in order to achieve valued goals, whereas satisfaction with a relationship reflects the perception that one's goals are being met. No matter how happy or unhappy people feel about their family or marriage, their reaction to another family member's behavior change will depend on the degree to which it disrupts their ability to attain valued goals, an impact that is likely to be greater in families with higher levels of interdependence.

The notion of action linkage, or interdependence, organizes and clarifies phenomena of close social relationships that otherwise are hard to explain. Interdependence explains why seemingly happy families with strong interpersonal bonds can be incapable of supporting a family member's efforts to change diet or exercise habits. Interdependence implies that families with many interlinked scripts will be more negatively affected, regardless of their level of happiness. When behavioral regimens appear to effect little visible improvement, those who persist in helping may become exhausted and depressed (Coyne, Ellard, & Smith, 1990).

Interdependence has important implications for establishing action goals in behavior change. First, success in behavior change may well depend on the extent to which the suggested changes disrupt important action sequences of persons with whom the subject is interdependent. Widely used measures of social support may fail to predict the degree of disruption as they measure relationship satisfaction rather than action linkage. Recently developed assessment approaches like the Relationship Closeness Inventory of Berscheid and her colleagues may prove more useful (Berscheid et al., 1989). Second, interdependence implies that other family members should be included in counseling designed to help them identify important goals and action sequences that are threatened by change, and to devise ways of being supportive that do not endanger access to important outcomes.

Although systematic study of action linkage in health care contexts has yet to be undertaken, recent research on coping with the illness of a spouse or with separation from a close family member has produced findings that suggest this is a promising area for investigation. In a study of women suffering from arthritis, Manne and Zautra (1989) found that wives who reported their husbands provided little coping support exhibited poorer adjustment as evidenced by activity restriction and pain indices. Husbands' lack of support was related to complaints about the ways their wives' condition had disrupted their daily routines or altered their lifestyles. In a study of young adults, the behavior of the one "most important person" in the subject's life explained most of the day-to-day variance in reports of subjective well-being, thus supporting the interdependence hypothesis (Ruehlman & Wolchik, 1988).

Useful applications of interdependence in health interventions require that two implications of the hypothesis be investigated further. The first is the notion that interconnected action sequences play a primary role in shaping family influences in long-term behavior change. Although excessive fears of illness (especially in contagious disease) and discrepant health beliefs may affect family members' desire to be supportive (Lichtman et al., 1984), the present model holds that the disruption or facilitation of linked action scripts has a more immediate and powerful impact on family members' proclivity to resist or even sabotage sustained diet and exercise changes. The degree of script linkage can be indexed by the number, frequency, and importance of family members' shared routines, making it possible to evaluate the relative importance of interdependence, illness fears, and health beliefs.

The second factor to investigate is the role of goal "congruence": Activity disruptions that prevent intimate others from attaining valued goals are expected to stimulate opposition, whereas interruptions that facilitate goal attainment should foster support. For example, where family members want to spend more time together, a walking program that facilitates this may engender more support than might a clinic-based program that does not. Measures of goal congruence (facilitation) could be obtained by having patient and partner rate the importance and self-consequences of the patient's engaging in recommended health protective activities. The interdependence model predicts that people who find that many of their *shared* routines are interrupted by behavior changes will report greater dysphoria and stress during self-change attempts and are likely to fail than are people who engage in (a) many shared activities that are *congruent* with change, or (b) health endangering behavior patterns that are not embedded in routines they share with important others.

Interdependence also implies that family structure may be a risk factor: Child compliance with diet or exercise changes should be affected by the degree to which action patterns are linked with those of siblings, or with the parent(s) who plays the dominant role in food selection and preparation. The number and type of activities shared with playmates also should affect compliance. Future intervention research could develop and evaluate techniques specifically designed to help parents and children "uncouple" vulnerable action sequences from shared, incongruent sequences, and to replace these with shared, congruent activities.

PROCESS MODEL OF HEALTH PROTECTIVE ACTION

The action state model identifies critical features of habitual health routines but fails to represent processes by which stable action states are created. Figure 11.2 presents a *process* model organizing present knowledge about how to establish new, self-sustaining action systems. This model supplements the negative feedback loop (Fig. 11.1) with "feedforward" processes that enable people to generate new action goals, strategies, and environments (Ford, 1987). The model rejects the widespread notion that changes in health behavior flow directly from changes in health knowledge, beliefs, attitudes, or contingencies of reinforcement. Instead, prolonged health behavior change is the product of sustained *problem solving*. Whereas motivation can be enhanced through skillfully crafted argument and appropriate reinforcement, habit change demands the redesigning of well-established scripts and routines, a task requiring some degree of creative thought. Problem solving is an ability in which people are known to differ and a skill they can be taught. The social action model holds that cognitive problem-

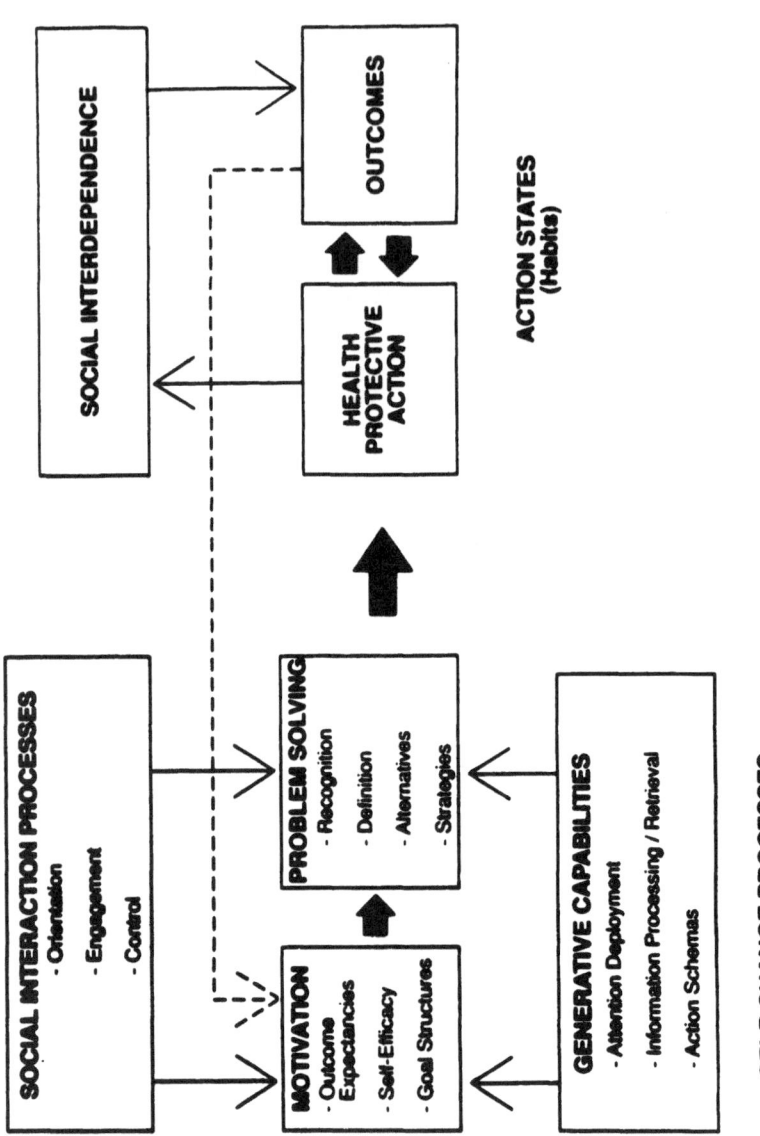

FIG. 11.2. *Process* (self-change) model of self-protective action. Habit change occurs only in the degree that motivational appraisal processes stimulate effective problem solving; motivation and problem solving both depend on the presence of personal generative capabilities and supportive social interactions. From Ewart (1991). Social action theory for a public health psychology. *American Psychologist, 46,* 931–946. Copyright (1991) by the American Psychological Association. Reprinted by permission.

solving activities are the *fulcrum* of the behavior change process; as indicated in Fig. 11.2, they *mediate* the relationship between motivation and behavior change. Efforts to change diet or exercise patterns will succeed only to the degree that they model and reward the extended application of a problem-solving approach.

Problem solving is stimulated by motivational appraisal processes, comprised of outcome expectations and perceptions of personal agency, as well as self-directive goal setting and evaluative activities. Yet these appraisals foster problem solving only if one posesses critical generative capabilities and if facilitative social interaction processes characterize one's interpersonal milieu. Generative skills and social interaction processes thus can be said to *moderate* the link between motivation to change and engagement in problem-solving activities needed to alter established patterns. Note also that proposed action processes are linked to action states (Action State Model) via the feedback function indicated by the broken line in Fig. 11.2. Disruption of an action state (e.g., by illness or injury) leads to reappraisal with potential for renewed problem solving, just as changes in appraisal can disrupt—via new problem-solving efforts—well-established action states.

Problem Solving

The need to change diet or exercise patterns confronts children and their families with many situations that demand a response for effective functioning, but for which no effective response is immediately apparent or available (D'Zurilla & Goldfried, 1971). Problem solving refers to the process by which families create new scripts, thereby discovering "solutions" to these problems. Research conducted over the past several decades reveals that children and adults display significant individual differences in their ability to generate new effective solutions to everyday problems, and that these skills can be enhanced through appropriate instruction (D'Zurilla, 1986; Nezu 1986; Nezu & Perri, 1989). Skill enhancement generally has involved teaching individuals to: (a) anticipate in advance situations where familiar scripts may prove inadequate; (b) generate a variety of ways to cope with anticipated threats; (c) use appropriate criteria to evaluate these alternatives; (d) select a coping strategy that is likely to work; and (e) decide on a specific course of action.

The success of dietary or other behavioral intervention depends on the degree to which training stimulates problem-solving activity. Including problem-solving training in behavioral treatment programs enhances weight reduction in obese adults (Black & Scherba, 1983) and children (Graves, Meyers, & Clark, 1988) more than does providing intervention without problem-solving instruction, or no treatment. In an evaluation of parent-administered treatments for obese children, weight reductions were correlated with posttreatment gains in parental problem-solving skill, supporting the view tha problem-solving competence affected the degree to which behavioral instruction and reinforcement interventions helped parents alter their childrens' eating habits. Research on problem-solving skills in children treated for high blood lipids reveals an association between adolescents' ability to solve hypothetical dietary problems and their adherence to lipid-lowering diets (Hanna, Ewart, & Kwiterovich, 1990).

In a different health context, a study of children with phenylketonuria (PKU) has shown that parents of children in good dietary control generated better solutions to hypothetical diet behavior problems than did parents of children in poor dietary control (Fehrenbach & Peterson, 1989). Other research in adults with Type II diabetes mellitus has disclosed that problem-solving skills predict adherence to exercise, glucose testing, and dietary regimens in diabetes self-care (Glasgow, Toobert, Riddle, Donelly, & Calder, 1989). Methods to assess dietary problem-solving skills have been developed for adults (Fehrenbach & Peterson, 1989; Glasgow et al., 1989), and for children and adolescents (Hanna, Ewart, & Kwiterovich, 1990), enabling researchers to identify individuals at risk for failure in behavior change and to assess the impact of problem-solving interventions. The social action model predicts that adding problem-solving training to motivational inducements will be especially helpful to persons whose dietary or exercise problem-solving skills initially are low.

Motivational Processes

People do not work very hard at solving problems unless they have compelling reasons to do so. In the present model, problem-solving efforts are stimulated by motivational appraisal processes, which include outcome expectancies, self-efficacy, and self-evaluative subprocesses.

Outcome Expectancies. Findings from a variety of research programs (Janz & Becker, 1984; Rogers, 1983) indicate that decisions to adopt health-protective behaviors are influenced by expectations concerning outcome *contingency*—the belief that an action will protect or enhance valued resources—and *value*—the importance accorded the outcome. These expectations involve anticipated intrinsic aspects of the activity itself, as well as its more extrinsic outcomes (Lepper & Greene, 1978). As Leventhal and his associates have demonstrated, outcome expectancies that shape health decisions often are based on misguided "personal theories of illness" (Bauman & Leventhal, 1985; Leventhal, Meyer, & Nerenz, 1980). Outcomes that are highly visible, affect valued resources, and are likely to occur immediately, or often, are more likely to prompt problem solving than are less visible, less important, more delayed, or infrequent outcomes.

Expectancies encouraged by health communications often lack power because they warn of outcomes children and adolescents perceive to be extremely delayed, uncertain, or remote from everyday experience. Often, young people are influenced more by such comparatively immediate outcomes as the opportunity to belong to a group that exercises together or tries out new foods, to look better, to feel more energetic, or to engage in new recreational pursuits. The reasons adults give for dropping out of exercise programs to enhance cardiovascular health tend to reflect immediate punishing experiences such as injury, fatigue, or difficulty getting to the exercise site, rather than the perception that risk reduction was not attainable through physical exertion (Oldridge, 1982). Children display individual differences in the extent to which their food choices are guided by nutritional expectations, with greater concern about nutrition appearing as children mature (Michela & Contento, 1986).

Self-Efficacy Appraisal. The mere belief that change is desirable does not necessarily stimulate problem solving; one must believe one is capable of taking the required action (Bandura, 1977, 1986a, 1986b, 1989). Self-perceptions of ability are specific: Confidence in one's ability to engage in jogging does not necessarily generalize to confidence in one's ability to lift weights (Ewart, Stewart, Gillilan, & Keleman, 1986a). Bandura (1977) has identified four major sources of information that shape self-perceptions of ability (i.e., self-efficacy). Listed in order of their power to influence actions, these sources include: (a) prior experiences performing similar behaviors, (b) opportunities to observe others similar to oneself performing the actions in question, (c) persuasion by a respected authority, and (d) feedback from internal physiologic states. Generally speaking, the most effective way to increase self-confidence for an activity is to have an individual perform it in gradually increasing doses while providing reassuring feedback and counseling.

In cardiovascular health, self-efficacy appraisals influence patients' motivation to resume normal routines including participating in rehabilitative exercise (Ewart, 1989b; Ewart et al., 1986a, 1986b; Ewart, Taylor, Reese, & DeBusk, 1983; Taylor, Bandura, Ewart, Miller, & DeBusk, 1985). Patients with higher initial confidence in their abilities have been shown to demonstrate greater strength gains following exercise training, suggesting higher initial self-efficacy fostered greater involvement in—and benefit from—the training tasks (Ewart et al., 1986a). Research on children's ability appraisals in behavior change is limited but suggestive. In a study of conduct-disordered children referred for therapy (Weisz, 1986), children's pretreatment perceptions of their ability to control problem situations at home and at school predicted reductions in behavior problems reported by parents after 6 months of therapy. The relationship between perceived self-competence and problem solving in therapy was strongest in 12- to 17-year olds, a finding compatible with other evidence suggesting that children do not fully comprehend the relationship between abilities and outcomes until about age 12 (Nicholls & Miller, 1984).

In adolescents with insulin-dependent diabetes mellitus, a positive relationship between measures of life stress and metabolic control indexed by averaged glycostated hemoglobin levels was attenuated in adolescents who reported high levels of confidence in their personal and social skills (Hanson, Henggeler, & Burghen, 1987), supporting a relationship between self-efficacy and regimen compliance in this age group. Given these encouraging results, an important question for further research concerns ways in which children's interactions with family members and peers shape their perceptions of their abilities in various domains, as well as the developmental sequence by which these perceptions come to exert increasing influence on health behavior.

Goal Appraisal. Although we often speak of health behaviors as if they were isolated responses, they usually are found to belong to larger "clusters" or structures of action sequences directed toward some greater goal. Smoking, avoiding exercise, eating fast foods, and experimenting with alcohol or drugs all may serve an adolescent's goal of belonging to an attractive peer group (Donovan, Jessor, & Costa, 1988). These structures, known variously as "projects" (Little, 1983) or "strivings" (Emmons, 1986), have important implications for subjective well-being and distress, with positive affect being related to the perception that important strivings are being fulfilled, and negative affect being associated with low expectations of striving success or with conflict among one's diverse strivings (Emmons, 1986; Ruehlman, 1985; Ruehlman & Wolchik, 1988). In the present model, these goal structures serve a *directive* function, guiding people into activities and environments that affect their ability to respond to behavior change inducements (Ford, 1987). Moreover, project goals contain *self-evaluative* criteria that influence one's sense of personal efficacy during behavior change attempts.

Health behavior changes that are seen to facilitate important strivings are more likely to be adopted than changes that are viewed as incompatible, even if the latter are considered desirable and feasible. People whose projects include strivings aimed at achieving physical attractiveness, popularity, athletic competence, or longevity should find diet or exercise changes easier to accommodate than people whose personal projects do not embody these strivings (Eiser & Gentle, 1988). Goals that appear incompatible sometimes can be resolved at a higher level of a goal hierarchy; for example, conflict between a career advancement project requiring that every available moment be spent on work, and a health project requiring regular jogging, might be resolved by viewing physical exercise as a source of energy needed to pursue one's professional goals. Methods to help people reflect upon their own projects and goal hierarchies are exemplified in the "values confrontation" method of Rokeach (1973). A recent experiment using values confrontation to support a dietary counseling intervention suggests the technique may facilitate clinic-based weight loss (Schwartz & Inbar-Saban, 1988).

In addition to developing directive goals, people formulate self-standards by which to evaluate the *adequacy* of their efforts. Research by social learning theorists has shown that children are more likely to emulate self-standards modeled by individuals they perceive to be similar to themselves (Bandura & Whalen, 1966), who consistently apply to themselves criteria they use to evaluate others, and who apply the same standard across a variety of tasks (Bandura & Mahoney, 1974).

An important question in designing health behavior interventions is how to create performance standards that will motivate involvement in behavioral tasks necessary to diet or activity change. The optimal rate of behavior change in a health-promoting intervention depends on the kind of superordinate goal the program is seen to serve. If a participant sees the intervention as serving projects aimed at achieving specific end states such as lowering disease risk indices, or altering physical appearance, then a progression of easy goals is recommended (Hyland, 1988). To the extent that the intervention is seen to serve an action goal such as increasing self-mastery or demonstrating self-control, moderately challenging goals are preferred (Atkinson, 1957; Bandura & Schunk, 1981; McClelland, 1951).

Hierarchical Integration of Motivational Influences

Outcome expectancies, self-efficacy, and goal structures can be viewed as interconnected processes in that changes in one motivational component can affect the functioning of the others. Self-efficacy perceptions are influenced by the degree of success one experiences in obtaining desired outcomes. Self-directive and evaluative goal structures are shaped by the amount and type of reinforcement one experiences in various activities, and by experienced ability to control important outcomes (self-efficacy). A social action analysis suggests, moreover, that personal projects will affect the degree to which self-efficacy appraisals influence actions, and beliefs about behavior–outcome contingencies will vary with differing perceptions of personal agency.

Generative Capabilities

Solving a problem, foreseeing the results of one's actions, or formulating a goal draw upon diverse forms of schematic knowledge or generative capabilities. Procedural skills and knowledge schemata enable one to attend to environmental and internal stimuli, formulate rules concerning behavior–outcome relationships, generate novel solutions to problems, and execute effective behavior sequences. Research on coping with cravings and discomforts that accompany health behavior change has shown that coping is enhanced by learning to attend to distracting stimuli, and to transform aversive stimuli into less threatening ones (Cioffi, 1991; McCaul & Malott, 1984). Self-motivation involves the ability to focus one's attention on positive outcomes of desired acts and negative outcomes of undesired behavior (Kanfer, 1980).

The importance of children's attention deployment skills in self-regulation is suggested by research on delay of gratification. In the paradigm studied, the child could choose to consume a small-sized food treat immediately or else wait to receive a larger food treat later. Preschooler's waiting time greatly decreases when the small treat remains in view during the waiting interval (Mischel & Ebbesen, 1970), but they delay longer when instructed to distract themselves (Mischel, Ebbesen, & Zeiss, 1972). Various delay strategies were evaluated in a series of experiments; the most effective was instructing the child to focus on the abstract ("cool") aspects of the treats, such as their shape. Focussing on "hot" aspects of the treats, such as their taste, substantially decreased the child's ability to wait for the larger reward (Mischel, 1984). Extension of this work to older children (6 to 12 years) with behavior problems disclosed that delay behavior was related to the attention deployment strategies used during delay, knowledge of delay rules, and intelligence (Rodriguez, Mischel, & Shoda, 1989). As the duration of the waiting interval and the frustrative aspects of the situation increased, children who spent a higher proportion of the time distracting themselves were able to delay longer. Attention deployment and delay rule knowledge each made signficant and unique contributions to delay time when age and intelligence were controlled.

These studies suggest that acquisition of delay skills may influence goals, self-efficacy, and outcome perceptions in motivation, while affecting one's ability to engage in reflective problem solving in the face of temptation. Support for this notion is found in population surveys of eating behaviors (Slater, 1989). Respondents' perceived ability to control distressing thoughts and ruminations ("cognitive control") predicted their self-efficacy for controlling eating behavior, and self-efficacy (but not cognitive control) predicted their eating habits. Experimental analyses of cognitions affecting self-efficacy on a laboratory task disclose that focussing one's attention on factors that could impair performance decreases self-efficacy, and that self-efficacy reductions subsequently impair performance (Cervone, 1989).

Other important generative skills are suggested by research on information processing: Decoding rules affect interpretation of events, thus influencing one's ability to predict important outcomes on the basis of internal and environmental stimuli (Bandura, 1986b). Studies of parent–child interactions have established that mothers who use few observational categories when describing their children's behavior problems are less accurate in detecting positive and deviant child behaviors apparent to an independent observer than are mothers who employ many categories (Wahler & Hann, 1984). A tendency to use few descriptive categories is associated with a tendency to respond inappropriately to prosocial and deviant behaviors in their children (Wahler & Dumas, 1989).

In addition to attention deployment and processing strategies, factual or "declarative" knowledge schemata (e.g., models of illness) influence peoples' ability to anticipate outcomes, appraise their capabilities, and formulate behavioral goals (Meyer, Leventhal, & Gutman, 1985; Weinstein, 1988) Knowledge sche mata can be changed through social modeling (Winett, King, & Altman, 1989) and by providing corrective information according to principles that facilitate cognitive encoding and retrieval (Ley, 1977). The present model asserts, however, that these interventions will alter health behavior only in the degree that they facilitate goal, self-efficacy, and outcome appraisals conducive to effective problem solving.

Social Interaction

The fact of social interdependence implies that self-change involves more than one's own capabilities and appraisals—it also depends on the capabilities of the social microsystems of which one is a part. With time, close interpersonal relationships come to be characterized by stable patterns of interaction that serve partners' goals; to promote self-change, it frequently is necessary to enhance the competence of the relationship system by fostering interaction processes that permit effective problem solving.

Orientation processes involve interactions that help participants apprehend each other's concerns, strivings, or projects. Problem solving is greatly facilitated when parties to a disagreement are able to identify the other's objectives, generate multiple relationship goals, separate conflict in one project context from other relationship goals and contexts, and endorse or "validate" at least some of the other's important strivings (Gottman, Notarius, Gonso, & Markman, 1976). Observational studies of distressed and nondistressed couples have shown that validation is facilitated by *engagement processes* including verbal and nonverbal behaviors to signal attentive listening, summarizing and paraphrasing the other to clarify communications and discern their true intent, and voicing complaints in terms of behavior patterns that can be changed instead of vague personality traits that cannot. There now is considerable evidence that familial conflict can be reduced by improving these skills (Jacobson & Holtzworth-Munroe, 1986). This research also demonstrates the value of strengthening relationship *control* processes by helping partners set clear and attainable goals, develop action plans, and monitor their implementation.

Most research relating family variables to health has relied on questionnaire measures of perceived family environment or support, rather than directly measuring or manipulating family interactions. Family members' reports that they feel free to express feelings and discuss problems, and that their family is supportive, have been positively related to compliance with treatment regimens in a variety of chronic diseases (Anderson, Miller, Auslander, & Santiago, 1981; Finney, Moos, & Mewborn, 1980; Hauser et al., 1985; Kirschenbaum, Harris, & Tomarken, 1984; Patterson, 1985).

Observational studies of family behavior provide a more direct test of processes envisaged in the social action model of personal change. This work reveals interaction processes affecting children and adults in ways detrimental to cardiovascular health. For example, frequent marital conflict has been found to make parents behave more punitively toward their children (Webster-Stratton, 1988), potentially undercutting efforts to secure compliance with diet and exercise changes. Parents who dictate menus and food choices during a family meal-planning task elicit more negative reactions to low-fat foods from their children than do parents who encourage their children to offer their own menu suggestions (Hanna, Ewart, & Kwiterovich, 1990). Familial conflict also may affect the cardiovascular system more directly; observation of marital conflict discloses that hostile communications during marital arguments increase blood pressure in hypertensive adults (Ewart, Burnett, & Taylor, 1983; Ewart, Taylor, Kraemer, & Agras, 1991), and that teaching couples to use positive engagement skills decreases cardiovascular reactivity during disagreements (Ewart, Taylor, Kraemer, & Agras, 1984).[3]

Social action theory predicts greater dietary and exercise compliance in families whose members are able to report shared goals and projects, who describe their conflicts in terms of specific situations and behaviors; and who often work together to set goals and evaluate their attainment. In these families, children and adults will be more likely to report that others support their change efforts, will report higher self-efficacy for behavior change, and will list fewer immediate negative consequences for changing than will children in families lacking the previously specified characteristics. Behavioral intervention to enhance these orientation, engagement, and control skills in families experiencing conflict related to diet and exercise changes represents a promising yet little studied approach to improving compliance.

CONTEXTUAL DETERMINANTS OF HEALTH PROTECTIVE ACTION

It is well known that one's ability to engage in health protective activities is affected by one's cultural environment and social class, one's biological condition, temperament, current mood, and level of maturation. The challenge to preventive intervention, however, is to explain how, when, and why these static structural categories exert their behavioral effects. This question is critical because within even the most socially or biologically disadvantaged groups there can be wide differences in personal willingness and ability to alter health-endangering behavior patterns.

In a social action view, biological and social structural factors create con-

---

[3]Omitted from the present discussion is Minuchin's application of family systems theory to anorexia nervosa. Although this treatment approach has been widely accepted by clinicians (Minuchin, Rosman, & Baker 1978), it is not well supported by research in heterogeneous groups of anorectic patients and their families (Kog, Vertommen, & Vandereyken, 1987).

textual influences that, by constraining or augmenting self-regulatory processes, can disrupt or facilitate self-sustaining action states. Contextual factors shown in Fig. 3.3 directly affect motivational appraisal, as well as generative capabilities and social interaction processes, thus influencing problem solving to achieve diet or exercise changes.

Social Settings and Relationships

Social settings include one's *physical* environment, *tasks* one routinely performs, and *people* with whom one interacts on a regular basis. By affecting access to recommended foods and to convenient, safe, and comfortable places to exercise, the physical environment of neighborhood or workplace affects expectations concerning possible outcomes of diet or exercise attempts. Noise, crowding, and extremes of temperature can detrimentally affect attentional control and related generative capabilities (Anderson, 1989). Social contacts in neighborhood or at work expose people to *social models* that exhibit behavior–outcome relationships ("values," "norms") and facilitate or inhibit actions such as exercising, eating, or smoking (Kniskern et al., 1983; Rosenthal & McSweeney, 1979). The nature of one's occupational or other routine tasks can affect perceptions of personal agency (Frese, 1982; Kohn & Schooler, 1982) and may induce cognitive sets that enhance or diminish one's ability to process health-relevant information (Lehman, Lempert, & Nisbett, 1988). The availability of supportive others affects the ways people construe and evaluate the consequences of health behavior change; families with limited incomes and few people to turn to are at greater risk of dropping out of behavioral parent training programs (Blechman et al., 1981). Although social resources in the form of people who can assist one's change efforts facilitate compliance (Sallis et al., 1987), receiving this support imposes the potentially demanding obligation to help one's helpers when they are in need (Riley & Eckenrode, 1986).

Biological Contexts

One's biological condition, including level of maturation, affects personal generative capabilities, shaping the ways children or adults perceive outcome contingencies, appraises their abilities, and generates self-change strategies (Hanna et al., 1991; Nicholls & Miller, 1984). Biologically based temperamental differences influence preferences for social interaction, tolerance of novel stimuli, and impulsivity, thus rendering some individuals more susceptible to social influences than others (Goldsmith et al., 1987).

Finally, the preceding biological and social influences interactively foster mood states reflecting combinations of energy level or "positive affect," and subjective distress or "negative affect" (Watson & Pennebaker, 1989). Moods affect one's ability to attend to novel health information, encode and retrieve it

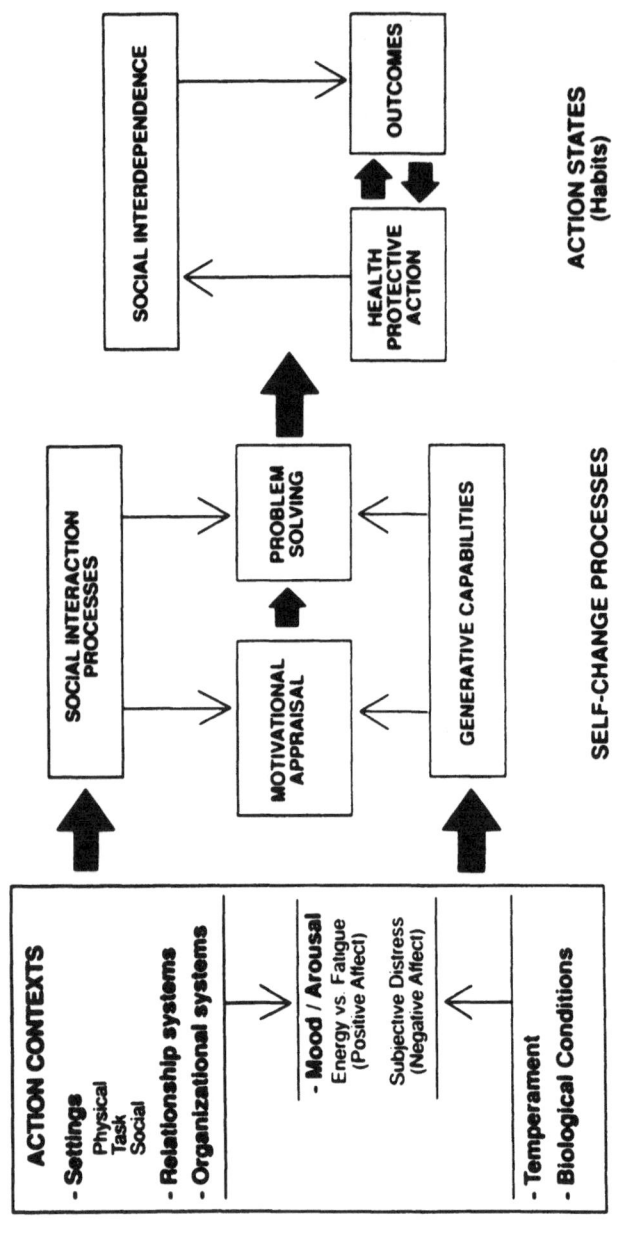

FIG. 11.3. *Contextual* model identifying social-environmental and biologic contexts that, by facilitating or inhibiting self-change processes, tend to foster or disrupt the maintenance of health-protective action states. From Ewart (1991). Social action theory for a public health psychology. *American Psychologist, 46,* 931–946. Copyright (1991) by the American Psychological Association. Reprinted by permission.

later, and may reduce one's ability to monitor one's behavior or appraise the long-term consequences of personal decisions (Jarvis, 1982; Petty & Cacioppo, 1986).

In specifying measurable *contexts* of behavior, the social action model identifies empirically testable pathways via which biological and social environments enhance or impede self-change efforts. The contextual model thereby enhances an intervention planner's ability to identify those persons within a particular social or health category who may be at greatest behavioral risk.

DEVELOPMENT OF COMPLIANCE CAPABILITIES

Social action theory provides a useful framework for understanding the development of behavioral compliance over the life span. Development is defined as the acquisition and use of self-protective capabilities; the course of development is determined by changes in biological and social environmental action contexts. These contextual changes facilitate or limit the degree to which individuals acquire core self-change competencies envisaged in the *process* model (Fig. 11.2); external agents (e.g., parents) can encourage healthy habits in others by manipulating situational cues and reinforcement contingencies, yet it is difficult for people to maintain these habits or create new ones if they lack needed self-regulatory goals and skills.

In a social action view, critical developmental events are those biological and social-contextual changes that enhance (or diminish) one's *generative capabilities* and that strengthen (or limit) the supportive competence of valued *interpersonal ties*. A contextual change of great significance in early life is the emergence of a capacity for concrete operations in thought, a transition that makes it possible for children to compare themselves to peers and appraise their personal capabilities more accurately. Improved self-comparison causes children to become less optimistic about their abilities, yet greater accuracy provides a more resilient basis for judgments of self-efficacy (Nicholls & Miller, 1984) and strengthens the child's ability to undertake and maintain new patterns of behavior. Moreover, an improved ability to form generalizations at this stage allows the child to use abstract categories such as "health" in anticipating outcomes and making behavioral choices, as when foods are selected for their strength-enhancing properties rather than for their sensory characteristics only (Michela & Contento, 1986).

As children enter adolescence they begin to encounter a wider range of social contexts and, as a result, begin to develop more differentiated conceptions of their abilities, preferences, and goals. These changes facilitate the creation of coherent personal projects that serve normative life tasks of making friends and formulating career plans. Although parents continue to influence the adolescent's choices with respect to fundamental moral values and long-term educational or occupational strivings, peers come to exert more influence on eating patterns and recreational pursuits. A project goal of winning peer acceptance may prove to be incompatible with health goals such as limiting high-fat food consumption or adhering to an exercise regimen.

Yet adolescence also sees important gains in generative capabilities needed to resolve goal conflicts and create coping strategies. The advent of formal operations thinking brings an enhanced ability to envisage hypothetical problem situations, to generate alternative strategies, and to weigh and select an effective course of action. Whereas involvement in a wider social network and range of settings has the potential to disrupt or inhibit health protective habits, improved cognitive capabilities permit the adolescent to create effective coping strategies if he or she is encouraged to learn and apply relevant social problem-solving skills (Hanna, Ewart, & Kwiterovich, 1990).

These developmental changes have implications for attempts to apply a social action model in behavioral intervention. Very young children cannot be expected to engage in self-change activities that would require them to appraise their capabilities accurately, formulate higher order goals, or engage in extensive cognitive problem-solving operations. Intervention in early childhood should aim at building favorable outcome expectancies by making healthy foods and activities as enjoyable as possible, and by exposing children to influential social models (e.g., parents and older siblings) whose health habits clearly exemplify the desired behaviors. In middle childhood, as children become more capable of making social comparisons and forming abstract categories, caregivers can impart fundamental self-regulatory skills by explaining behavior–outcome relationships, by providing explicit self-standards for desired health behaviors, by teaching children to set appropriate behavioral goals, and by providing supportive feedback and praise for goal attainment (Ewart & Cunningham, 1990). In adolescence, increased capacity for abstract thought makes it possible to teach and encourage the use of problem-solving skills for avoiding or managing difficult social situations. Due to the importance of peer-oriented goals and projects, problem-solving training with adolescents is more successful when provided in a peer group setting without parents present (Ewart, 1989a).

The ability to engage in self-protective activities is not stable in adulthood but changes as people pursue careers, raise families, and undertake other normative life tasks. Each task entails new projects with the potential to alter social contexts of behavior; these contextual changes can undermine or facilitate the creation and maintenance of desired action states. Important contextual changes also occur as a result of biological events such as illness, injury, or processes of aging. Whereas a full developmental account of self-protective capabilities is beyond the scope of this chapter, this brief overview should give the reader an idea of how the social action model may help explain variations in compliance behavior over the life span.

IMPLICATIONS

In a social action view, *compliance* is best understood as a process of acquiring and enhancing self-protective capabilities. The social action framework integrates disparate social, psychological, and behavioral perspectives in a tripartite model that clarifies self-change processes while suggesting new intervention approaches, hypotheses, and experiments. An action *state* perspective generates behavioral objectives for interventions to encourage sustained self-protective action. A model of self-change processes offers a blueprint for intervention planning by organizing the problem solving, motivational, cognitive skill, and social interactive components of self-change. Finally, a *contextual* model aids the planner in identifying social and biological structural factors that could impede critical self-change processes, thus making it easier to target vulnerable population subgroups.

The present approach represents a move away from narrowly individualistic conceptions of self-regulation that have characterized psychology, toward a more social-contextual perspective. Thus the notion of action linkage in social interdependence, and the emphasis on social interaction processes, focus attention on the interconnectedness of people's action goals and scripts, as well as the interactive "competence" of their relationship systems. Not only do these influences shape people's health outcome beliefs; they also affect their sense of personal agency, their goals, and their readiness to engage in practical problem-solving activities that translate motivation into sustained patterns of health protective behavior. The task of explaining how social-contextual processes operate to affect compliance at different points in the life span provides a stimulating and potentially fruitful agenda for compliance research.

ACKNOWLEDGMENT

Preparation of this chapter was supported in part by grant RO1–HL36298 from the National Heart, Lung, and Blood Institute.

REFERENCES

Abelson, R. P. (1981). Psychological status of the script concept. *American Psychologist, 36*, 715–729.

Anderson, B., Miller, J. P., Auslander, W., & Santiago, J. (1981). Family characteristics of diabetic adolescents: Relationship to metabolic control. *Diabetes Care, 4*, 586–594.

Anderson, C. A. (1989). Temperature and aggression: Ubiquitous effects of heat on occurrence of human violence. *Psychological Bulletin, 106*, 74–96.

Atkinson, J. W. (1957). Motivational determinants of risk-taking behavior. *Psychological Review, 64*, 359–372.
Averill, J. R. (1982). *Anger and aggression: An essay on emotion.* New York: Springer–Verlag.
Baer, D. M. (1981). The imposition of structure on behavior and the demolition of behavioral structures. In H. E. Howe, D. J. Bernstein, & R. G. Wahler (Eds.), *Nebraska Symposium on Motivation, 1981: Response structure and organization* (pp. 217–254). Lincoln: University of Nebraska Press.
Bandura, A. (1977). Self-efficacy: Toward a unifying theory of behavioral change. *Psychological Review, 84*, 191–215.
Bandura, A. (1986a). Self-efficacy mechanism in physiological activation and health-promoting behavior. In J. Madden IV, S. Matthysse, & J. Barchas (Eds.), *Adaptation, learning, and affect.* New York: Raven.
Bandura, A. (1986b). *Social foundations of thought and action.* Englewood Cliffs, NJ: Prentice–Hall.
Bandura, A. (1989). Human agency in social cognitive theory. *American Psychologist, 44*, 1175–1184.
Bandura, A., & Mahoney, M. J. (1974). Maintenance and transfer of self-reinforcement functions. *Behavior Research and Therapy, 12*, 89–97.
Bandura, A., & Schunk, D. H. (1981). Cultivating competence, self-efficacy, and intrinsic interest through proximal self-motivation. *Journal of Personality and Social Psychology, 41*, 586–598.
Bandura, A., & Whalen, C. K. (1966). The influence of antecedent reinforcement and divergent modeling cues on patterns of self-reward. *Journal of Personality and Social Psychology, 3*, 373–382.
Baumann, L. J., & Leventhal, H. (1985). "I can tell when my blood pressure is up, can't I?" *Health Psychology, 4*, 203–218.
Berscheid, E. (1983). Emotion. In H. Kelley, E. Berscheid, A. Christensen, J. H. Harvey, T. L. Huston, G. Levinger, E. McClintock, L. A. Peplau, & D. R. Peterson (Eds.), *Close relationships.* New York: Freeman.
Berscheid, E., Snyder, M., & Omoto, A. M. (1989). The relationship closeness inventory: Assessing the closeness of interpersonal relationships. *Journal of Personality and Social Psychology, 57*, 792–807.
Black, D. R., & Scherba, D. S. (1983). Contracting to problem solve versus contracting to practice behavioral weight loss skills. *Behavior Therapy, 14*, 100–109.
Blechman, E. A., Budd, K. S., Christopherson, E. R., Szykula, S., Wahler, R., Embry, L. H., Kogan, K., O'Leary, K. D., & Riner, L. S. (1981). Engagement in behavioral family therapy: A multisite investigation. *Behavior Therapy, 12*, 461–472.
Cervone, D. (1989). Effects of envisioning future activites on self-efficacy judgments and motivation: An availability heuristic interpretation. *Cognitive Therapy and Research, 13*, 247–261.
Cioffi, D. (1991). Beyond attentional strategies: A cognitive-perceptual model of somatic interpretation. *Psychological Bulletin, 109*, 25–41.
Coyne, J. C., Ellard, J. H., & Smith, D. A. F. (1990). Social support, interdependence, and the dilemmas of helping. In B. R. Sarason, I. G. Sarason, & G. R. Pierce (Eds.), *Social support: An interactional view* (pp. 129–149). New York: Wiley.
DiClemente, C. C., Prochaska, J. O., Fairhurst, S. K., Velicer, W. F., Velasquez, M. M., & Rossi, J. S. (1991). The process of smoking cessation: An analysis of precontemplation, contemplation, and preparation stages of change. *Journal of Consulting and Clinical Psychology, 59*, 295–304.
Donovan, J. E., Jessor, R., & Costa, F. M. (1988). Syndrome of problem behavior in adolescence: A replication. *Journal of Consulting and Clinical Psychology, 56*, 762–765.
D'Zurilla, T. J. (1986). *Problem solving therapy: A social competence approach to clinical intervention.* New York: Springer.

D'Zurilla, R. J., & Goldfried, M. R. (1971). Problem solving and behavior modification. *Journal of Abnormal Psychology, 78,* 107–126.

Eiser, R. J., & Gentle, P. (1988). Health behavior as goal-directed action. *Journal of Behavioral Medicine, 11,* 523–535.

Emmons, R. A. (1986). Personal strivings: An approach to personality and subjective well-being. *Journal of Personality and Social Psychology, 51,* 1058–1068.

Ewart, C. K. (1989a). Changing dietary behavior: A social action theory approach. *Clinical Nutrition, 8,* 9–16.

Ewart, C. K. (1989b). Psychological effects of resistive weight training: Implications for cardiac patients. *Medicine and Science in Sports and Exercise, 21,* 683–689.

Ewart, C. K. (1991). Social action theory for a public health psychology. *American Psychologist, 46,* 931–946.

Ewart, C. K., Burnett, K. F., & Taylor, C. B. (1983). Communication behaviors that affect blood pressure: An A–B–A–B analysis of marital interaction. *Behavior Modification, 7* (3), 331–344.

Ewart, C. K., & Cunningham, S. (1990). Elevated blood pressure. In A. M. Gross & R. S. Drabman (Eds.), *Handbook of clinical behavioral pediatrics.* New York, Plenum Press.

Ewart, C. K., Stewart, K. J., Gillilan, R. E., Kelemen, M. H. (1986a). Self-efficacy mediates strength gains during circuit weight training in men with coronary artery disease. *Medicine and Science in Sports and Exercise, 18,* 531–540.

Ewart, C. K., Stewart, K. J., Gillilan, R. E., Keleman, M. H., Valenti, S. A., Manley, J. D., & Kelemen, M. D. (1986b). Usefulness of self-efficacy in predicting overexertion during programmed exercise in coronary artery disease. *American Journal of Cardiology, 57,* 557–561.

Ewart, C. K., Taylor, C. B., Kraemer, H. A., & Agras, W. S. (1984). Reducing blood pressure reactivity during interpersonal conflict: Effects of Marital communication training. *Behavior Therapy, 15,* 473–484.

Ewart, C. K., Taylor, C. B., Kraemer, H. A., & Agras, W. S. (1991). High blood pressure and marital discord: Not being nasty matters more than being nice. *Health Psychologist, 10,* 155–163.

Ewart, C. K., Taylor, C. B., Reese, L. B., & DeBusk, R. F. (1983). The effects of early post myocardial infarction exercise testing on self-perception and subsequent physical activity. *American Journal of Cardiology, 51,* 1076–1080.

Fehrenbach, A. M. B., & Peterson, L. (1989). Parental problem-solving skills, stress, and dietary compliance in phenylketonuria. *Journal of Consulting and Clinical Psychology, 57,* 237–241.

Finney, J., Moos, R., & Mewborn, R. (1980). Post-treatment experiences and treatment outcome of alcoholic patients six months and two years after hospitalization. *Journal of Consulting and Clinical Psychology, 48,* 17–29.

Ford, D. H. (1987). *Humans as self-constructing living systems: A developmental perspective on personality and behavior.* Hillsdale, NJ: Lawrence Erlbaum Associates.

Frese, M. (1982). Occupational socialization and psychological development: An underemphasized research perspective in industrial psychology. *Journal of Occupational Psychology, 55,* 209–224.

Glasgow, R. E., Toobert, D. J., Riddle, M., Donnelly, J., & Calder, D. (1989). Diabetes-specific social learning variables and self-care behaviors among persons with Type II diabetes. *Health Psychology, 8,* 285–303.

Goldsmith, H. H., Buss, A. H., Plomin, R., Rothbart, M. K., Thomas, A., Chess, S., Hinde, R. A., & McCall, R. B. (1987). Roundtable: What is temperament? Four approaches. *Child Development, 58,* 505–529.

Gottman, J. M., & Levenson, R. W. (1986). Assessing the role of emotion in marriage. *Behavioral Assessment, 8,* 31–48.

Gottman, J., Notarius, C., Gonso, J., & Marksman, H. (1976). *A couple's guide to communication.* Champaign, IL: Research Press.

Graves, T., Meyers, A. W., & Clark, L. (1988). An evaluation of parental problem solving training

in the behavioral treatment of childhood obesity. *Journal of Consulting and Clinical Psychology, 56,* 246–250.
Hanna, K. J., Ewart, C. K., & Kwiterovich, Jr., P. O. (1990). Child problem solving competence, behavioral adjustment, and adherence to lipid-lowering diet. *Patient Education and Counseling, 16,* 119–131.
Hanson, C. L., Henggeler, S. W., & Burghen, G. A. (1987). Social competence and parental support as mediators of the link between stress and metabolic control in adolescents with insulin-dependent diabetes mellitus. *Journal of Consulting and Clinical Psychology, 55,* 529–533.
Hauser, S., Jacobson, A., Wertlieb, E., Brink, S., & Wentworth, S. (1985). The contribution of family environment to perceived competence and illness adjustment in diabetic acutely ill adolescents. *Family Relations, 34,* 99–108.
Hyland, M. E. (1988). Motivational control theory: An integrative framework. *Journal of Personality and Social Psychology, 55,* 642–651.
Jacobson, N. S., & Holzworth-Munroe, A. (1986). Marital therapy: A social learning-cognitive perspective. In N. S. Jacobson & A. S. Gurman (Eds.), *Clinical handbook of marital therapy* (pp. 29–70). New York: Guilford Press.
Janz, N. K., & Becker, M. H. (1984). The health belief model: A decade later. *Health Education Quarterly, 11,* 1–47.
Jarvis, I. L. (1982). Decision making under stress. In L. Goldberger & S. Breznitz (Eds.), *Handbook of stress: Theoretical and clinical aspects* (pp. 69–87). New York: Free Press.
Jeffery, R. W. (1989). Risk behaviors and health: Contrasting individual and population perspectives. *American Psychologist, 44,* 1194–1202.
Kanfer, F. H. (1980). Self-management methods. In F. H. Kanfer & A. P. Goldstein (Eds.), *Helping people change* (2nd ed., pp. 334–389). New York: Pergamon.
Kazdin, A. E. (1982). Symptom substitution, generalization, and response covariation: Implications for psychotherapy outcome. *Psychological Bulletin, 91,* 349–365.
Kazdin, A. E. (1984). *Behavior modification in applied settings.* The Dorsey Press.
Kirschenbaum, D. S., Harris, E. S., & Tomarken, A. J. (1984). Effects of parental involvement in behavioral weight loss therapy for preadolescents. *Behavior Therapy, 15,* 485–500.
Klinger, E. (1975). Consequences of commitment to and disengagement from incentives. *Psychological Review, 82,* 1–25.
Kniskern, J., Biglan, A., Lichtenstein, E., Fry, D., & Bavry, J. (1983). Peer modeling effects in the smoking behavior of teenagers. *Addictive Behaviors, 8,* 129–132.
Kog, E., Vertommen, H., & Vandereyken, W. (1987). Minuchin's psychosomatic family revisited: A concept validation study using a multitrait–multimethod approach. *Family Process, 26* (2), 235–253.
Kohn, M. L., & Schooler, C. (1982). Job conditions and personality: A longitudinal assessment of their reciprocal effects. *American Journal of Sociology, 87,* 1257–1286.
Kristeller, J. L., & Rodin, J. (1984). A three-stage model of treatment continuity: Compliance, adherence and maintenance. In A. Baum, S. Taylor, & J. Singer (Eds), *Handbook of psychological aspects of health.* Hillsdale, NJ: Lawrence Erlbaum Associates.
Lehman, D. R., Lempert, R. O., & Nisbett, R. E. (1988). The effects of graduate training on reasoning: Formal discipline and thinking about everyday events. *American Psychologist, 43,* 431–442.
Lepper, M. R., & Greene, D. (Eds.). (1978). *The hidden costs of reward.* Hillsdale, NJ: Lawrence Erlbaum Associates.
Leventhal, H., Meyer, D., & Nerenz, D. (1980). The common-sense representation of illness danger. In S. Rachman (Ed.), *Medical psychology* (Vol. 2). New York: Pergamon.
Leventhal, H., Zimmerman, R., & Gutman, M. (1984). Compliance: A self-regulation perspective. In W. D. Gentry (Ed.), *Handbook of behavioral medicine* (pp. 369–436). New York: Guilford.
Ley, P. (1977). Psychological studies of doctor–patient communication. In S. Rachman (Ed.), *Contributions to medical psychology* (Vol. 1). Oxford: Pergamon Press.

Lichtman, R., Taylor, S., Wood, J., Bluming, A., Dosik, G., & Leibowitz, R. (1984). Relations with children after breast cancer: The mother–daughter relationship at risk. *Journal of Psychosocial Oncology, 2,* 1–19.
Little, B. R. (1983). Personal projects: A rationale and method for investigation. *Environment and Behavior, 15,* 273–309.
Mandler, G. (1975). *Mind and emotion.* New York: Wiley.
Manne, S. L., & Zautra, A. J. (1989). Spouse criticism and support: Their association with coping and psychological adjustment among women with rheumatoid arthritis. *Journal of Personality and Social Psychology, 56,* 608–617.
McCaul, K. D., & Malott, J. M. (1984). Distraction and coping with pain. *Psychological Bulletin, 95,* 516–533.
McClelland, D. C. (1951). *Personality.* New York: Sloane.
Meyer, D., Leventhal, H., & Gutman, M. (1985). Common-sense models of illness: The example of hypertension. *Health Psychology, 4,* 115–135.
Michela, J. L., & Contento, I. R. (1986). Cognitive, motivational, social, and environmental influences on children's food choices. *Health Psychology, 5,* 209–230.
Minuchin, S., Rosman, B. L., & Baker, L. (1978). *Psychosomatic families: Anorexia nervosa in context.* Cambridge, MA: Harvard University Press.
Mischel, W. (1984). Convergences and challenges in the search for consistency. *American Psychologist, 39,* 351–364.
Mischel, W., & Ebbesen, E. B. (1970). Attention in delay of gratification. *Journal of Personality and Social Psychology, 16,* 329–337.
Mischel, W., Ebbesen, E. B., & Zeiss, A. R. (1972). Cognitive and attentional mechanisms in delay of gratification. *Journal of Personality and Social Psychology, 21,* 204–218.
Nezu, A. M. (1986). Efficacy of a social problem-solving therapy approach for unipolar depression. *Journal of Consulting and Clinical Psychology, 54,* 196–202.
Nezu, A. M., & Perri, M. G. (1989). Social problem-solving therapy for unipolar depression: An initial dismantling investigation. *Journal of Consulting and Clinical Psychology, 57,* 408–413.
Nicholls, J. G., & Miller, A. T. (1984). Development and its discontents: The differentiation of the concept of ability. In J. G. Nicholls (Ed.), *The development of achievement motivation* (pp. 185–218). Greenwich, CT: JAI Press.
Oldridge, N. B. (1982). Compliance and exercise in primary and secondary prevention of coronary heart disease: A review. *Preventive Medicine, 11,* 56–70.
Patterson, G. R. (1982). *A social learning approach to family intervention, Volume 3: Coercive family process.* Eugene, OR: Castalia.
Patterson, J. (1985). Critical factors affecting family compliance with home treatment for children with cystic fibrosis. *Family Relations, 34,* 79–89.
Petty, R. E., & Cacioppo, J. T. (1986). *Communication and persuasion: Central and peripheral routes to attitude change.* New York: Springer-Verlag.
Prochaska, J. O., & DiClemente, C. C. (1983). Stages and processes of self-change of smoking: Toward an integrative model of change. *Journal of Consulting and Clinical Psychology, 51,* 390–395.
Riley, D., & Eckenrode, J. (1986). Social ties: Subgroup differences in costs and benefits. *Journal of Personality and Social Psychology, 51*(4) 770–778.
Rodriguez, M. L., Mischel, W., & Shoda, Y. (1989). Cognitive person variables in the delay of gratification of older children at risk. *Journal of Personality and Social Psychology, 57,* 358–367.
Rogers, R. W. (1983). Cognitive and physiological processes in fear appeals and attitude change: A revised theory of protection motivation. In J. T. Cacioppo, R. E. Petty, & D. Shapiro (Eds.), *Social psychophysiology: A sourcebook.* New York: Guilford.
Rokeach, M. (1973). *The nature of human values.* New York: Free Press.

Rosenthal, B., & McSweeney, F. K. (1979). Modeling influences on eating behaviors. *Addictive Behaviors, 4,* 205–214.

Ruehlman, L. S. (1985). Depression and affective meaning for current concerns. *Cognitive Therapy and Research, 9,* 553–560.

Ruehlman, L. S., & Wolchik, S. A. (1988). Personal goals and interpersonal support and hindrance as factors in psychological distress and well-being. *Journal of Personality and Social Psychology, 55,* 293–301.

Sallis, J. F., Grossman, R. M., Pinski, R. B., Patterson, T. L., & Nader, P. R. (1987). The development of scales to measure social support for diet and exercise behaviors. *Preventive Medicine, 16,* 825–836.

Schwartz, G. E. (1983). Disregulation theory and disease: Applications to the repression/cerebral disconnection/cardiovascular disorder hypothesis. *International Review of Applied Psychology, 32,* 95–118.

Schwartz, S. H., & Inbar-Saban, N. I. (1988). Value self-confrontation as a method to aid in weight loss. *Journal of Personality and Social Psychology, 54,* 396–404.

Seeman, J. (1989). Toward a model of positive health. *American Psychologist, 44,* 1099–1109.

Shaver, P., Schwartz, J., Kirson, D., & O'Connor, C. (1987). Emotion knowledge: Further exploration of a prototype approach. *Journal of Personality and Social Psychology, 52,* 1061–1086.

Slater, M. D. (1989). Social influences and cognitive control as predictors of self-efficacy and eating behavior. *Cognitive Therapy and Research, 13,* 231–245.

Stokes, T. F., & Baer, D. M. (1977). An implicit technology of generalization. *Journal of Applied Behavior Analysis, 10,* 349–367.

Stokes, T. F., & Osnes, P. G. (1989). An operant pursuit of generalization. *Behavior Therapy, 20,* 337–355.

Taylor, C. B., Bandura, A., Ewart, C. K., Miller, N. H., & DeBusk, R. F. (1985). Exercise testing to enhance wives' confidence in their husband's capability soon after clinically uncomplicated myocardial infarction. *American Journal of Cardiology, 55,* 636–628.

Timberlake, W., & Allison, J. (1974). Response deprivation: An empirical approach to instrumental performance. *Psychological Review, 81,* 146–164.

Wahler, R. G., & Dumas, J. E. (1989). Attentional problems in dysfunctional mother–child interactions: An interbehavioral model. *Psychological Bulletin, 105,* 116–130.

Wahler, R. G., & Hann, D. M. (1984). The communication patterns of troubled mothers: In search of a keystone in the generalization of parenting skills. *Education and Treatment of Children, 7,* 335–350.

Watson, D. W., & Pennebaker, J. W. (1989). Health complaints, stress, and distress: Exploring the central role of negative affectivity. *Psychological Review, 96,* 234–254.

Webster-Stratton, C. (1988). Mothers' and fathers' perceptions of child deviance: Roles of parent and child behaviors and parent adjustment. *Journal of Consulting and Clinical Psychology, 56,* 909–915.

Weinstein, N. D. (1988). The precaution adoption process. *Health Psychology, 7,* 355–386.

Weisz, J. R. (1986). Contingency and control beliefs as predictors of psychotherapy outcomes among children and adolescents. *Journal of Consulting and Clinical Psychology, 54,* 789–795.

Winett, R. A., King, A. C., & Altman, D. G. (1989). *Health psychology and public health.* New York: Pergamon.

V INTERVENTION

Norman A. Krasnegor

This section explores the topic of intervention approaches designed to improve compliance in children who are afflicted with chronic disease. Three chapters are offered. Two of the three focus on a particular disease (asthma and diabetes) and use the research reviewed to elucidate the unique compliance problems raised by the disease for the affected children. The third chapter employs a health compliance research example, associated with medicine taking to reduce cholesterol level in an adult population. Important conclusions can be drawn from each of the chapters concerning general principles that can guide strategies for intervening with health compliance behaviors over a developmental range that covers childhood through adolescence.

The first chapter in this section, "Adherence Intervention Research: The Need for a Multilevel Approach" by W. Stewart Agras, has as its focus an overview of the factors that must be addressed when approaching research on interventions for influencing adherence to health regimens. Agras first probes the question of who should be studied. He points to the fact that not only the patient but, depending on his or her developmental stage, the family, school/worksite, community, and national economy might have to be taken into consideration. The other elements that must be included are the health care professionals and the patient's contact with the health care system, and the finding of only weak relationships between level of adherence and clinical outcome.

Agras identifies the difficulties in conducting adherence interventions in pediatric populations given the different stages through which children pass from birth to adulthood. Thus, theoretical approaches may have to shift in emphasis and in the constructs that are deemed important depending on the developmental stage of the patients being studied. Theories about interventions for infants may really be about parents, whereas theories of health adherence interventions for adolescents require quite a different perspective (e.g., social learning model). As a child develops its contact with the environment broadens dramatically, requiring different theoretical and operational strategies to adequately deal with a chronic disease that may span infancy to adulthood.

Agras employs the Coronary Primary Prevention Trial (CPPT) as a heuristic device to illustrate the needs for identifying and dealing with the multiple factors necessary to engender a successful compliance intervention. The trial involved a randomized design to test the efficacy of cholestyremine, a drug designed to lower cholesterol in patients whose cholesterol levels were above 265 mg/dl. The compliance goals of the trial included the following: (a) remaining an active participant for 7–10 years; (b) attending all trial visits; (c) fasting at each visit; (d) accurate adherence to the medication regime; (e) accurate adherence to the dietary recommendations; (f) maintaining the double-blind code, and so on. Medication packet count was the primary index of adherence.

Agras, who was in charge of the adherence part of the trial, indicates that he and his staff had to make the transition from recruitment phase to the following of patients. This required strict staff organization and education. He and his colleagues had to develop methods for enhancing adherence and monitoring clinic performance in relation to adherence to detect problems. He employed the social learning model of Bandura as the framework for conducting the study. Agras found that using medication packets as the index of adherence (bioassay was not available due to the double blind nature of the study) led to many problems because the relationship between the measure and the medication's effects changed over time even though the same adherence was being reported. This meant that either the drug's physiological effect changed over time or the adherence measure was less indicative of the patients' behaviors.

Steps were taken to enhance adherence. For example, newsletters were published across clinics to foster group cohesiveness. Clinics sponsored social events that involved family members (e.g., spouse). Medication dispensers were employed (see Rudd, this volume). Methods were devised to enhance staff performance. These included special campaigns to highlight motivation among staff and patients to focus on the need to adhere to the prescribed regimens. Adherence was better during the first year among those on placebo compared with those patients taking the drug. The differences were most likely due to the side effects of the drug.

The next chapter, "Medication Compliance and Childhood Asthma," by Thomas L. Creer, provides an overview of asthmatic children's compliance to medication regimes for controlling their illness. Although this chapter focuses on a specific disease, many of the points made have applicability to the wider issue of interventions designed to improve compliance in chronically ill children. The chapter is divided into three parts: (a) scope of the problem (prevalence of compliance), (b) methods for measuring compliance, and (c) intervention strategies for improving compliance.

Creer points out that asthma is the leading diagnosis for children admitted to hospitals in the United States, and such hospital stays are often connected with medication compliance problems. For example, data from studies where biological markers have been used to estimate compliance reveal a wide range of between 2% to 100%.

As others in this volume have discussed, Creer too points out that there are two basic ways to assess compliance. These are: (a) biological assays or markers of drug in body fluids, or (b) patient reports, medication counts, instrumentation, and treatment outcome. Creer's review of the various methods for assessing compliance provides the reader with an excellent overview of the strengths and weaknesses of different approaches to the problem of compliance measurement.

Creer next summarizes intervention procedures that have been tried to enhance compliance for taking asthma medication. These include: (a) patient education, (b) altering treatment regimes (i.e., making medication taking as convenient as possible for the patient, and (c) behavioral techniques. Creer's review of these three areas is a thorough and detailed analysis based on results of published research. The examination of the different techniques under each respective rubric provides the reader with a sense of the range of possibilities and the state of the art.

Creer articulates two recent trends relating to interventions designed to enhance compliance. First he notes that practitioners have begun to recognize that compliance is not a simple problem. Patients, particularly children, are not automatically going to follow advice simply because the doctor says to do this. This trend is reflected by the fact that there is a move to change the term *compliance* to *adherence*. This shift represents a recognition that patients can and often do disagree with their physicians, and patients change doctors if there is an authoritarian approach rather than a dialogue in connection with medical advice. The second trend is the emerging idea that there are two behavioral components associated with compliance: preventive behaviors and attack behaviors. The former category includes the administration of maintenance medications for some children with asthma. The latter category relates to how children, and physicians, react to the advent of an asthma attack. A number of self-regulatory behaviors can be acquired that can ward off attacks, because life-threatening breathing problems often come with warning days before a major attack ensues.

The final chapter in this section, "Compliance Interventions for Children with Diabetes and Other Chronic Diseases" by Alan M. Delamater, is concerned with intervention strategies to improve compliance in children who are chronically ill with diabetes. As with the previous chapter, although the focus is on a specific disease, the principles raised in the discussion can be generalized to health compliance problems in other diseases.

Dalamater outlines the factors that influence regimen compliance. These are: (a) age effects—developmental stage does seem to interact with compliance particularly during adolescence; (b) knowledge and skills—knowledge about the disease is assumed to aid compliance but the data does not bear out this putative relationship; (c) health beliefs—this factor seems to be relevant for older children; (d) family factors—there is good evidence that family interaction patterns influence metabolic control of diabetic children; and (e) peers—this factor does influence compliance particularly in the developmental stage of adolescence.

Dalamater provides an overview of compliance interventions studies conducted and breaks down the research reviewed into two categories. The first of these is the *single case design* approach. The results of his analysis reveals that behavioral intervention strategies are efficacious in improving compliance among children from ages 9–18. The second category of studies can be placed under the heading of *randomized group designs*. Delamater reviews 14 studies reported in the literature and provides the reader with an in-depth analysis.

Delamater also addresses compliance research conducted on other chronic diseases. He reviews studies on children who have cystic fibrosis, end-stage renal disease, hemophilia, and myelomeningocele. Whereas some studies have been conducted on children's compliance associated with each of these diseases, the scope of the research is much reduced in comparison with that carried out on diabetes or asthma.

12 Adherence Intervention Research: The Need for a Multilevel Approach

W. Stewart Agras
Stanford University School of Medicine

This chapter serves as an introduction to compliance intervention research in pediatric populations, first discussing some of the problems facing the field, and then presenting an overview of the compliance intervention strategies used in the Coronary Primary Prevention Trial (CPPT), as a clinical example of a multilevel compliance intervention.

One of the first questions facing the researcher, or indeed the clinician, in addressing a compliance problem is at whom should the intervention be aimed? The obvious answer is the patient with the problem. On reflection this answer is, however, rather facile. It is evident, for example, in a pediatric population that the parent must also be the intervention target and is the only target in the case of the infant or very young child. Parental behavior must be changed to affect compliance in the infant or young child. Taking an even broader view, the health care system and the economy of the country also affect compliance in the individual patient and in turn are affected by poor compliance. For example, if a child does not receive adequate treatment by virtue of poor compliance and hence develops a chronic condition that may lead to more than average ill health, the health care system will have to absorb higher treatment costs, an employer may eventually have to pay larger insurance premiums and may also have to absorb the costs of absenteeism due to ill health.

There are, then, a number of possible organizational levels for compliance intervention research. These include: the patient, the patient's family, the worksite, the community, and the national economy on the one hand; the health care worker, the treatment team, the immediate clinical environment, and the larger institutional environment on the other. The vast majority of compliance intervention research has focused on the patient, and to a lesser extent, on the patient's family. Much less is known about the effects of intervention at other levels.

Whereas with few exceptions the intervention targets have been too narrowly defined, the field of compliance intervention research has other problems. First, it has often been noted that physicians in particular, and health care workers in general, do not pay enough attention to compliance problems in their patients (e.g., Pendelton, 1983). There are several good reasons why this might be so. A critical problem in the clinic is the recognition of poor adherence. It has been demonstrated over and over again that physicians recognize adherence problems at a level that is no better than chance, when their estimates are compared with a more objective measure (Blackwell, 1973; Caron & Roth, 1968). Moreover, physicians tend to overestimate adherence. If the problem is not recognizable, then physicians will not take any steps to remediate the problem. What is needed is a simple yet accurate method to assess adherence in the patient's own environment that can display data in a form that is immediately understandable to both the health care worker and the patient. As noted in the chapter by Rudd (this volume), there are some encouraging developments along these lines, although no practical method to objectively assess adherence behavior in the clinic presently exists.

A further difficulty is that patients with compliance problems tend to disappear from the clinic because they do not keep appointments. Thus, there is a tendency for the worst compliance problems to drop out of sight. Finally, it may be easier for physicians to alter the treatment regimen than to deal with a compliance problem. For the patient not responding in terms of a biologic measure (e.g., blood pressure) to a particular medication, it is relatively easy to switch to a new medication that may have fewer side effects. In this way compliance to the initial medication is never addressed, although it should be noted that there may or may not have been a compliance problem in the first place.

The relative neglect of the problem of compliance by health care workers may be one reason why interest in the field of compliance intervention research appears to be waning. As Blackwell (1989) points out, the field emerged in the early 1970s stimulated by workers from McMaster University (e.g., Haynes et al., 1976). The field quickly gathered adherents and the main outlines of knowledge concerning degree of compliance, the numerous determinants of poor compliance, and compliance intervention were filled in by research over the next decade. Although there have been some advances in our knowledge concerning the remediation of compliance problems, there have been relatively few developments that have resulted in practical methods to enhance compliance in the clinical setting, and the diffusion of such methods into the clinic has been less than adequate. Such limited accomplishment has led a number of researchers to leave the field, and as a consequence interest in the area has declined. One index of the decreasing interest in the field is that publication of the *Journal of Compliance in Health Care* has been discontinued. The present volume implicitly addresses the question as to whether the field should or can be revived. One possibility is that there should not be a separate field of compliance research. The issue of compliance is an aspect of all clinical outcome research. Perhaps the two fields should be merged. Outcome researchers are beginning to tackle the problem of maintaining long-term behavior change and preventing relapse (Brownell, Marlatt, Lichtenstein, & Wilson, 1986), although experimental knowledge in this area is still quite meager. Clearly, research concerned with the maintenance of behavior change overlaps with compliance intervention research.

A final problem with the field of compliance intervention research is the relatively weak relationship between poor compliance and treatment outcome. This is exemplified by a recent study in which participants were randomly allocated to three different weight loss programs: a hand-held computer with and without group support, and a traditional behavior therapy program led by a therapist (Agras, Taylor, Feldman, Losch, & Burnett, 1990). The adherence to self-monitoring, a behavior that has been shown to be correlated with outcome in weight control programs (e.g., Wilson & Dubbert, 1983) is shown in Fig. 12.1. Notice that the two computer groups demonstrated similar adherence patterns until the 10th week of treatment, when the group using the computer without support showed a sharp decline. The behavior therapy group demonstrated a similar pattern to the two computer groups until the sixth week of treatment when it demonstrated a rapid decline in the use of self-monitoring that corrected slightly until the 11th week of treatment before falling off to equal the computer alone group. The computer treatment with group support participants were adhering at 70% in the final week of treatment, whereas the other two groups were at 29% adherence in the same week. Despite this large and clearly clinically significant difference in the use of an important component of weight loss programs, there was no difference between the groups in weight loss either at the end of treatment or at 6-month follow up. Correlations between the use of self-monitoring and outcome in terms of weight loss were, on the other hand, approximately 0.3 and were statistically significant for two of the groups.

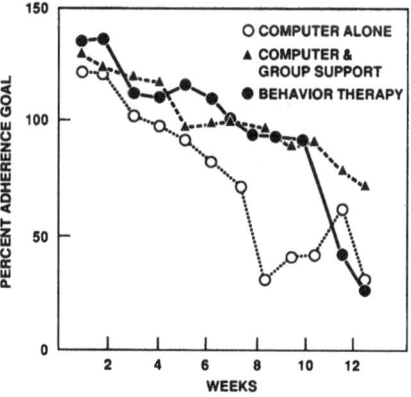

FIG. 12.1. Adherence to self-monitoring in three groups of overweight women treated with different weight loss methods over a 12-week period.

This finding, of a relatively weak relationship between adherence level and clinical outcome is not surprising; indeed, it tends to be the rule rather than the exception (see Epstein, this volume, for a fuller discussion of this issue). Moreover, it is quite understandable from a theoretical viewpoint. In the case of either medication or behavior change procedures, therapeutic outcome is controlled by a number of variables over and above the treatment regimen. In the case of weight loss, for example, caloric intake, activity levels, binge eating, and the resting metabolic rate all affect the rate of weight loss and may be more powerful determinants of weight loss than any behavior change procedure in many individuals (Agras, 1989a). In addition most treatments target several behaviors; hence, compliance with one behavior may not generalize to other behaviors important for therapeutic success. Nonetheless, the weak relationship between compliance with a therapeutic intervention and outcome dictates that the remediation of compliance will not usually be associated with large gains in therapeutic outcome, although large gains may be obtainable in some individuals. Thus, the field may be doomed to relatively weak effects, a state of affairs unpopular with both researchers and journal editors.

Although there are examples of successful outcome research in the area of compliance both in adults and in children, as described in the following chapters, we know very little about the process of compliance. The data in Fig. 12.1 suggest that, at least for weight loss, there is initial overcompliance, followed by a brief period of full compliance, followed by a persistent decline. The factors associated with each of these phases are almost totally unexplored. The initial overenthusiasm may be related to unrealistic expectations of success. Perhaps the reality of relatively slow weight loss gradually dawns and the individual loses interest in the behavior change procedures with a resultant drop in adherence and presumably a weakening of therapeutic effect. Put another way, the reinforcement for continued practice of the behaviors associated with weight loss is not sufficient over the long run to maintain those behaviors. We need to know a great deal more about such influences on the process of adherence if we are to advance the field of compliance intervention research.

DEVELOPMENTAL ASPECTS OF COMPLIANCE

The pediatric population spans several developmental stages from infancy through adolescence, posing a more difficult problem for both researcher and clinician than for those who work with populations less affected by developmental processes. Although the exemplar used in this chapter stems from an adult population, one in which developmental processes were not a major influence, many of the themes are relevant to pediatric compliance research. For example, the theories guiding intervention research may have differential applicability across the developmental span applicable to pediatrics. In young children, for example, a relatively simple environmental control model may suffice, because the child's environment is relatively constrained and hence responsive to straightforward reward systems. In the infant, when dealing with the family, or in adolescence, a more complex social learning model may be needed, taking into account not only environmental influences but also social influences and cognitive processing. Hence, theoretical models may have to shift depending on developmental stage.

Issues concerning the effect of the clinic, including clinic organization, on adherence are clearly relevant across the developmental span, although at one stage it is the family that is most affected, whereas later in life it is both the family and the child who are directly affected by their contacts with the clinic and clinic staff. Behavioral consistency, which may be an important factor in adherence, may vary markedly across developmental stages from infancy through adolescence, posing different challenges to research at each level. Observations from the Coronary Primary Prevention Trial suggest that patterns of medication taking within the same adherence level may vary widely as a result of varying interactions with the medication or the environment. As the child's contact with the environment broadens, variation within adherence category may also become more pronounced and may be particularly marked during adolescence. The importance of this observation is that totally different behaviors may underly apparently similar adherence levels, hence demanding very different behavior change approaches for apparently similar problems. Hence, both the phenomenon of adherence and adherence intervention approaches will vary across the developmental span, although in general one might hypothesize that there is increasing complexity at every level of adherence concern from infancy through adolescence. Even though the Coronary Primary Prevention Trial experience was with middle-aged men, many of the themes noted before are relevant to pediatric adherence research, particularly the necessity to consider adherence from a multilevel perspective. Moreover, the findings are clearly applicable to multicenter pediatric trials that offer an excellent medium for the examination of compliance issues.

Compliance in the Coronary Primary Prevention Trial

The problem set for compliance by the CPPT provides an example of the need to consider compliance as a process affected by factors at multiple levels. The CPPT was designed to test the hypothesis that cholesterol lowering in asymptomatic men 35 to 59 years old with cholesterol values above 265 mg/dl would reduce the morbidity and mortality associated with coronary heart disease. Eligible participants were allocated at random to either cholestyramine (24 gms/day) or placebo, and both groups were placed on a protocol-specified prudent diet providing a daily intake of 400 mg cholesterol and a polyunsaturated/saturated fat ratio of approximately 0.8. The daily dose of study medication was six packets and was usually taken three times each day mixed with fluid into a suspension. Thus, the mode of administration was not convenient for the participant, requiring, for example, mixing the medication at work. A total of 3,810 men with a mean age of 47.7 years were entered into the study and were followed on treatment for a minimum of 7 years (Lipid Research Clinics 1983, 1984). There were 12 participating centers, 11 in the United States and 1 in Canada. The number of participants at each of these Lipid Research Clinics (LRCs) ranged from 236 to 403. These differences were based largely on the ability of the clinics to recruit suitable participants.

Because it was clear that both recruitment and adherence to the medication regimen over such a long period would pose difficulties, shortly after the trial began a recruitment and adherence coordinating center (RAC) composed of behavioral scientists was formed at the Stanford University School of Medicine. The function of this group was to maximize both recruitment to the trial and the subsequent adherence of participants to the trial requirements.

Among the compliance goals set by the trial were the following: remaining an active participant for between 7 and 10 years; attendance at all scheduled trial visits; fasting at each visit; accurate adherence to the trial medication; accurate adherence to the dietary recommendations; maintaining the double-blind; and reporting endpoints, illness, etc. The goal of accurate adherence to medication was complicated by the double-blind nature of the trial, so that neither the treatment team nor the participants had access to their cholesterol levels for the duration of the trial. Thus, the biological measure was not available as a partial guide to clinical management. For this reason the packet count, based on the number of unused packets of medication returned by participants at each visit, was the prime measure of adherence to the trial medication. Because this measure would be sensitive to reinforcement (i.e., participants could bring back fewer packets than they had consumed), interventions such as providing reinforcement contingent on packet count levels could not be used.

A number of issues needed to be addressed throughout the course of the trial in order to maintain optimal trial-wide adherence. The first of these concerned the transition from the recruitment phase of the trial to the different longer term effort of following participants and maintaining adherence. This required attention to the staff organization at each clinic, a task that continued throughout the trial. A second issue was that of educating staff members concerning the type of adherence difficulties that might be expected during the course of the trial and training staff members in adherence intervention methods. Third, there was a need to develop specific methods to enhance or maintain participant adherence. Finally, methods to monitor overall clinic performance in relation to adherence and to detect particular problems within a clinic needed to be developed and refined over the course of the trial.

The Theoretical Model. The theoretical approach to adherence espoused by the behavioral science group was based on a social learning model (Bandura,

1978, 1986). Social learning theory arose in part from dissatisfaction with earlier models of psychological processes, such as conditioning or reinforcement theories, which were viewed as being too simplistic to reflect the complexities of human behavior. Social learning theory postulates a reciprocal determinism of behavior in which environmental influences, particularly the social environment, shape behavior, and in which the individual perceiving the influence can in turn alter his or her personal environment to maximize or minimize the effect. Among the determinants of such decisions are cognitive processes encompassing beliefs and expectations. Thus, the social environment, cognitive processes, and the behavioral performance itself interact to modulate behavior. In different circumstances, and with different individuals, one or another of these three determinants may predominate (Agras, 1989b). Aspects of this model were applied both in understanding particular compliance problems and in intervention attempts. The model also provided a consistent framework that served as a basis for staff training throughout the trial.

As noted earlier, relatively simple reinforcement or environmental control models may suffice to explain adherence and may be used to alter adherence, early in life. On the other hand, when dealing with parents or the older child or adolescent, the more complex social learning model will prove more useful.

Initial Approaches. The recruitment phase of the CPPT began in July 1973 and extended for 37 months (Agras, Bradford, & Marshall, 1982). During this time nearly half a million men were screened. This extensive recruitment drive required much effort from a specialized clinic staff. As the LRCs accrued trial participants, the attention of the staff had to shift from recruitment to adherence. This shift required staff with different skills and a different type of organizational structure. Because research had demonstrated that adherence is better if the patient sees the same health care worker over time (Becker, Drachman, & Kirscht, 1972), it was felt necessary to develop a consistent caretaker model within the clinics. The person fulfilling this role was called an adherence counselor. The professional selected as the adherence counselor varied from clinic to clinic and included nurses, persons with a counseling background, and at one center, physicians.

Clinic Organization. The difference between high- and low-performing clinics in a multicenter trial is often threefold. Dropout rates have been the most investigated variable in this context. In the Hypertension Detection and Follow-up Study (HDFP), for example, center exerted a statistically significant influence on drop out rates (Smith, Hardy, Cutter, Curb, & Hawkins, 1980). In a related trial, the dropout rates between four centers varied from a high of 35.4% to a low of 10.7% (Goldman, Holcomb, Perry, Schnaper, Fitz, & Frohlich, 1982). Among the factors affecting clinic performance is the mode of staff organization. In turn, organizational factors influence the relationship between the participant and the clinic, and personnel efficiency through processes such as clarity of roles and lines of communication within the clinic, both of which affect the counselor–participant interaction and the supervision of counselors. In the early days of the trial, LRC physicians were also brought together to impart current knowledge concerning adherence and its remediation.

The basic organizational model that was eventually decided on included the role of adherence coordinator. This person, often a key individual within the clinic, for example, the chief clinic nurse, was responsible for the day-to-day organization of all the adherence activities within the clinic. Adherence counselors reported to the adherence coordinator, who in turn reported to the trial director. The latter two individuals worked closely together in planning adherence strategies. Thus, the lines of communication were clear, as were the respective roles of trial director, adherence coordinator, and adherence counselor. In addition to attending to the organizational framework of the LRCs, the physical facilities at each of the clinics were examined for adequacy, including parking access, adequate and comfortable waiting room space, and private space for adherence counseling sessions. Where necessary, space improvements were made.

These considerations are relevant to any pediatric therapeutic trial and are particularly relevant to multicenter trials in which attention to these variables may reduce the variance in outcome that may be a problem in the analysis and interpretation of trial results. As noted earlier, physicians typically do not have the time to attend to adherence problems in the necessary detail. Hence, the model of the adherence counselor working within a well-organized clinic appears to be an excellent approach for any trial in which adherence will become a major issue.

Counselor Training. Because there were no individuals with existing skills as adherence counselors when the CPPT entered the adherence phase, the staff of each LRC had to be trained as counselors. Moreover, because over the duration of the trial staff were lost and new problems demanding different solutions emerged, staff training became an ongoing concern. The initial decision was that training should be trial wide and that all counselors should receive the same training program in national workshops. Various models were used over the course of the trial, although the most common was to bring all the trial adherence staff to one location where they were taught basic skills in lectures and small groups. Occasionally, regional workshops were used with three or so clinics participating. In the early days of the trial, LRC physicians were also brought together to impart current knowledge concerning adherence and its remediation.

For the most part, two areas were focused on in teaching adherence counseling: basic relationship and counseling skills, and specific adherence counseling skills. The model used for adherence counseling included the formation of a supportive relationship, a simple data-gathering and feedback process, the use of appropriate social reinforcement for progress in maintenance, and the use of problem solving and goal setting. Interim telephone calls between visits were also used as a counseling technique in problem cases, and the rudiments of telephone interviewing were also taught.

In the middle phase of the trial two additional educational methods were used. The first included local supervision of adherence counselors using behavioral scientists at each of the participating centers. This allowed for follow-up of the national training workshops and for more detailed teaching of counseling skills in very small groups. These behavioral scientists attended trial-wide meetings from time to time so that they were aware of the trial-wide counseling model and could add their experience to the further development of adherence methods. The second method of adherence training was more complex and involved certification of adherence counselors based on the completion of a standard program of training and the demonstration of a certain level of proficiency. Such certification, which was useful to many of the adherence counselors for their future careers, also helped to improve the standards of counseling within the trial by remotivating counselors during the last half of the trial to expand their skills. The training program was comprised of several modules including: basic information concerning the CPPT and adherence; interviewing skills; medication-taking behavior assessment; behavioral counseling; precision counseling (an advanced version of adherence counseling); and guidelines for newsletter preparation. New modules were added to this basic package as new issues developed within the ongoing trial.

Some Basic Problems. As noted earlier in this chapter, the basic measure of adherence available to the clinic staff was the packet count. Because this measure was a variation of self-report, it would be expected that it would not provide a completely accurate account of adherence. Although the relationship between adherence and cholesterol lowering in the active medication group was essentially linear (The Lipid Research Clinic's Program, 1984), there was a sizeable difference in cholesterol lowering at 7 years between those at 95% adherence and those at 100% adherence. There was also more than a four-fold difference in LDL lowering between the 95% and 100% adherers between clinics, suggesting that clinic factors (e.g., differential adherence rates between clinics) may have been responsible for this phenomenon. In addition, the LDL lowering in the first year of the trial for participants taking at least five packets of medication was 33%, whereas in the seventh year of the trial, LDL lowering was only 26% for the same adherence level. This suggested that either the physiologic effect of medication was waning over time, or that the packet count became a less accurate measure of adherence over time.

All this suggested that there were individuals whose packet count marked them as excellent adherers, but whose cholesterol levels suggested that they were imperfect adherers (i.e., they were over reporting their adherence level). Individuals adhering above the 90% level could be divided into consistent and inconsistent adherers, depending on the variation in packet count over the 7 years of the trial. Consistent good adherers demonstrated greater cholesterol lowering than inconsistent adherers even though their overall packet count levels were identical. Thus, behavioral consistency appears to be an important factor in adherence.

When the characteristics of these two groups of adherers were examined, it was found that inconsistent adherers had a statistically significant higher level of gastrointestinal symptoms before beginning the study medication than consistent adherers, and a nonsignificant higher level after beginning medication. However, because these individuals may have been taking less medication to avoid side effects, the number of side effects in these individuals would have been reduced. Moreover, inconsistent adherers were also more likely to smoke cigarettes at the end of the trial (41.9%) than consistent adherers (24.5%), a statistically significant difference. This suggests that individuals less concerned about activities that risk ill health are likely to be poor adherers to a preventive regimen.

These data analyzed at the end of the trial suggest that there were some risk factors for poor adherence including symptoms in the same organ system as that affected by the study medication, in this case gastrointestinal symptoms and engaging in behaviors that promote health risk. This latter finding may have important implications for pediatric compliance research, because the level of understanding of health risks, and the type of risk taking behaviors in which individuals engage, will vary over the developmental span. In particular, adolescence would appear to be a time of particular difficulty in terms of risk-taking behaviors and inability to process information concerning long-term outcomes. Hence, adherence approaches to the adolescent may have to focus on these issues.

Although the packet count was useful to ascertain a basic level of adherence and for the recognition of gross adherence problems, it was not useful for more precise problem solving. When a more precise assessment of adherence was required, a combination of more detailed interviewing and self-monitoring was used. Self-monitoring focussed on medication-taking patterns over more than 1 week and was based on the observation that a packet count of 50% could represent one of several behavior patterns, as indicated in Fig. 12.2.

In the top graph, the participant takes three packets of medication on each of 8 days. Because the prescribed dose of the trial medication was six packets daily, this participant's adherence is 50%. The most likely cause for such an adherence pattern (i.e., excellent adherence to a reduced dose) is intolerance of medication side effects. The intervention strategy, if any, would be to increase dosage while treating any emergent side effects. The middle pattern is evidently more complex. One possibility is that this participant can take four packets per day but forgets to take either a morning or an evening dose quite frequently. This possibility would be investigated by further self-monitoring of each dosage occasion and the circumstances surrounding the dosage. The intervention strategy would

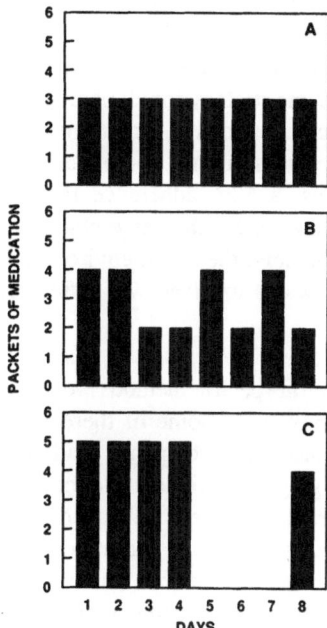

FIG. 12.2. Three diagrams of different ways in which individuals could have adhered to 50% of their medication dose over an 8-day period. The prescribed dosage in the Coronary Primary Prevention Trial was six packets of medication daily.

be to use stimulus control procedures to enhance adherence. For example, if the morning dose was forgotten in the rush to leave for work, the family breakfast pattern might be carefully examined, and the participants spouse might agree to prepare the medication and serve it with breakfast. An evening missing dose might be dealt with through the use of a reminder built into some other repetitive activity, for example, toothbrushing. The medication packets might be placed such that they are accessed when reaching for a toothbrush. The final pattern illustrates another possible problem. Here the participant takes a reasonable dose of the trial medication on some days, followed by a pattern in which no medication is taken, followed by restarting medication at a lower dose. This pattern is typically seen on trips where the participant either forgets to take medication along or is too embarrassed to take medication, or at weekends when the participant does not wish to take medication, perhaps because of side effects interfering with leisure activities, or where the participant forgets to take medication because of a schedule different from that of weekdays. The intervention strategies might differ for each of these eventualities. For travel, a compact medication carrying and mixing kit might solve the problem. A changed schedule might be dealt with using stimulus control procedures specifically aimed at the different weekend schedule; whereas not wishing to take medication at weekends would demand the skilled use of persuasion techniques.

The complexity of the adherence problem is nicely illustrated by these graphs examining just one facet of adherence, namely, patterning of medication intake.

Several different remediation strategies are called for in response to each of these problems. Clearly, no one intervention strategy would be successful with each of these individuals. Yet the most common approach to intervention research is to use one strategy for all poor adherers, a tactic not likely to succeed. This problem is compounded in long-term studies in pediatric populations where developmental issues further complicate the meaning of a particular adherence number. Thus, a 50% adherence for a child of 10 years may involve very different behaviors for the same child in adolescence, because the range and variety of behaviors, the social environment controlling those behaviors, and the cognitive processes involved will differ between the two ages.

Specific Methods to Enhance Compliance. During the course of the trial several specific methods were introduced across all the LRCs in order to enhance compliance. Some of these procedures, such as newsletters and special clinic events for participants, had been used in previous trials and were aimed at forging a continued relationship between the clinic and the trial participants. Newsletters were published by each clinic at regular intervals throughout the trial. A trial-wide committee was formed to delineate guidelines for the production of newsletters. Among the chief objectives were: the fostering of group cohesiveness among participants; providing a contact with the clinic between visits; providing information to maintain and enhance compliance; and providing information regarding the progress of the trial, heart disease in general, and the importance of research especially the CPPT. Clinics were free to publish newsletters at any given frequency. In 1980 a survey revealed that clinics published newsletters at between 3- and 4-month intervals, and that the average number per clinic was 3.5, with a range from 1:8. About 25% of each newsletter dealt directly with medication compliance issues.

Clinic events were of two main types, educational and social, often involving the participant's spouse, because the family was felt to have a major influence on compliance. Among the educational events were cooking demonstrations illustrating the preparation of diets that would meet the LRC prescribed diet, seminars on the purpose of the CPPT and on heart disease and diet, and on the study medication. A special educational event was held midway through the trial at which both the clinic director and the NIH research director for the CPPT reported on the status of the trial with the aim of increasing motivation for adherence in this long trial. A wide variety of social events was held. Attendance at these events varied widely, being between 8 and 570 including participants' family members.

As part of the data-based approach to adherence within the CPPT, clinics analyzed the effects of these events by comparing adherence figures before and after the event for those who attended and those who did not attend. The overall experience was that such events did not directly affect compliance with the medication regimen. As is often the case, there was a trend for those attending such events to show superior compliance before the event (i.e., better compliers tend to be participants who are more involved in all the clinic activities).

Other more specific interventions used during the trial included the use of medication dispensers, because research had demonstrated the utility of these devices in enhancing adherence (e.g., Moulding, 1961). These dispensers were used on a trial-wide basis being specifically designed for the CPPT. The dispenser carried a 1-week supply of medication with each day separated and was hung on a wall in a prominent place in the home. In this way the dispenser acted as a reminder concerning both daily dosage of medication and planning medication taking for the week ahead. The medication dispenser was provided to all participants in the CPPT. (The use of such devices is considered in detail in the chapter by Rudd, this volume.) Other interventions were applied to a subset of individuals who had been identified as problems. An example of this was the introduction of a shaping procedure to raise the medication taking of poor adherers who suffered from side effects from the medication, despite medical interventions aimed at ameliorating such side effects. The basis of this procedure was a slow incremental addition of small amounts of medication over a relatively long period of time with supportive counseling and careful medical management of increases in side effects.

Methods to Enhance Staff Performance. Several approaches were taken to enhance and maintain staff performance in relation to adherence. Basic to these approaches was a decision to take a data-based approach to adherence within the trial. At meetings of the CPPT intervention committee, data on packet count and, later in the trial, general information concerning the relationship between cholesterol lowering and packet count, and clinic ranking on cholesterol reduction were introduced. Each clinic could see where they stood in relation to the other LRCs and where in general their problems lay. Such data were presented in various ways (e.g., cross-sectionally for specific intervals), or over time, or addressing specific adherence levels (e.g., dropouts). These data were used to elucidate and present both successes and trial-wide problem areas. These data presentations led to detailed discussions at meetings of the intervention committee, as well as at counselor training sessions, and were often followed by attempts at one or more clinics to remediate the problem. Such attempts were analyzed and successful protocols were then promoted at all the clinics.

Early in the trial it was realized that, if clinics were to be able to use their own packet count data, these data would have to be computerized. Each center was encouraged to develop a computerized data collection and analysis system to allow rapid use of their data in problem solving. Several innovative methods of displaying adherence changes were developed by the LRCs and were then promoted on a trial-wide basis.

An example of one of these data displays is presented in Fig. 1.3. The participant who suffered from side effects to the medication and whose dosage of

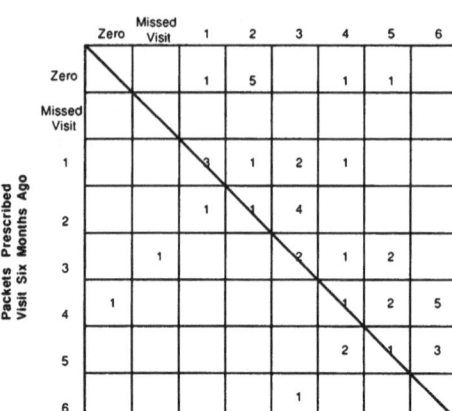

FIG. 12.3. A prescription matrix designed to facilitate the tracking of adherence over time in groups of patients. The vertical axis represents the amount of medication prescribed 6 months ago. The horizontal axis represents the amount of medication prescribed at the last visit.

medication was then reduced represented, as noted earlier, a particular problem to the trial. The matrix shown in Fig. 12.3 demonstrates a method for clinics to compare data for two periods of time for all those patients in an LRC with a reduced dose of medication, in this case 6 months ago. The improvement over a 6-month period is easy to see in this case. Such grids were used to detect various problems (or successes) within an LRC over varying periods of time, for example, from month to month. Such data were examined frequently by the adherence staff, and any trends within a clinic that signalled a problem could then be dealt with by a clinic-wide approach.

The annual site visits to each clinic were also used to analyze particular clinic problems, to consider the organization of the clinic and to suggest any needed changes, and to examine the adequacy of adherence counseling, and so on. Frequent contacts were also maintained between the RAC and the adherence coordinator and often adherence counselors at the various LRCs. These took the form of weekly telephone conversations examining current adherence data, and attempting to solve current problems. Thus, a multilevel problem identification and feedback system was in effect throughout the duration of the trial.

The importance and effect of the the wider social milieu on compliance is usually neglected in studies of adherence. In pediatric research the different development phases through which children pass would seem likely to induce differential interaction with the clinical milieu, just as a differential interaction with the family occurs over time. It would seem important in future research to begin to document the differential effects of aspects of the clinical milieu on children at different developmental stages.

Trial-Wide Campaigns.   Several trial-wide campaigns were held during the course of the CPPT. An example of such a campaign was that held during the final 18 months of the trial called "The Final Lap Campaign." In general, the aims of all campaigns were to inform participants concerning specific salient issues, to help motivate participants to comply more accurately, to help motivate adherence staff, and to provide them with a new vehicle to augment counseling.

The Final Lap Campaign was aimed at maintaining adherence during the final year of the trial to ensure that there would be no letdown in adherence. In addition, the campaign was aimed at preparing participants and staff for the end of the trial. Such preparations included special training for the adherence counselors concerning the variety of expected emotional responses to termination and separation from the CPPT. More specific preparations were also made for unblinding the participants and for dealing with reactions to the knowledge that a participant had or had not been on the active medication. Specific counselor sessions were orchestrated both around maintaining adherence and for the unblinding sessions. Mechanisms for disseminating information to participants included lectures by the trial director or clinic director, newsletter information, and direct contacts with the adherence counselors. Each of these activities were orchestrated so that they were mutually reinforcing and so that they were introduced in the correct sequence.

Adherence Results. It is, of course, impossible to know in the absence of a controlled trial whether or not the adherence strategies used in the CPPT were successful. Indeed, it is unlikely that such a study of a multilevel approach to adherence will ever be undertaken. At the most, some of the elements of the multilevel package might be tested in smaller studies. Given the initial expectation that adherence to a medication with marked side effects over a considerable period of time without either staff or participants knowing whether they were benefitting would be difficult, the long-term adherence results were quite encouraging (The Lipid Research Clinics' Program, 1984). In the first year of the trial the average adherence for the group on active medication was 70% and for those on placebo 81.7%. The difference between the two groups is most likely explicable by the greater prevalence of side effects in the medication group. Thus, 68% of participants in the cholestyramine group reported gastrointestinal side effects compared with 43% of the placebo group in the first year of the trial. During the seventh year of the trial adherence in both groups had declined somewhat to 63% in the cholestyramine group and 76.7% in the placebo group. These differences in packet count were paralleled by the changes in LDL–C. In the first year of the trial the diet led to a 3.4% fall in LDL-C, whereas the addition of cholestyramine led to a further 14% reduction. By the seventh year of the trial this differential had dropped to 9.6%, a 31% decline over a 7-year period. It should be remembered that adherence data tends to be distributed in a J-shape at any one time. The CPPT was no exception in this regard, with some half of the participants adhering 90% or better and 15%–20% taking no medication. Thus, many participants continued to be excellent adherers throughout the entire course of the trial. Over time, one would expect the J-shape to become more U-shaped as the percentage of nonadherers grows.

Large-scale controlled trials such as the CPPT offer an excellent opportunity to test the effectiveness of adherence procedures in small controlled substudies. Such studies should be of the additive variety (i.e., adding a new procedure to the ongoing program so that adherence will not be diminished in the experimental group), thus protecting the power of the main study. Procedures that enhance adherence can then be applied trial wide. In multicenter trials the generalizability of successful strategies across centers can be examined, exploiting a relatively unique situation. Thus, research and clinical application can proceed hand in hand.

CONCLUSIONS

The thesis of this introduction to the chapters on compliance intervention is that factors at multiple levels of the medical system and the patients life affect compliance with the medical regimen. This is further complicated in the pediatric domain by the likelihood of differential interactions among the infant, child, or adolescent, and their families as a consequence of different stages of maturation. Very different sets of behaviors will be associated with compliance problems at different ages. A comprehensive approach to compliance maintenance and remediation demands a consideration of the effect of each of these levels on the patient behaviors associated with compliance. As exemplified by the CPPT, these included the national level in terms of the NIH program office involved with the trial, because this office set policy and maintained funding priorities that could affect adherence by, for example, altering staffing levels in a particular way. At the next level were the physicians involved in the trial, particularly the LRC and trial directors. These key investigators needed to be aware of the technical problems involved in compliance and the potential solutions to such problems, so that they could adapt their clinic staffing to meet the demands involved in maintaining compliance. At the next level came the organization of the LRC, whether this involved a particular staffing pattern, or the provision of an adequate environment for the participant, or of access to computers for the adherence staff. The latter staff were also key individuals over the duration of the trial. The critical decision here was to adopt an adherence counselor model, to provide national and later local training for such counselors, and eventually to provide certification. The development of a data-oriented decision-making system and the use of specific counseling strategies were important developments at this level. All this provided the framework for the important continuing relationship between the counselor and participant, and the participant's family.

ACKNOWLEDGMENT

This chapter was completed while I was a Fellow at the Center for Advanced Study in the Behavioral Sciences. I am grateful for the support provided by the John D. & Catherine T. MacArthur Foundation.

REFERENCES

Agras, W. S. (1989a). Obesity, bulimia, and anorexia nervosa. In E. Rubenstein & D. D. Federman (Eds.), *Scientific American medicine.* New York: Scientific American.

Agras, W. S. (1989b). Understanding compliance with the medical regimen: The scope of the problem and a theoretical perspective. *Arthritis Care and Research, 3,* S2-8.

Agras, W. S., Bradford, R. H., & Marshall, G. D. (1982). Recruitment for clinical trials: The Lipid Research Clinics Coronary Primary Prevention Trial Experience, its implications for future trials. American Heart Assocation Monograph, Number 93. *Circulation, 66,* Suppl IV.

Agras, W. S., Taylor, C. B., Feldman, D. E., Losch, M., & Burnett, K. F. (1990). Developing computer-assisted therapy for the treatment of obesity. *Behavior Therapy, 21,* 91–110.

Bandura, A. (1978). The self-system in reciprocal determinism. *American Psychologist, 33,* 344–358.

Bandura, A. (1986). *Social foundations of thought and action: A social cognitive theory.* Englewood Cliffs, NJ: Prentice-Hall.

Becker, M. H., Drachman, R. H., & Kirscht, J. P. (1972). Predicting mother's compliance with pediatric medical regimens. *Journal of Pediatrics, 81,* 843–845.

Blackwell, B. (1973). The drug defaulter. *New England Journal of Medicine, 289,* 249–252.

Blackwell, B. (1989). Compliance—measurement and intervention. *Current Opinion in Psychiatry, 2,* 787–789.

Brownell, K. D., Marlatt, G. A., Lichtenstein, E., & Wilson, G. T. (1986). Understanding and preventing relapse. *American Psychologist, 41,* 765–782.

Caron, H. S., & Roth, H. P. (1968). Patients' cooperation with a medical regimen: Difficulties in identifying the noncooperator. *Journal of the American Medical Association, 203,* 120–124.

Goldman, A. I., Holcomb, R., Perry, H. M., Schnaper, H. W., Fitz, A. E., & Frohlich, E. D. (1982). Can dropout and other noncompliance be minimized in a clinical trial? *Controlled Clinical Trials, 3,* 75–89.

Haynes, R. B., Sackett, D. L., Gibson, E. S., Taylor, D. W., Hackett, B. C., Roberts, R. S., & Johnson, A. L. (1976). Improvement of medication compliance in uncontrolled hypertension. *Lancet, 1,* 1265–1268.

Moulding, T. (1961). Preliminary study of the pill calender as a method of improving the self-administration of drugs. *American Review of Respiratory Disease, 84,* 284–287.

Pendelton, D. (1983). Doctor–patient communication: A review. In D. Pendelton & J. Hasler (Eds.), *Doctor–patient communication.* New York: Academic Press.

Smith, E. O., Hardy, R. J., Cutter, G. R., Curb, J. D., & Hawkins, C. M. (1980). Application of survival analysis techniques to evaluation of factors affecting compliance in a clinical trial of hypertension control. *Controlled Clinical Trials, 1,* 59–69.

The Lipid Research Clinics Program. (1983). Pre-entry characteristics of participants in the Lipid Research Clinics' coronary primary prevention trial. *Journal of Chronic Disease, 36,* 467–479.

The Lipid Research Clinics' Program. (1984). The Lipid Research Clinics' Coronary Primary Prevention Trial Results. I. Reduction in the incidence of coronary heart disease. *Journal of the American Medical Association, 251,* 352–364.

Wilson, G. T., & Dubbert, P. M. (1983). Failures in behavior therapy for obesity: Causes, correlates, consequences. In E. Foa & P. M. G. Emmelkamp (Eds.), *Failures in behavior therapy.* New York: Wiley.

13 Medication Compliance and Childhood Asthma

Thomas L. Creer
Ohio University

In the past two decades, a number of effective medications have been introduced for the treatment of asthma. Advances with theophylline, beta agonists, cromolyn sodium, and inhaled corticosteroids have greatly expanded the arsenal of drugs available to physicians in tailoring a treatment regimen for a child with asthma (Ellis, 1988). The burst of newer and more efficacious medications was accompanied by the widespread dissemination of technologies that provided more objective measurement of the degree of compliance in patients with asthma. Ironically, it was the development of technologies, particularly high-pressure chromatography for assessing serum theophylline, that generated much of the research on compliance in the past decade. It had long been suspected that asthmatic patients did not comply with prescribed medication regimens, but the report by Eney and Goldstein (1976), which showed that only 11% of their sample of asthmatic children had therapeutic levels of theophylline in their blood, jolted many physicians as to the extent of the problem of noncompliance, and to the reality that better medications did not necessarily insure improved management of asthma.

In the 15 years since Eney and Goldstein (1976) published their article, a number of studies and reviews have focused on the topic of medication compliance in patients, particularly children, with asthma (Dirks & Kinsman, 1982; Jerome, Wigal, & Creer, 1987; Spector, 1985; Spector et al., 1986; Voyles & Menendez, 1983). The general conclusion is that medication compliance is best conceived of as a continuum ranging from total compliance to total noncompliance. There is always uncertainty about compliance in that, even if a test reveals a patient is correctly taking medications as prescribed, his or her behavior may not remain consistent over time (Spector et al., 1986). In addition, a number of variables contribute to the complexity of medication compliance in children, including: (a) the schedule of medications (e.g., whether prescribed medications are taken daily on a maintenance basis or on an as-needed basis); (b) the duration of a medication dose (e.g., whether a given drug lasts 6, 8, 12, or 24 hours); (c) route of delivery (e.g., whether a medication is taken orally, injected, or inhaled); (d) multiple doses of medications (e.g., whether one or more doses are required to either maintain the patient's health or to manage an attack); and (e) multiple medications (e.g., whether more than one drug is required to control a child's asthma).

The present review focuses on three topics: First, there is a review of the prevalence of noncompliance in children with asthma when a biochemical assay or marker is used to measure the behavior. Second, there is a review of both direct and indirect methods employed to assess compliance in children with asthma. Direct methods include blood serum assays, tracers or markers, and observation; indirect methods include patient reports, pill and liquid medication measurement, mechanical instruments, and treatment outcomes. Finally, strategies for improving medication compliance are discussed. These include patient education, altering treatment regimens, and the application of behavioral techniques.

Prevalence of Medication Compliance in Children with Asthma

Asthma is the leading diagnosis of children admitted to hospitals in the United States (Reed, 1986), an outcome likely related to widespread medication noncompliance. Table 13.1 depicts the percentage of compliance found in nine studies in which a biochemical marker was used as a major dependent variable. These differences show a broad range of compliance in children with asthma ranging from 2% to 100%. Methodological differences and patient characteristics account for much of the variance in these studies. For example, Sublett, Pollard, Kadlec, and Karibo (1979) randomly selected 50 children from nearly 500 walk-in patients at the emergency room of a children's hospital; only 2% of these youngsters were considered as compliant in that the amount of theophylline levels in their blood was within the acceptable therapeutic range of 10 to 20 $\mu g/ml$. The percentage of compliance may seem low, but it is consistent with current estimates of compliance in children with asthma reported by physicians in many emergency rooms in metropolitan areas. Furthermore, the results reported by Sublett and his colleagues (1979) are not that disparate from findings obtained when children appeared for asthma treatment at walk-in or ambulatory clinics (Eney & Goldstein, 1976; Miller, 1982). At the other end of the spectrum, the study by Baum and Creer (1986) revealed another problem: Investigating only patients who volunteer for a medication compliance study may result in an artificially inflated estimate of compliance. In this double-blind study, only 20

TABLE 13.1
Studies using Biochemical Assays or Markers to Assess Medication Compliance in Children with Asthma

Author(s)	Number and Age Range of Subjects	Criteria of Compliance	Results
Sublett et al. (1979)	50 0.8 - 14 yrs	<10 µg/ml theophylline level	2%
Miller (1982)	21 12 - 17 yrs	<10 - 20 µg/ml theophylline level	10%
Eney and Goldstein (1976)	43 3 - 16 yrs	<10 - 20 µg/ml theophylline level	11%
Cluss et al. (1984)	22 7 - 12 yrs	<80% theophylline level riboflaven tracer	50%
Christiaanse et al. (1989)	38 7 - 17 yrs	<5 mg/dl theophylline level	56%
LeBaron et al. (1985)	31 6 - 17 yrs	cromolyn sodium spot urine test	57.75% (T) to 66.50% (C)
Wood et al. (1985)	111 1 - 20 yrs	<5 µg/ml theophylline level	66%
Radius et al. (1978)	80 0.9 - 17 yrs	lab data theophylline level	66.3%
Smith et al. (1984)	37 3 - 15 yrs	(<70%) theophylline level	67.9%
Baum and Creer (1986)	20 6 - 16 yrs	<10 - 20 µg/ml theophylline level	100%

out of a population of 86 children volunteered to participate; 12 of the sample of 20 agreed to allow blood serum levels to be drawn on four separate occasions. It was only at the conclusion of the study that the physicians reported that the blood samples of all children, no matter the condition to which they were assigned, indicated they were compliant both before and during the study. A similar ceiling effect, in that compliant children were mainly recruited for the study, was reported by LeBaron, Zeltzer, Ratner, and Kniker (1985); it could account for why greater compliance was observed in their control group throughout the study. Expectations about whether medication compliance will be assessed is a variable that could account for much of the differences between studies that reported low versus high compliance (Baum & Creer, 1986; Renne & Creer, 1985); the variable, however, has not been investigated with respect to compliance in childhood asthma.

Measurement Issues

A number of approaches have been taken to assess medication compliance in children with asthma. These are of two major types: (a) those that directly assess compliance by measuring the presence of a drug in the bloodstream, add tracers or makers with the taking of medications, or that observe the patients' performance; and (b) those that indirectly assess medication compliance through patient reports, reported pill and liquid medication consumption, mechanical in-

TABLE 13.2
Strengths and Weaknesses of Direct Measures Used in Assessing Medication Compliance

Strengths	Weaknesses
Blood Serum Assays	
1. Objective	1. Pharmacokinetic interactions with other medications
2. Direct	2. Pharmacologic variations according to drug interactions
3. Yields quantifiable data	3. Timing of assays
	4. Long- versus short-term medications
	5. Pain and inconvenience to patients
	6. Specialized equipment required
	7. Lack of standardized criteria for judging compliance
Tracers or Markers	
1. Objective	1. Timing of testing
2. Direct	2. Specialized equipment required
3. Yields quantifiable data	3. Marker or tracer may interact with other substances
Observation	
1. Objective	1. Obtrusive
2. Direct	2. Reactivity may occur
3. Yields quantifiable data	3. Observer may become involved
4. Superior to patient or physician estimates	4. Requires training of observers
5. Family members may provide observation	5. Not feasible for physician use over extended periods of time

struments, and treatment outcomes. Strengths and weaknesses of the direct approaches used in assessing compliance are enumerated in Table 13.2; each is briefly described.

DIRECT METHOD

Blood Serum Assays

Blood serum assays are common methods used to assess compliance in children with asthma, particularly those who take theophylline drugs (Ellis, 1988). There are three advantages to performing blood serum assays: First, serum assays provide an objective way to assess compliance. Reliable and valid data can be obtained; these findings reveal what are regarded as safe levels of theophylline in the blood (Hendeles & Weinberger, 1985). Second, blood serum assays permit direct assessment at or within a specific time period. If multiple measurements occur, serum assays provide an objective index of compliance that is independent of self-report (Jerome et al., 1987). Third, methods for quantifying serum theophylline levels appear to be reasonably sensitive and specific (Weinberger, 1978). When individual differences in absorption, distribution, metabolism, and secretion are considered, serum theophylline levels provide an accurate estimate of medication intake.

There are, however, six potential weaknesses to using blood serum assays to measure medication compliance in children with asthma: First, pharmacokinetic interactions occur when two drugs taken concurrently accelerate or retard the metabolism of one of the drugs. This is common with theophylline preparations. Reed (1991) recently noted that while such drugs as Allopurinol, Cimetidine, Cipofloxacin (and other quinolone antibiotics), Erythromycin, Propranolol, and Troleandomycin retard theophylline metabolism, other drugs, including Carbamazepine, Nicotine, Phenobarbital, Phenytoin, and Rifampin, accelerate theophylline metabolism.

Second, pharmacologic interactions occur when two drugs produce either similar or antagonistic effects on the same tissue, thus producing a magnified or no physiological response (Kelly, 1991). According to Kelly, the most obvious examples of these two mechanisms are the combination of two classes of bronchodilators to produce an additive effect and combining a receptor antagonist with an agonist.

Third, the time testing occurs relative to taking a medication is significant. If testing occurs when the drug is at its peak in the blood, the patient will be classified as compliant; if testing occurs when the drug is at its lowest point (such as prior to taking a prescribed medication), equivocal findings emerge and the patient may be regarded as noncompliant.

Fourth, whether a patient is taking a short- versus long-lasting preparation must be considered, as well as the fact that there are differences in the extent and rate of absorption of available medications of a given class of drugs.

Fifth, blood levels are more accurate indices of theophylline levels than saliva levels (Hendeles & Weinberger, 1985). However, the discomfort of having blood drawn may persuade children or their parents not to permit this measure to be regularly used to evaluate medication compliance (Baum & Creer, 1986).

Sixth, specialized equipment for performing blood assays are required. A number of relatively inexpensive and accurate methods have been developed for assessing the level of theophylline in the blood (Ellis, 1988); equipment for assessing the other three types of medications used to treat childhood asthma—cromolyn sodium, corticosteroids, and β-agonists—are not as readily available.

Finally, there is no standardized criteria for judging whether a patient is compliant. In most studies of theophylline, compliance is defined as serum levels in the range of 10 to 20 μg/ml. Not all investigators subscribe to this criterion, however, in that some accept serum levels as low as 5 μg/ml. The number of blood serum measurements, as well as the time frame within which they are taken, also varies across studies. Some investigators consider a single measure as indicative of compliance, although the representativeness of a solitary sample for assessing long-term compliance has no empirical basis (Jerome et al., 1987).

Tracers or Markers

Cluss, Epstein, Galvis, Fireman, and Friday (1984) and Cluss and Epstein (1985) described the use of a riboflavin tracer to accurately assess compliance in asthmatic children. The method has several strengths, including the fact that the procedure is direct, objective, and produces quantifiable data. Weaknesses are similar to those discussed with blood assays. Despite its potential, there is also little empirical evidence for the use of tracers in assessing compliance in childhood asthma.

Observation

Direct observation of patient compliance can be made by either a member of a child's family or treatment team. Strengths of observation are that it is direct, objective, provides quantifiable data, and is more valid and reliable than estimates of compliance made by either clinicians or patients (Jerome et al., 1987). Observations can also be made by members of a child's family (Rapoff & Christophersen, 1982). There are several weaknesses to observation, however:

1. Observation may be obtrusive in that it disrupts the normal routine of children and their families. This seems particularly the case when observation occurs in a child's home (Renne & Creer, 1985).
2. Reactivity can occur. The knowledge that someone is monitoring the child may change his or her behavior. This is a task-confounding variable that affects conclusions made by the observer.
3. It is sometimes difficult to teach others to observe and not interfere with children. There is the possibility that the observer, particularly a child's parent, may wish to provide instruction or even badger the patient into complying with medication instructions (Rapoff & Christophersen, 1982).
4. Observers require training and constant monitoring. The lack of training and monitoring of observers can result in invalid information.
5. Observational procedures are not feasible for extended use by physicians. It would be far more economical, from both a time and a cost viewpoint, for other medical personnel to observe and record information on patients.

INDIRECT MEASURES

Strengths and weaknesses of indirect measures used to assess medication compliance in children with asthma are enumerated in Table 13.3. Several of these strengths or weaknesses were previously noted by Rapoff and Christophersen (1982). Each type of measure is briefly described.

Patient Self-Reports

Self-reports are the most commonly used method used to assess compliance in patients with asthma. Jerome and colleagues (1987) point out that two approaches have been followed: The most widely used approach is to ask all patients, during regular appointments with their physicians, if they are compliant with medication instructions. The approach is followed by most physicians, although some are more systematic in gathering such information than are others. The second approach is to teach patients self-management skills, including self-monitoring and recording, of data related to their compliance. This technique, as is noted, is an extremely valuable procedure for assessing medication compliance. There are four strengths to using self-report data.

First, self-report data represents the best data that can be gathered from patients with asthma. Only the patient knows whether he or she has complied with all medication instructions; furthermore, only patients know of all the attacks they may have experienced. If they are reliable observers of their behavior, they can provide a wealth of valid and reliable information to those who treat their asthma. (On the other hand, patients may be lax in gathering information on themselves and their asthma. In these cases, any data may not only be worthless, but it can mislead the patient's physician into making erroneous treatment decisions.)

Second, the collection of data can be tailored to the competencies of individual patients. Usually, children are asked to gather information on (a) peak flow values; (b) asthma medications, as well as specific doses, taken; (c) the schedule on which the medications are taken; (d) and whether a patient experienced an asthma attack. Instruction, sometimes involving shaping, can be used to teach children these skills (Creer, 1979).

Finally, data can be easily obtained; physicians can assist patients by preparing diaries and other materials to help patients gather data on their medication use.

Weaknesses of self-report data include the following:

1. The major problem with self-reports is that many patients overestimate the self-administration of their medications (Jerome et al., 1987). They report

TABLE 13.3
Strengths and Weaknesses of Indirect Measures Used in Assessing Medication Compliance

Strengths	Weaknesses
Patient Reports	
1. Provides accurate information 2. Easily tailored for individual patient 3. Easily obtained information	1. Overestimated compliance 2. Underreports noncompliance 3. Generally less accurate than other methods 4. Requires patient training 5. Requires external check 6. Memory distortion 7. Physician skill in eliciting information
Pill and Liquid Medications Assessment	

1. Easily obtained
2. Inexpensive
3. Superior to patient or physician estimates
4. Complements other procedures
	1. Relies on patients' motivation and efforts
	2. Overestimates compliance
	  a. pills may be removed but not ingested
	  b. does not delineate consumption patterns
	  c. pills may be taken by other family members
	3. Inherent difficulties occur in measuring liquid medications
	4. Physicians and medical personnel find pill counting and weighing canisters to be boring and tedious

Mechanical Instruments	
1. Objective 2. Technically sophisticated 3. Yields quantifiable data	1. Assesses use of dispensers, not medication use 2. Requires expensive equipment 3. Instrument breakdown
Treatment Outcomes	

1. Identifies noncompliance patients
2. Readily available to clinician
	1. Lacks validity
	2. Influenced by such factors as:
	  a. misdiagnosis
	  b. incorrect treatment
	  c. spontaneous remission of symptoms

they took prescribed medications when other measurement techniques, such as serum assay methods, indicate otherwise.

2. Patients often underreport noncompliance. Many children will not admit to their physicians that they did not follow their advice. However, as noted by Jerome and co-workers (1987), less compliant patients are often more likely to accurately report their behavior because they are aware of the

degree of deviation between their performance and their prescribed regimen.
3. Self-report data are often less accurate than are other, more direct methods of assessing medication compliance.
4. The gathering of accurate self-report data requires patients' training and the constant monitoring of their progress. Asthma diaries must be carefully reviewed with the patient; thereafter, there must be regular monitoring of his or her performance.
5. There is need for an external check to monitor the progress of children. A proven solution with asthmatic children is to have a parent verify the data collected by children on their asthma (Creer et al., 1988).
6. Memory can influence the accuracy of self-reports (Dunbar & Agras, 1980). Children must remember what occurred long enough to record their observations; any delay between the taking of medications and the recording of the performance increases the likelihood that the patient will forget what he or she did.
7. The skills of the physician at eliciting information may influence the accuracy of self-reports (Dunbar & Agras, 1980). These physician skills affect such variables as the type of information collection, the motivation of the patient in gathering such information, and the transmission of information between the patient and the physician.

Pill and Liquid Medication Assessment

There are several strengths to incorporating pill count and liquid medication measures into medication assessment. These strengths include the fact that such assessment is easy to perform, inexpensive, and superior to both patient and physician estimates; the result can be reliable and valid data (Jerome et al., 1987). Rapoff and Christophersen (1982) suggest that pill and liquid assessment complement other measures of medication compliance.

There are several weaknesses to assessing pills and liquid medications in children with asthma, however (Jerome et al., 1987). These weaknesses include: First, the accuracy of the procedures ultimately rests on the patient. Despite their expressed willingness to bring their medications to their medical appointments, many patients fail to do so. In these instances, no assessment can take place.

Second, pill count and liquid assessment overestimate compliance. This occurs with pill count because the number of pills counted does not necessarily mean that the patient took the pills; he or she could have easily taken some out of the bottle and ditched them on the way to a medical appointment. The same behavior may occur with taking inhaled liquid medications; instead of taking the medication, the child can blast off a few doses into the air. These illustrations point out that consumption patterns cannot be determined from pill count and liquid assessment alone. The overestimation of compliance by counting pills and weighing canisters of inhaled liquid medications is also influenced by family members other than the patient who takes the medications. This often occurs with adolescents in the family because they have heard they can get "high" off some asthma medications, particularly those that contain theophylline.

Third, there are problems inherent in determining the exact dose of liquid medications. A study by Leistyna and Macauley (1966) examined the teaspoons used by a group of patients to take liquid medications. The results indicated that the teaspoons held volumes of medications ranging from 2.8 to 4.2 ml.

Finally, pill count and inhaled liquid medication assessment are unpopular with physicians and other members of a child's treatment team. They not only dislike counting a patient's pills, but they find weighing canisters to be a time-consuming and tedious approach to assessing medication compliance.

Mechanical Instruments

A number of instruments have been developed in the past few years for assessing medications. One is the Chronolog (Spector, 1985). The Chronolog encircles any commercial nebulizer like a glove; it is small, lightweight, and easily fits into a pocket or purse. Each inhalation triggers a microswitch. The memory unit of the instrument measures each actuation to within 4 minutes of actual use; up to 256 actuations, gathered over several months, can be stored at one time. A separate piece of equipment, the interpreter, reads out the memory of the Chronolog; a printer produces a printout of the exact times of usage. The instrument has been widely used in asthma. A second instrument, the Medication Event Monitoring System (MEMS), consists of a container with a computer chip embedded into its cap. When the cap is removed, the chip records the day and time. The cap may then be inserted into a translator and printer to provide a printout to the physician. The MEMS has only been used in clinical trials, although it has potential for use in childhood asthma.

The strengths of these mechanical instruments are that they are objective, technically sophisticated, and yield quantitative information. Data gathered with the instruments can be valid and highly reliable. A weakness of the instruments is that they may assess use of the dispensers, not medication use. Hence, as was described for pill count and liquid assessment, a value depicting usage does not necessarily mean that the patient took the medication. He or she could have easily discarded pills or discharged doses of an inhaled medication into the air. The equipment, including both the measuring devices and translating equipment, is expensive. Finally, there has been a high rate of mechanical unreliability reported for the Chronolog. Gong, Simmons, Clark, and Tashkin (1988) lauded the effectiveness, accuracy, and ability of the Chronolog to monitor daily nebulizer use. At the same time, however, 53% of the instruments they used developed a malfunction during the course of their study.

Treatment Outcomes

There are two strengths to the use of treatment outcomes in assessing compliance (Jerome et al., 1987). First, the physician is often the first to suspect noncompliance when, despite the best treatment regimen that can be tailored for a patient, no control is established over a patient's asthma. Although other variables may account for this lack of control, many experienced clinicians will consider patient noncompliance. Second, the technique is frequently employed by physicians because it is the most readily accessible procedure for them to use. There are two weaknesses to the use of treatment outcomes for assessing medication compliance in asthmatic children (Jerome et al., 1987). First, treatment outcomes often lack validity in that, whereas patient noncompliance may be singled out as the culprit for the lack of control over a child's asthma, it may be the wrong variable. Thus, by itself, treatment outcome is not a robust measure of medication noncompliance; other assessment procedures should be performed to buttress treatment outcome. Second, there are a number of other factors that can influence treatment outcome that are independent of compliance. These factors include: (a) a misdiagnosis of asthma, (b) an incorrect treatment regimen that is incapable of establishing control over a child's asthma, and (c) the fact that asthma can spontaneously remit independently of treatment. The latter is a confounding variable anytime treatment outcome is considered in asthma, including the use of the procedure as a method for drug assessment.

Despite the problems presented by treatment outcome as a measure of medication compliance, greater attention has been focused on this variable by asthma investigators. Representative of these investigations are those that have assessed medication compliance as a result of introduction of longer lasting medications, closer patient monitoring, and self-management.

Longer Lasting Medications. Tinkelman, Vanderpool, Carroll, Page, and Spangler (1980) evaluated compliance between administration of theophylline at 6- and 12-hour intervals in 20 asthmatic children; the study featured a crossover design. They found compliance, as assessed by pill count, was significantly better with longer lasting tablets than with shorter acting tablets. The treatment outcome was a more enduring improvement in the pulmonary functioning of the youngsters taking the sustained-release drug. Tabachnik and colleagues (1982) also found improved compliance, as measured by pill count, in 40 children who received sustained-released theophylline in a crossover design study. The treatment outcome reported by the authors was that more patients had a significantly greater percentage of wheeze-free days while on the longer lasting medication.

Monitoring. In the first study to assess serum and salivary levels of theophylline, Eney and Goldstein (1976) found only 11% of a sample of 43 children were compliant. Compliance improved to 42% with closer monitoring of a second group of 47 children. The authors stated there was an improvement in the pulmonary functions of the children in the second group who were more compliant. Weinstein and Cuskey (1985) used monitoring, as well as behavioral counseling, to improve compliance to theophylline regimens in 39 asthmatic children. The authors reported that their procedure improved medication compliance as assessed by blood serum assays; this compliance, in turn, resulted in fewer wheezing episodes and improved pulmonary function. However, cautioned Weinstein and Cuskey, the lack of a control group limits interpretation of their data.

Cluss and colleagues (1984) assessed compliance to theophylline medication with a riboflavin tracer method. Of 22 asthmatic children, 11 were classified as compliant and 11 were classified as noncompliant. The authors described a number of significant changes in that the children who were noncompliant reported a higher number of days when they wheezed, greater variability in their pulmonary functions as measured by peak flow meters, and lower peak flow rates. There was also a higher proportion of noncompliant children who wheezed during the end-of-screening visit with the experimenter.

Education and Self-Management. Almost 2 dozen educational and self-management programs for childhood asthma have been developed and evaluated during the past 15 years (Wigal, Creer, Kotses, & Lewis, 1990). Several have included measures of medication compliance in their programs, and most have reported positive findings. This was clearly reflected in the report of a program, *Living with Asthma,* by Creer and colleagues (1988). In this study, children recorded whether they were compliant to all medications on a weekly asthma diary. As they participated in the program, they indicted they were compliant. Whereas compliance cannot be separated from other self-management skills, it was emphasized that the positive results obtained in the study would not have been obtained had the children been noncompliant. These results included significant improvement in the following outcome variables: (a) peak flow values, (b) number of attacks, (c) school attendance, and (d) attitudes towards asthma. In addition, the experimenters analyzed self-report measures to determine the likelihood of a patient experiencing an asthma attack if he or she missed a dose of medications. Using Bayesian procedures, it was found that the probability of an attack occurring by missing medications ranged from 0 (no effect) to 1.00 (an attack). This procedure offers a quantitative method of predicting attacks in individual patients when they are noncompliant with medication instructions.

STRATEGIES FOR INCREASING COMPLIANCE

There have been three major approaches taken to improve medication compliance in children with asthma: (a) patient education, (b) altering treatment regimens, and (c) applying behavioral techniques. Each approach is described separately.

Patient Education

There are a number of suggestions, many of which are similar to those used to increase compliance in youngsters with other chronic disorders, on how patient education can improve medication compliance in children with asthma. There is often, however, little formal evaluation of a particular educational technique in improving compliance. This is why some reviews suggest that educational efforts alone may fail with asthmatic patients (Moran, 1987); patient education should be used, it is suggested, in combination with other intervention procedures (Spector et al., 1986). This is generally the case. Those methods found to be of value in the education of children with asthma are enumerated in Table 13.4.

Instruction About Asthma and its Treatment. The basis for any approach taken to increase or maintain medication compliance is that the patient have an understanding of asthma and how it is treated. The latter should include a discussion of any prescribed drugs and their side-effects, with pharmacokinetics often emphasized (Moran, 1987). The physician or other medical personnel must be able to communicate verbally what he or she wants the child to do. This can be a difficult task for many physicians and may result in incomplete patient instruction or poor physician–patient communication. The latter were regarded by Sublett and his colleagues (1979) as two factors contributing to non-compliance in children with asthma. A number of experts (e.g., Spector et al.,

TABLE 13.4
Patient Education

I. Instruction about asthma and its treatment
    A. Use of educational materials to increase patients' and parents' knowledge of asthma
        1. use verbal materials
        2. use written and audiovisual materials
    B. Carefully explain importance of compliance to patients
    C. Relate possible side-effects of prescribed medications
II. Use basic vocabulary with clear, short sentences
    A. Emphasize practicality of compliance
    B. Avoid medical jargon
    C. Communicate in language of patient
    D. Physician should be warm and empathetic, and provide ample active interaction with patient
III. Categorize information with respect to:
    A. Prevention of attacks
    B. Management of attacks
IV. Demonstrate instrument use
    A. Incorporate behavioral procedures when possible
V. Constant follow-up
    B. Assess comprehension and recall by having patient repeat what has been told to him or her
VI. Provide constant support and reinforcement

1986) have suggested that written materials be used to augment verbal instruction. The use of single-sheet handouts from tear-off pads, provided by such groups as the American Medical Association and pharmaceutical companies, are useful in this regard. They are well conceived and written for any audience, including those who speak Spanish.

Spector (1985) has pointed out the importance of stressing the necessity of patients taking medications as prescribed. By taking maintenance medications, a child may either avoid an attack or prevent the episode from increasing in severity; by taking PRN medicines, the patient can help establish control over the attack. A number of investigators (e.g., Creer, 1979; Spector et al., 1986; Sublett et al., 1979) have emphasized the importance of describing possible side effects that may accompany the taking of asthma medications. The side effects of these drugs are often reported by patients as a reason for their noncompliance; they either have experienced such side effects or they have read of them. In many instances, patients or their parents make a conscious choice that they would rather experience asthma than the side effects that may accompany use of the medications taken to control the disorder (Creer, 1979). Discussing potential side effects with patients also permits the physician to determine if the patient is wrongly blaming his or her asthma medications for some physical or psychological change not produced by the drug.

Use of Basic Vocabulary. A well-publicized assumption is that patients understand medical jargon (Moran, 1987). In some instances, this may be the case; there are patients who are very knowledgeable about asthma. At other times, particularly with children, they may have no inkling as to what the physician is saying to them. Under these circumstances, patients may believe that they would be better off attempting to manage asthma in their own manner. This approach is likely to exclude medication compliance. Communicating in the language of the patient is a way to avoid misunderstanding. Finally, it is imperative that physicians and other medical personnel provide ample opportunity for patients to interact with them with respect to compliance. If a patient does not understand the purpose of a drug and his or her questions are answered in a condescending or sarcastic manner, why should the patient comply? He or she may not only be skeptical about the proposed treatment, but about the physician who has suggested it. Patient–physician communication patterns appear as a significant variable contributing to either compliance or noncompliance in children with asthma (Jerome et al., 1987; Sublett et al., 1979).

Categorize Information. There are a number of ways to categorize the information about medications presented to children with asthma, but perhaps the simplest way is to describe the drugs in terms of whether they are designed to prevent or abort an attack. Some medications taken by children with asthma, including cromolyn sodium and inhaled steroids, are prophylactic drugs that are useful only in preventing attacks; they have no value in treating asthma episodes and can actually intensify an ongoing attack. Other drugs, such as adrenergic preparations, may be the medicines of choice for patients during an acute attack (Ellis, 1988). Depending on the combination of medications prescribed for a patient, he or she must recognize their purpose and role in either preventing or in managing asthma.

Demonstrate Instrument Use. Many asthma medications are dispensed via an inhaler. Although inhalers may seem an easy instrument to operate, this has not proven to be the case with many children. A number of studies have been devoted to developing techniques to teach younger children to properly inhale their asthma medications; these are depicted in Table 13.5. As noted, the techniques range from use of items readily available in the homes of many children with asthma (e.g., disposable coffee cups; Henry, Milner, & Davies, 1983, and freezer bags; Lee & Evans, 1984, to instruments designed and marketed by pharmaceutical companies, particularly various types of spacers). As noted, many of the devices have been particularly helpful with younger children. Various types of spacers have recently been introduced by pharmaceutical companies throughout the United States. Depending on the preference of the physician, a child may use a tube-like aerosol holding chamber, the same chamber with a mask, a solid, plastic holding chamber, or a collapsible metered dose inhaler for use in inhaling nebulizer asthma medications. In all cases, children need instruc-

TABLE 13.5
Methods Used to Dispense Medications to Younger Children with Asthma

Author(s)	Number and Age Range of Subjects	Methods	Results
Ellul-Micallef et al. (1980)	12 7-11 yrs	Spacer Terbutaline	Significant PEFR change
Lee & Evans (1984)	20 3-6 yrs	Freezer bag Albuterol	Significant PEFR change
Pedersen (1983)	20 6-12 yrs	Tube spacer Terbutaline	Significant FEV1 change
Russell & Frame (1986)	15 3-10 yrs	Nebuhaler Terbutaline	Significant PEFR change
Gleeson & Price (1988)	11 7-14 yrs	Nebuhaler Terbutaline	Significant PEFR change
Croft (1989)	20 1.9-2.9 yrs	Tube spacer Salbutamol	15 or 20 children modeled mother; 40% used spacer correctly
Henry et al. (1983)	12 3.7-7.8 yrs	Disposable coffee cup Salbutamol	Significant PEFR change

tion in such steps as holding the nebulizer, pressing down the container to release the medication, correctly inhaling the nebulized drug, and any other behavior required to insure that the medication reaches the airways of a youngster.

Constant Follow-up. In his review of noncompliance in patients with asthma, Moran (1987) pointed out that physician instructions are frequently forgotten or misunderstood. Indeed, the major excuse for missing a medication is that the patient claims he or she forgot to take it as instructed. Spector (1985) employed several aids to insure that patients remember to comply with their medication program. These included: (a) having the patient recite what he or she has just been told by the physician or other medical personnel; (b) the physician asking to see both prescribed medications and other drugs taken by the patient; and (c) the use of medication charts.

Weinstein (1987) advocated providing patients with a written summary of their asthma medications. Advantages to a youngster of such a summary are: (a) it makes it possible for the child's asthma to be treated promptly; (b) it reduces the uncertainty and panic often associated with an attack; (c) it specifies the proper dosage and timing of each of the child's medications, as well as the order in which they should be taken; (d) it emphasizes the potential side effects of each medication; (e) it reminds the child of what medications should be avoided; and (f) it specifies the exact point in the attack when the youngster or his or her parents should notify the child's physician. These instructions are not only useful in helping the children remember their treatment regimen, but written instructions serve as a cue or reminder as to the behaviors they should perform to achieve compliance.

Provide Constant Support and Reinforcement. A common theme woven throughout reviews on medication compliance in children with asthma was the need to provide constant support and reinforcement to patients (Jerome et al., 1987; Spector et al., 1986; Voyles & Menendez, 1983). Compliant behavior is often overlooked and nonrewarded, in part because the physician tends to concentrate on patients who are noncompliant (Jerome et al., 1987). However, as with most behaviors, the maintenance of compliance rests upon periodic reinforcement from a child's physician or a member of his or her staff.

Altering Treatment Regimens

Reviewers of medication compliance argue that a way to improve compliance is to alter the treatment regimen so that it is as convenient as possible to the patient. Those who have discussed medication compliance in asthmatic children make such a case. Specific actions suggested to achieve compliance include steps outlined in Table 13.6.

TABLE 13.6
Altering Treatment Regimens

I. Drop ineffective medications
II. Decrease complexity of medications
    A. Prescribe as few medications as possible
    B. Medications should be taken as few times per day as necessary
        1. Use longer-lasting preparations
    C. Simplest or easiest to administer medications should be introduced first, followed by additional or more complex tasks (shaping)
III. Decrease duration of medication use
    A. Shift from maintenance to as-needed (PRN) medications if possible
IV. Start with medications causing fewest side-effects
V. Negotiate times for patients to take medications. Attempt to fit taking medications into patient's established routine
VI. Use cues and reminders, e.g., pill containers, calenders, stickers, etc.
VII. Minimize number of lifestyle changes
VIII. Help reduce costs of medications to patients.

Drop Ineffective Medications

In the course of monitoring what medications are taken by the patient, Spector (1985) suggested dropping ineffective medications. Because their parents have seen products advertised, children with asthma will often take over-the-counter medications that have little or no value for them. At times, these drugs, including cough syrups and antihistamines, may interfere with prescribed medical treatment (Plaut, 1988). With any new prescription, a youngster may not require other drugs he or she has been taking to help manage asthma. These drugs, Spector (1985) points out, should also be dropped from the patient's regimen with an explanation as to why they are no longer necessary.

Decrease Complexity of Medication Regimen

Williams (1980) noted that as a general principle of therapy physicians should "employ as much medication as is necessary to produce and maintain improvement, and then to reduce the intensity of treatment when symptoms subside" (p. 315). This philosophy is followed by most physicians treating childhood asthma who, in general, have attempted to control a child's asthma while permitting him or her to live as normal a life as possible (Chai & Newcomb, 1973). This has meant most physicians attempt to fit a treatment regimen to the characteristics of a child and, for a given point in time, to his or her asthma. Sometimes, the child may be on a lean regimen and require only PRN medications; at other times, the child may require both maintenance and PRN drugs. In general, it has been found that the more complex the treatment regimen, the greater the probability that noncompliance will occur (Jerome et al., 1987).

Prescribe Few Medications. Earlier, it was noted that Spector (1985) advocated a regular review of what medications a patient takes, not only for his or her asthma but for any other health concern. In the course of such reviews, any unnecessary medications can be eliminated from the child's regimen. This might be achieved by dropping one medication and increasing the dosage of a second medication. Keeping the number of other treatments to a minimum is also a way to improve compliance (Spector et al., 1986). The fewer times a child takes drugs per day is another way to enhance compliance (Spector et al., 1986; Voyles & Menendez, 1983). In the past, many children required theophylline every 6 hours for their asthma to be controlled. The result often was that at least one dose, usually that taken in the middle of the night, was omitted (Creer, 1979). This changed with the introduction of 12- and 24-hour theophylline doses; the child and his or her parents no longer had to wake up for the youngster's late night medications but could rely on drugs with effects lasting 12 or 24 hours. As noted, the result of these longer lasting preparations was improved compliance (e.g., Tinkelman, Vanderpool, Carroll, Page, & Spandler, 1980). Introducing the child to the simplest or easiest medication to administer, with positive reinforcement following shortly, is referred to as a shaping procedure by Voyles and Menendez (1983). Adding and evaluating the effects of medications one at a time should also enhance the acquisition of compliance behaviors.

Decrease Duration of Use

Compliance is often found to decrease when medications are taken over a period of time (Garfield, 1982). This certainly is the case with chronic childhood asthma: The longer a child is required to take drugs to control his or her asthma, the more likely he or she is to become noncompliant. This particularly becomes prominent in adolescents with asthma. Many will test to determine whether they actually require medications by missing doses and observing what happens. Their behavior may be reinforced if no attack occurs; this can lead to even greater noncompliance that may end with a severe attack. However, even the latter event may not alter noncompliant behavior because many adolescents become convinced that their behavior is independent, which it may be to some extent, of the frequency and severity of the attacks of asthma they experience (Creer, 1979, 1983a). The adolescent's behavior may then become more difficult to change. Thus, most physicians make every effort to alter a child's treatment regimen from a maintenance to an as-needed basis whenever possible.

Start with Medications Causing Fewest Side Effects

In prescribing drugs for childhood asthma, a physician will initiate treatment with the safest agents, such as theophylline and adrenergic aerosols, and then escalate the therapy, if necessary, by increasing doses and adding more powerful, albeit more dangerous, medications, including corticosteroids (Williams, 1980). The principle of matching treatment with severity of the disorder guides the physician in drug selection (Ellis, 1988). Medication usage is reduced in the reverse manner by withdrawing the more powerful drugs first, reducing doses of medications, etc. (Plaut, 1988). Of the four classes of asthma medications, cromolyn sodium has the fewest side effects. Unfortunately, it is often most effective only with children who have mild asthma (Ellis, 1988); as noted earlier, it also has no value in treating asthma episodes. Theophylline is a useful drug for the treatment of mild and moderate attacks, as well as a daily preventative medication. There are a number of common side effects, including overactivity, nervousness, upset stomach, nausea, vomiting, headache, and loss of appetite; these are most pronounced during the initial days a youngster is on the medication (Plaut, 1988). As noted by Reed (1991), theophylline can also interact with a number of substances, which can either increase or decrease the potency of theophylline.

Most physicians use an adrenergic drug as their first choice in the treatment of an asthma episode; these medications can be given by injection, taken by mouth, or inhaled directly into the lungs (Plaut, 1988). Side effects include shakiness, rapid or pounding heart beat, and nausea; these common effects are not considered to be dangerous, however. Plaut (1988) opined that adrenergic pills are particularly useful for children under 3 years of age. A recent study by Sears and colleagues (1990) has brought into question the efficacy of regular inhaled beta-agonist treatment in bronchial asthma. This investigation has not only sparked considerable controversy but is bound to generate a number of future studies on the role of this class of medications in the treatment of asthma.

The final class of asthma medications are corticosteroids. These can be invaluable in the treatment of severe asthma, particularly when inhaled and when taken for only brief periods of time. There are a long list of potential side effects, ranging from weight gain to the formation of posterior subcapsular cataracts. Most of these adverse effects, dose and dosing-interval related, can be avoided by the use of an alternate-day regimen or aerosolized agents (Ellis, 1988).

Negotiate Times for Medication Use

Compliance can be improved by having the child take his or her medications in accordance with appropriately timed events that are consistent with his or her schedule. Thus, if the patient is instructed to take a pill or inhalation three times a day, it is best to prescribe such treatment "with each meal" if the youngster has three appropriately timed meals, rather than prescribing it "three times a day" (Spector et al., 1986). The times a medication is taken should always be discussed with children and their parents. Through such interactions, a physician or other medical personnel can determine if negotiation is necessary in order for the patient to be compliant to medical and medication instructions.

Use Cues and Reminders

Several investigators (Spector, 1985; Spector et al., 1986; Voyles & Menendez, 1983) suggested that reminders and cues be used to improve compliance in asthmatic patients. Cues that might prove useful with children include calenders, stickers, and daily dispensers. These not only provide feedback to the youngster that he or she has taken prescribed medications, but they provide a record for the child's physician (Voyles & Menendez, 1983). Daily asthma or medication diaries are useful (Spector, 1985); these techniques have become, as noted later, a staple of self-management programs for childhood asthma.

Minimize Lifestyle Changes

Fitting the medication schedule to naturally occurring events in the child's environment is one approach to minimizing lifestyle changes. A problem that may occur with adolescents is that they begin to smoke. This behavior cannot only precipitate attacks, but it can have an effect upon theophylline medications taken by the patient. In the case of smoking, physicians and other personnel may need to devise a program, including smoking cessation efforts, for the adolescent. The physician must also be aware of illicit mood-altering drugs that are taken by some adolescents with asthma (Creer, 1987). Barbituates can inhibit theophylline metabolism, thus producing a marked elevation in serum theophylline concentration. Phencyclidine and amphetamines can elicit such adverse effects as arrhythmias, lower seizure thresholds, irritability, and apprehension. The latter may be misinterpreted as toxicity related to theophylline or adrenergic bronchodilators (Szefler, Rogers, & Strunk, 1984). Inhaled agents, particularly glue, present a risk of hypoxia and suffocation; the unsupervised use of tranquilizers, antidepressants, or minor sedatives can increase the risk of seizures, arrhythmias, and hypoxia. Marijuana can produce short-term bronchodilation, but it is well documented that use of the substance is associated with accelerated theophylline metabolism. Furthermore, as Szefler and his colleagues (1984) conclude, the long-term use of marijuana can affect pulmonary functions and result in asthmatic symptoms, laryngitis, pharyngitis, bronchitis, coughing, and hoarseness. Because the adolescent is apt to be exposed to such illicit substances, his or her physician should be alert to possibly solve more potential problems than medication compliance.

Reduce Costs

There are a number of practical approaches that can be taken by physicians to reduce the costs of asthma medications (Creer, 1979). These include: (a) teaching families to do comparative shopping for medications, (b) instructing families to seek health insurance that defrays some portion of medication expenses, (c) prescribing generic medications when feasible, and (d) tailoring the child's drug regimen to fit the pocketbook of his or her parents. Many physicians assist children by providing office samples of medications; in addition, a physician may obtain spacers for the child to use in taking inhaled drugs. Finally, for the truly indigenous patient, the physician may refer him or her to governmental programs (e.g., Social Security) that may help with the expenses of asthma.

BEHAVIORAL TECHNIQUES

Behavioral techniques used to improve medication compliance in children with asthma include (a) shaping, (b) negotiation and contracting, (c) modeling, (d) monitoring, and (e) self-management. Later it becomes apparent that recent emphasis has been placed on monitoring and self-management procedures.

Shaping

Shaping entails the training of successive approximations of a target response. Two methods of shaping discussed earlier involve addition of one medication at a time, and the introduction of the simplest to take medications (e.g., oral liquid medications), followed by the more difficult to administer drugs (e.g., inhaled medications) that require eye–hand coordination on the part of the child. Two investigations have employed shaping with asthmatic children: Marion, Creer, and Burns (1983) targeted behaviors required to correctly use a hand-held inhaler. By using an intervention composed of shaping, modeling, and reinforcement, children with asthma were taught to correctly use the nebulizer during attacks. Because many medications are dispensed via this route, Marion and his colleagues suggested that the method could be used with any asthmatic child, regardless of his or her age. In a second study, Renne and Creer (1976) observed that a number of children with asthma did not use a compressor-driven nebulizer correctly. It was observed that the children must coordinate three responses—diaphragmatic breathing, attending to the apparatus, and inhaling the dispensed medication properly—in order for the apparatus to achieve its goals. By employing a multiple baseline design, shaping was carried out with each of these behaviors; training, in most instances, involved a single 30- to 40-minute session. The results demonstrated that, once they were taught to use the equipment, the youngsters not only required less medication to control their attack—there was an 100% improvement in the efficacy of medications administered—but a procedure was developed that was readily used by nurses and respiratory therapists to teach patients to use the equipment correctly. Finally, most self-management programs developed for children with asthma have incorporated shaping by introducing easier to learn skills, reinforcing the performance of the youngsters, and then teaching them additional skills for managing their asthma.

Negotiation and Contracting

Spector and his colleagues (1986) repeatedly noted the value of negotiation with asthmatic patients with respect to the medications they were to take and when they were to take them. In particular, they stressed the need to achieve a negotiated plan with respect to the schedule of when asthma drugs are taken. The outcome of negotiation between patients and medical personnel should be a written agreement or contract. With medication compliance, the contract would stipulate the reinforcement contingency the patient would receive in return for his or her performing the stipulations of the contract. An example of such a contract with children with asthma and their physicians was that employed at the National Asthma Center in Denver (Creer, 1979, 1987; Jerome et al., 1987). A contract was negotiated with all residents several weeks before they were considered for discharge from the facility. The behavior expected from the children was that they manage their own medications by taking their prescribed medications in the proper dose according to the appropriate schedule. The reinforcement offered by the physicians was discharge from the facility and return to their homes. The procedure outlined in the contract became the backbone of successfully teaching medication compliance skills to the youngsters before they performed these skills in their homes. Although no systematic evaluation was made of the procedure, it has been suggested that low mortality rates in children discharged from the facility may have resulted from such training (Creer, 1986).

Modeling

Modeling has been used to teach children to use nebulized medications correctly (Croft, 1989; Marion et al., 1983). An example of such an approach was an investigation reported by Croft (1989). In his study, he had the mothers of 20 two-year-old children model correct usage of a tube spacer. Croft reported that 15 of the 20 children learned to imitate the responses of their mother; this resulted in 8 of the children using the spacer correctly to inhale their medication. Modeling has also been an integral component of many self-management programs for children with asthma. Perhaps the best illustration is provided in *Living with Asthma* (Creer, Backial, Ullman, & Leung, 1986). In this program, children are taught to model the behaviors of a mythical youngster, Marvin Marvelous, and his physician, Dr. Quackenbush (or Dr. Q).

Monitoring

Methods used in monitoring medication compliance in children with asthma include those that follow.

Use Prepared Checklists of Medication Charts. Many experts advocate the use of prepared checklists or medication charts by asthmatic children and/or their parents (Spector, 1985; Weinstein & Cuskey, 1985). These devices simplify data collection for the patient and provide uniformity in information obtained (Jerome et al., 1987). Asthma diaries are also useful in monitoring medication compliance. As part of an asthma diary completed by children each day, Creer and co-workers (1988) not only had youngsters list the medications they took, but also mark how accurate they were in adhering to the schedule of drug use. The diary also served as a reminder to the children to take their medications as prescribed. Diaries completed by the children offer an additional advantage (Creer et al., 1988): if a child is taught to monitor and record information about his or her behavior, the youngster's parents can serve as a reliability check for the information that is collected.

Regular Telephone Calls. Weinstein and Cuskey (1985) used weekly telephone calls to monitor medication compliance in children with asthma. They indicated this was not only a useful way of monitoring patient's behavior, but that such calls served as prompts to encourage compliance. A weekly telephone call also permits physicians or members of his or her staff to reiterate key elements of treatment. This point cannot be overemphasized, particularly with respect to a disorder in which the child may be asymptomatic for long periods of time (Jerome et al., 1987).

See all Medications Taken by Child. Spector (1985) recommended that medical personnel periodically ask a patient to bring in all medications he or she takes, including vitamins, so they can be reviewed. This is a sound tactic for several reasons: First, it can be determined if the child's parents have actually had a prescription filled. As pointed out by Sublett and his co-workers (1979), failure to have a prescription filled is a significant factor contributing to medication noncompliance in asthmatic children. Second, the physician can determine if the patient, especially a youngster, is taking a substance that could interfere with his or her asthma medication. Perhaps the best illustration is the child who, while taking a theophylline drug product prescribed by one physician, receives a prescription for erythromycin from a second physician. This type of drug interaction can be avoided by regular monitoring of the medications taken by the asthmatic child. Finally, a periodic audit permits the physician to determine if a youngster can discontinue taking a particular drug. As noted earlier, this is an easy and effective way to simplify a child's medication regimen (Spector, 1985).

Introduce Instruments for Assessing Compliance. Procedures and instruments described earlier can be introduced to more closely monitor medication compliance in children with asthma. Investigators might select such techniques as weighing canisters, counting pills, performing serum or salivary assays, or adding a tracer or marker to the taking of an asthma drug. Devices such as the Chronolog or the MEMS may also be used to more closely assess compliance.

Provide Feedback. Spector and his colleagues (1986) suggested feedback on test results (e.g., theophylline testing) should be provided to patients with asthma to reward compliance when it is high and to stimulate compliance when it is low. This would be part of an ongoing effort to assess compliance each time the patient has an appointment with his or her physician. The procedure appears to have merit, although there is always the possibility that a patient may comply only for those times preceding an office visit. Such feedback is not provided in clinical trials because it is believed that such information could compromise other data collected in a study.

Introduce Closer Monitoring. There are times when children with asthma may consciously ditch their medications. Spector (1985), for example, noted his experience with this illustration: "One patient simply threw her pills down the toilet, others hid them in shirt pockets, bras, or other orifices other than the mouth. A few would be chewing gum when they received the pills so that both would land in the waste basket" (p. 552). These are common behaviors observed in children institutionalized for their asthma (Creer, 1979). The only way these behaviors can be corrected is through close monitoring and, as suggested by Spector and his colleagues (1986), an occasional review of the noncompliant behavior of the children with their physician.

Add Parental Support and Reminders. Parental support and reminders are useful when a child is placed on asthma medications. Parents cannot only serve as a cue for medication taking, but they may answer questions that the child has about the purpose of such treatment. After awhile, however, parental support and reminders should be faded from the program. The reasons for this are because many youngsters, particularly older children and adolescents, begin to resent their parents for what they view as an intrusion into their lives, and because such parental behavior can defeat attempts to teach self-management skills to the youngsters (Creer et al., 1988).

Constantly Reiterate Key Elements. Spector (1985) repeatedly emphasized the need to carefully explain the importance of medication compliance to patients, including children, with asthma.

Continually Reinforce Child for Appropriate Behaviors. A theme stressed in reviews of medication compliance in patients with asthma (Spector, 1985; Spector et al., 1986; Voyles & Menendez, 1983) is the need to reinforce patients for complying with medical and medication instructions.

Self-Management of Childhood Asthma. As noted, there have been close to two dozen programs developed and evaluated for the self-management of childhood asthma (Wigal, Creer, Kotses, & Lewis, 1990). The importance of each of the self-management skills used to control childhood asthma includes (Creer et al., 1988) information gathering, information processing, decision making, and self-instruction.

Information Gathering. There are two components to gathering information regarding one's performance: (a) self-monitoring and (b) self-recording. Self-monitoring refers to a child observing or monitoring any changes related to his or her asthma. With medications, the child must monitor two aspects of his or her performance: (a) the usage of any maintenance medications required to prevent attacks; and (b) the usage of medications required on a PRN basis. The former aspect becomes routine to many children; they realize that maintenance medications, when prescribed, are taken with the hope that the number and severity of the patient's attacks can be reduced. The latter aspect is far more complex: The patient must detect any changes in his or her breathing that could signal either an impending attack or the increased intensity of an ongoing episode. Failure to discriminate these changes could produce delays in seeking treatment and an intensification in an ongoing attack.

Self-recording refers to the act of recording any observations made through self-observation (Kanfer, 1980). Two strategies seem invaluable: First, it is useful to have the youngster complete a daily diary with such information as peak flow rates, medication usage, and whether he or she had an attack. Each asthma episode should be described on a separate asthma attack form. The latter form not only provides more detailed information, but it serves as a check on diary data. Second, the youngster should be taught to monitor and record information relating to his or her asthma. When this occurs, the youngster's mother and/or father can serve as a reliability check on the accuracy of any recorded information. These self-reports assume greater significance with the recognition that, in many instances, the frequency and severity of attacks, as well as any self-treatment initiated, is known only by the child (Creer & Winder, 1986).

Information Processing and Evaluation. Children must analyze the information they collect to determine if any potential problems exist that require action, and to evaluate a problem so it can be solved. With children with asthma, this entails that they collect information about their breathing, continually analyze the information to detect any changes, determine if any changes signal an attack, and decide how any asthma flareups are to be treated. Information processing and evaluation can be complex for a child with asthma. A variety of factors operate in symptom discrimination ranging from a lack of hypoxic drive, which physically signals an attack, to contextual cues that serve to distract the child from attending to what is occurring with his or her asthma (Creer, 1983b).

Decision Making. After the child realizes that he or she has a problem, the youngster must select what, potentially, is the most appropriate solution from among available options. In deciding how to manage an attack, a number of variables can come into play, including patient knowledge, experience, and the context within which the decision is made. The best choice usually represents a set of events agreed upon beforehand by the child and his or her physician; however, the context within which the youngster is operating may dictate the decision he or she makes (Creer et al., 1988). The latter can influence whether or not a patient wants to use a nebulized medication, particularly in the presence of others. Children with asthma must remember that decision making is a dynamic matter in which alternative solutions may be generated. Different solutions may be warranted with (a) new environments or contexts, (b) changes in treatment, and (c) past failure of the child to bring about the desired solution (Kanfer & Busemeyer, 1982).

Self-Instruction. Self-instruction refers to the statements children make to themselves to prompt, direct, and maintain compliance. The exact sequence of steps followed by a youngster will not only be a function of a given asthma attack, but of the management strategy he or she has worked out beforehand with his or her physician. An example of such a sequence tailored for children with asthma was provided by Creer and Kotses (1983):

> From the outset, they were taught to conceive of asthma management as a chain of responses. Each link in the response chain occurs in sequence so that the patient performed one response, then a second, and so on until control was established over the episode. By working in conjunction with the physician, a patient and his or her family could develop a coherent script that could be performed by the patient in the event of an attack. Management of asthma is more readily achieved when a patient follows a predetermined sequence of responses; self-instruction, in turn, becomes the core of the subsequent recall and performance of such a sequence. (p. 1032)

Two other aspects of self-instruction are as follows:

1. *Self-Induced Stimulus Change.* Self-induced stimulus change refers to the youngster changing aspects of his or her environment in order to prevent or abort an asthma attack. The child may prevent or abort attacks by avoiding or escaping from known precipitants of an attack. The child can also make stimulus changes that enhance compliance by placing cues and other stimuli around the environment to remind him or her to take medications as prescribed.

2. *Self-Induced Response Change.* Self-induced response change refers to the youngster changing aspects of his or her performance in order to prevent or avoid respiratory distress. Taking PRN medications would be an example of response change initiated by the child; based upon the steps previously outlined, he or she would determine if a dose or additional doses of a prescribed medication are required to halt the flareup.

Self-Reaction. Bandura (1986) defined self-reaction influences as the development of evaluative standards and judgmental skills. These internal standards establish the child's capability for self-evaluation and, in turn, produce self-reactions. Based upon the outcome of his or her performance, the youngster may recognize that his or her behavior led to control being established over an attack. The child is reinforced, and the outcome should provide feedback to strengthen self-management skills. If the youngster is not reinforced, however, there may be a weakening of self-management skills; additional training in self-management with respect to medication compliance is then necessary.

DISCUSSION

This chapter has reviewed the topic of medication compliance in childhood asthma. Three topics were discussed in detail: the prevalence of compliance, assessment of the behavior, and strategies taken to improve compliance in asthmatic youngsters. In describing strategies, various methods used to assess compliance were enumerated. There have been two recent trends with respect to compliance and childhood asthma. First, although noncompliance is an old problem, there has been increased recognition among practitioners of both the prevalence and complexity of the problem. It can be safely stated that there are few asthmatic patients, including children, who are always compliant; regardless of the severity of a patient's disorder, he or she will, at times, be noncompliant. There are many reasons for this outcome, many of which have been discussed in earlier reviews (Creer, 1979; Jerome et al., 1979; Spector et al., 1986; Sublett et al., 1979; Voyles & Menendez, 1983), ranging from specific characteristics of asthma to medication side effects. The increased recognition of noncompliance has led to an abandonment of any simplistic notion that a patient is merely a robot who will automatically fulfill the physician's instructions. There are even suggestions that the term *compliance* should be replaced by the term *adherence*. An example is contained in a statement by Falliers (1983): 'Compliance' is a rather authoritarian term. Patients have a right to disagree with their physicians and, at times, they are inclined to change doctors because they dislike following instructions without discussion" (p. 416). This statement embodies the recognition that compliance is not only the result of assessment and application of treatment strategies, but the context created by medical and behavioral scientists acting in cooperation with patients. The context not only dictates the reliability and validity of patient data, but the efficacy of any strategy taken to increase and enhance compliance.

The second trend is the realization that compliance is composed of two types of behavior: preventative behaviors and attack behaviors. The former class includes taking maintenance medications required by some children with asthma. These drugs are prescribed with the hope that they may prevent an attack from occurring; in addition, some of these drugs (e.g., cromolyn sodium) have fewer side effects than other asthma medications. Medication compliance can be weakened by such factors as the length of time over which these drugs are required, and because the consequences that result from missing a dose or doses of medication may be perceived as distal from the noncompliant action. Most patients miss occasional doses without any noticeable consequence, although failure to take a prophylactic medication may increase the likelihood of their experiencing an acute attack that requires hospital care (Canny et al., 1989).

A major problem with medication compliance in childhood asthma occurs with respect to the management of attacks. As was noted earlier, the management of an attack involves a number of steps by the patient beginning with symptom detection and ending with the termination of the episode. There are a number of compliant behaviors that can be observed during an attack (e.g., the child taking an inhaled medication). In addition, it is possible to assess treatment outcomes of the child's behavior (e.g., a diminuition of symptoms, improved performance in respiratory testing, etc.). It is in the area of cognitive patient skills that uncertainty occurs, because knowledge regarding information processing and evaluation, decision making, and self-reaction can be obtained only through self-reports of the patient. At the present time, not enough patients know these self-management skills and are able to communicate their actions to others. As a result, patients encounter difficulties when they could be avoided. For example, FitzGerald and Hargreave (1989) recently proclaimed that "Most emergency visits, hospital admissions and life-threatening exacerbations are preventable because severe asthma usually develops over days and there is time to increase treatment to reverse them before they become severe" (p. 892). For various and sundry reasons, patients, including children, do not process information about what is occurring to their breathing, make management decisions based on this information, and communicate their needs to medical personnel. The matter becomes even more serious with respect to asthma mortality. A number of reports, including those that investigated mortality in children (e.g., Carswell, 1985), have found that deaths often result from severe asthma that is inadequately assessed and treated by the child and the medical staff alike. Future efforts must be directed towards teaching self-management skills to children with asthma; along with increased knowledge, effective ways to assess cognitive self-management skills, public only through self-report, must be developed. Increased performance of these self-management skills is ultimately the key to medication compliance and, in turn, to the successful control of childhood asthma.

ACKNOWLEDGMENTS

Preparation of this chapter was supported, in part, by Grant No. HL 32538 from the National Heart, Lung, & Blood Institute. I am indebted to Raymond E. Tobey, MD and John A Winder, MD for their advice, and to Harry Kotses, PhD for his comments concerning the manuscript.

REFERENCES

Bandura, A. (1986). *Social foundations of thought and action: A social cognitive theory.* Englewood Cliffs, NJ: Prentice-Hall.

Baum, D., & Creer, T. L. (1986). Medication compliance in children with asthma. *Journal of Asthma, 23,* 49-59.

Canny, G. J., Reisman, J., Healy, R., Schwartz, C., Petrou, C., Rebuck, A. S., & Levison, H. (1989). Acute asthma: Observations regarding the management of a pediatric emergency room. *Pediatrics, 83,* 507-512.

Carswell, F. (1985). Thirty deaths from asthma. *Archives of Disease in Childhood, 60,* 25-28.

Chai, H., & Newcomb, R. W. (1973). Pharmacologic management of childhood asthma. *American Journal of Diseases of Children, 125,* 757-765.

Christiaanse, M. E., Lavigne, J. V., & Lerner, C. V. (1989). Psychosocial aspects of compliance in children and adolescents with asthma. *Journal of Developmental Behavioral Pediatrics, 10,* 75-80.

Cluss, P. A., & Epstein, L. H. (1985). The measurement of medical compliance in the treatment of diseases. In P. Karoly (Ed.), *Measurement strategies in health psychology* (pp. 403-432). New York: Wiley.

Cluss, P. A., Epstein, L. H., Galvis, S. A., Fireman, P., & Friday, G. (1984). Effect of compliance for chronic asthmatic children. *Journal of Consulting and Clinical Psychology, 52,* 909-910.

Creer, T. L. (1979). *Asthma therapy: A behavioral health care system for respiratory disorders.* New York: Springer.

Creer, T. L. (1983a). Respiratory disorders. In T. G. Burish & L. A. Bradley (Eds.), *Coping with chronic diseases: Research and applications* (pp. 313-336). New York: Academic Press.

Creer, T. L. (1983b). Response: Self-management psychology and the treatment of childhood asthma. *The Journal of Allergy and Clinical Immunology, 72,* 607-610.

Creer, T. L. (1986). Psychological factors and death from asthma. Creation and critique of a myth. *Journal of Asthma, 23,* 261-269.

Creer, T. L. (1987). Psychological and neurophysiological aspects of childhood asthma. In D. G. Tinkelman, C. J. Falliers, & C. K. Naspitz (Eds.), *Childhood asthma: Pathophysiology and treatment* (pp. 341-371). New York: Marcel Dekker.

Creer, T. L., Backial, M., Burns, K. L., Leung, P., Marion, R. J., Miklich, D. R., Morrill, C., Taplin, P. S., & Ullman, S. (1988). Living with asthma. I. Genesis and development of a self-management program for childhood asthma. *Journal of Asthma, 25,* 335-362.

Creer, T. L., Backial, M., Ullman, S., & Leung, P. (1986). *Living with asthma. Part 1. Manual for teaching parents the self-management of childhood asthma. Part 2. Manual for teaching children the self-management of asthma* (NIH Publicaiton No. 86-2364). Washington, DC: U.S. Government Printing Office.

Creer, T. L., & Kotses, H. (1983). Asthma: Psychologic aspects and management. In E. Middleton Jr., C. E. Reed, & E. F. Ellis (Eds.), *Allergy: Principles and practice* (2nd ed., pp. 1016-1035). St. Louis: Mosby.

Creer, T. L., & Winder, J. A. (1986). Asthma. In K. A. Holroyd & T. L. Creer (Eds.), *Self-management of chronic disease: Handbook of clinical interventions and research* (pp. 269-303). Orlando, FL: Academic Press.

Croft, R. D. (1989). 2 year old asthmatics can learn to operate a tube spacer by copying their mothers. *Archives of Diseases in Childhood, 64,* 742-743.

Dirks, J. F., & Kinsman, R. A. (1982). Nondichotomous patterns of medication usage: The yes-no fallacy. *Clinical Pharmacology and Therapeutic, 31,* 413-423.

Dunbar, J. M., & Agras, W. S. (1980). In J. M. Ferguson & C. B. Taylor (Eds.), *The comprehensive handbook of behavioral medicine* (Vol. 3, pp. 115-145). New York: Spectrum.

Ellis, E. F. (1988). Asthma in infancy and childhood. In E. Middleton Jr., C. E. Reed, & E. F. Ellis (Eds.), *Allergy: Principles and practice* 3rd ed., pp. 1037–1061). St. Louis: Mosby.

Ellul-Micallef, R., Moren, F., Wetterlin, K., & Hidinger, K. C. (1980). Use of a special inhaler attachment in asthmatic children. *Thorax, 35,* 620–623.

Eney, R. D., & Goldstein, E. O. (1976). Compliance of chronic asthmatics with oral administration of theophylline as measured by serum and salivary levels. *Pediatrics, 57,* 513–517.

Falliers, C. J. (1983). Comments. *Journal of Asthma, 20,* 416.

FitzGerald, J. M., & Hargreave, F. E. (1989). The assessment and management of acute life-threatening asthma. *Chest, 95,* 888–894.

Garfield, E. (1982). Patient compliance: A multifaceted problem with no easy solution. *Current Comments, 37,* 5–14.

Gleeson, J. G. A., & Price, J. F. (1988). Nebuhaler technique. *British Journal Diseases of Chest, 82,* 172–174.

Gong, H. Jr., Simmons, M. S., Clark, V. A., & Tashkin, D. P. (1988). Metered-dose inhaler usage in subjects with asthma: Comparison of Nebulizer Chronolog and daily diary recordings. *Journal of Allergy and Clinical Immunology, 82,* 5–10.

Hendeles, L., & Weinberger, M. (1985). Theophylline produce and dosing interval selection for chronic asthma. *Journal of Allergy and Clinical Immunology, 76,* 285–291.

Henry, R. L., Milner, A. D., & Davies, J. G. (1983). Simple drug delivery system for use by young asthmatics. *British Medical Journal, 286,* 2021.

Jerome, A., Wigal, J. K., & Creer, T. L. (1987). A review of medication compliance in children with asthma. *Pediatric Asthma, Allergy, & Immunology, 1,* 193–211.

Kanfer, F. H. (1980). Self-management methods. In F. H. Kanfer & A. P. Goldstein (Eds.), *Helping people change: A textbook of methods* 2nd ed., pp. 334–389). New York: Plenum Press.

Kanfer, F. H., & Busemeyer, J. R. (1982). The use of problem solving and decision making in behavior therapy. *Clinical Psychology Review, 2,* 239–266.

Kelly, H. W. (1991). Pharmacologic problems in the allergic patient with multiple medical problems. *Immunology and Allergy Clinics of North America, 11,* 17–29.

LeBaron, S., Zeltzer, L. K., Ratner, P., & Kniker, W. T. (1985). A controlled study of education for improving compliance with cromolyn sodium (Intal): The importance of physician–patient communication. *Annals of Allergy, 55,* 811–818.

Lee, H., & Evans, H. E. (1984). Aerosol bag for administration of bronchodilators to young asthmatic children. *Pediatrics, 73,* 230–232.

Leistyna, J., & Macaulay, J. (1966). Therapy of streptococcal infections: Do pediatric patients receive prescribed oral medications? *American Journal of Diseases of Children, 111,* 22–26.

Marion, R. J., Creer, T. L., & Burns, K. L. (1983). Training asthmatic children to use a nebulizer correctly. *Journal of Asthma, 20,* 183–188.

Miller, K. A. (1982). Theophylline compliance in adolescent patients with chronic asthma. *Journal of Adolescent Health Care, 3,* 177–179.

Moran, M. G. (1987). Treatment noncompliance in asthmatic patients: An examination of the concept and a review of the literature. *Seminars in Respiratory Medicine, 8,* 271–277.

Pedersen, S. (1983). Aerosol treatment of bronchoconstriction in children, with or without a tube spacer. *New England Journal of Medicine, 308,* 1328–1330.

Plaut, T. F. (1988). *Children with asthma: A manual for parents.* Amherst, MA: Pedipress.

Radius, S. M., Becker, M. H., Rosenstock, I. M., Drachman, R. H., Schuberth, K. C., & Teets, K. C. (1978). Factors influencing mothers' compliance with a medication regimen for asthmatic children. *Journal of Asthma Research, 15,* 133–149.

Rapoff, M. A., & Christophersen, E. R. (1982). Improving compliance in pediatric practice. *Pediatric Clinics of North America, 29,* 339–357.

Reed, C. E. (1986). New therapeutic approaches in asthma. *Journal of Allergy and Clinical Immunology, 77,* 537–543.

Reed, C. E. (1991). Pharmacologic basis of the treatment of the allergic patient. *Immunology and Allergy Clinics of North America, 11,* 1–15.
Renne, C. M., & Creer, T. L. (1976). The effects of training on the use of inhalation therapy equipment by children with asthma. *Journal of Applied Behavior Analysis, 9,* 1–11.
Renne, C. M., & Creer, T. L. (1985). Asthmatic children and their families. In M. L. Wolraich & D. K. Routh (Eds.), *Advances in developmental and behavioral pediatrics* (pp. 41–81). Greenwich, CT: Jai Press.
Russell, G., & Frame, M. (1986). Terbutaline by nebuhaler in young children. *The Practitioner, 230,* 1043–1046.
Sears, M. R., Taylor, D. R., Print, C. G., Lake, D. C., Li, Q., Flannery, E. M., Yates, D. M., Lucus, M. K., & Herbison, G. P. (1990). Regular inhaled beta-agonist treatment in bronchial asthma. *The Lancet, 336,* 1391–1396.
Smith, N. A., Searle, J. P., & Shaw, J. (1984). Medication compliance in children with asthma. *Australian Paediatric Journal, 20,* 47–51.
Spector, S. L. (1985). Is your asthmatic patient really complying? *Annals of Allergy, 55,* 552–556.
Spector, S. L., Lewis, C. E., Feldman, C. H., Haynes, R. B., Hindi-Alexander, M., Kinsman, R. A., Menendez, R. A., & Sbarbaro, J. A. (1986). Workshop 6: Compliance factors. *Journal of Allergy and Clinical Immunology, 78,* 529–533.
Sublett, J. L., Pollard, S. J., Kadlec, G. J., & Karibo, J. M. (1979). Non-compliance in asthmatic children: A study of theophylline levels in a pediatric emergency room population. *Annals of Allergy, 43,* 95–97.
Szefler, S. J., Rogers, R. J., & Strunk, R. C. (1984). Drug abuse and the asthmatic patient: A case report. *Journal of Allergy and Clinical Immunology, 74,* 201–204.
Tabachnik, E., Scott, P., Correia, J., Isles, A., MacLeod, S., Newth, C., & Levison, H. (1982). Sustained-release theophylline: A significant advance in the treatment of childhood asthma. *The Journal of Pediatrics, 100,* 489–492.
Tinkelman, D. G., Vanderpool, G. E., Carroll, M. S., Page, E. G., & Spangler, D. L. (1980). Compliance differences following administration of theophylline at six- and twelve-hour intervals. *Annals of Allergy, 44,* 283–286.
Voyles, J. B., & Menendez, R. (1983). Role of patient compliance in the management of asthma. *Journal of Asthma, 20,* 411–418.
Weinberger, M. (1978). Theophylline for the treatment of asthma. *Journal of Pediatrics, 92,* 1–7.
Weinstein, A. M. (1987). *Asthma: The complete guide to self-management of asthma and allergies for patients and their families.* New York: McGraw-Hill.
Weinstein, A. G., & Cuskey, W. (1985). Theophylline compliance in asthmatic children. *Annals of Allergy, 54,* 19–24.
Wigal, J. K., Creer, T. L., Kotses, H., & Lewis, P. S. (1990). A critique of self-management programs for childhood asthma: Part I. The development and evaluation of the programs. *Pediatric Asthma, Allergy & Immunology, 4,* 17–39.
Williams, M. H. Jr. (1980). Clinical features. *Seminars in Respiratory Medicine, 1,* 304–314.
Wood, P. R., Casey, R., Kolski, G. B., & McCormick, M. C. (1985). Compliance with oral theophylline therapy in asthmatic children. *Annals of Allergy, 54,* 400–404.

14 Compliance Interventions for Children With Diabetes and Other Chronic Diseases

Alan M. Delamater
University of Miami School of Medicine

The purpose of this chapter is to review studies of interventions to improve compliance to medical regimens in children with chronic diseases. Although studies of factors affecting regimen compliance in this population have increased in recent years, few controlled studies of the effects of compliance interventions have been reported in the literature. Relatively more studies of children with diabetes have been conducted than of other patient groups. This review therefore focuses on diabetes, not only because there is a larger literature, but also because diabetes can be considered a model chronic disease to investigate. The diabetic regimen requires compliance to a variety of health behaviors, including insulin administration, glucose testing, diet, exercise, and timing of all these regimen components, which impact on child and family life and have significant developmental effects. After reviewing the literature concerning factors affecting compliance and studies of compliance interventions for diabetic youths, intervention studies in other chronic diseases, including cystic fibrosis, renal disease, hemophilia, and myelomeningocele, are considered. Future research issues are then discussed, followed by summary and conclusions.

DIABETES

Factors Affecting Regimen Compliance

Regimen compliance has been assumed to be a key determinant of metabolic control of patients with diabetes. Some empirical studies have shown that compliance is predictive of metabolic control (e.g., Brownlee-Duffeck et al., 1987;

Kuttner, Delamater, & Santiago, 1990; Schafer, Glasgow, McCaul, & Dreher, 1983), although it is clear that other variables impact on metabolic control. Because metabolic control may be important to long-term health outcomes, recent research has sought to identify predictors of regimen compliance and develop interventions to improve these health behaviors. Compliance is best considered a multidimensional construct with six distinct behavioral factors (exercise, injection, diet type, diet amount, testing, and eating frequency), as demonstrated by a factor-analytic study of health compliance behaviors (Johnson, Silverstein, Rosenbloom, Carter, & Cunningham, 1986; Johnson, Tomer, Cunningham, & Henretta, 1990). In general, studies indicate that compliance problems to various aspects of the regimen are common among young patients (e.g., Christensen, Terry, Wyatt, Pichert, & Lorenz, 1983; Johnson et al., 1986; Wing, et al., 1985).

Age Affects. Several studies have shown that age is a significant correlate of regimen compliance. For example, in a study of 168 patients, adolescents exhibited poorer compliance than younger children to injection, exercise, dietary, and glucose testing prescriptions (Johnson et al., 1986). In a study of situational aspects of dietary compliance, older adolescents reported more compliance problems than younger patients with afternoon snacking, while alone, and with parents (Delamater, Smith, Kurtz, & White, 1988). Some aspects of the regimen, however, show improved compliance (or at least the potential of improvements) with increased age. With greater cognitive maturity, older adolescents were more likely to engage in self-adjustment of insulin doses than were younger, less cognitively mature patients (Ingersoll, Orr, Herrold, & Golden, 1986). In general, however, studies have shown that compliance to a variety of regimen behaviors deteriorates with increasing age.

Knowledge and Skills. Disease-specific knowledge and skills are of obvious importance to regimen compliance. Johnson et al. (1982) demonstrated that diabetic children and their parents have substantial deficits in knowledge and skills, with older children being better informed than younger, and knowledge in one area unrelated to knowledge in another area. Additionally, skill levels for various regimen behaviors were only moderately correlated (Harkavy et al., 1983). Patients and their mothers evidenced significant deficits in dietary knowledge and skills and could recall on average only 50% of dietary prescriptions (Delamater et al., 1988); furthermore, dietary skills were unrelated to self-reported dietary compliance. Another study of dietary skill and compliance in young patients found similarly high rates of problems (Lorenz, Christensen, & Pichert, 1985). Skills deficits have also been reported for the glucose testing (Delamater et al., 1989; Wing, Koeske, New, Lamparski, & Becker, 1986) and insulin administration (Johnson et al., 1982) components of the regimen.

Increasing diabetes knowledge and skill through education programs has been assumed to lead to better compliance and metabolic control. Studies have shown, however, that improvements in knowledge do not necessarily lead to improved compliance and metabolic control (Etzwiler & Robb, 1972). In fact, studies suggest that patients in poor metabolic control actually have higher levels of knowledge than those in good control (Hamburg & Inoff, 1982). Thus, the available data indicates that diabetes-specific knowledge and skills appear to be necessary but not sufficient to predict performance of health compliance behaviors.

Health Beliefs. Health beliefs and attributions have also been considered to be important determinants of regimen compliance. In a study of adult patients, those who believed that their self-care behaviors could result in decreased probability of long-term complications were more likely to engage in appropriate self-care behaviors (Sanders, Mills, Martin, & Horne, 1975). Few studies of these cognitive factors have been conducted with diabetic youths, however. In a study of adolescent patients, Brownlee-Duffeck and colleagues (Brownlee-Duffeck et al., 1987) found health beliefs to be significant predictors of both regimen compliance and metabolic control. In other recent studies with diabetic adolescents, self-efficacy (Grossman, Brink, & Hauser, 1987) and learned helplessness (Kuttner et al., 1990) were associated with metabolic control, but not with measures of regimen compliance. Although more study of these factors is needed, there is some evidence that health beliefs contribute to the performance of health behaviors; however, these effects are probably significant only for older children and adolescents.

Family Factors. Fairly strong evidence exists for the important role of family factors in relationship to metabolic control of diabetic children. In particular, family conflict has consistently been associated with poor metabolic control of children (Anderson, Miller, Auslander, & Santiago, 1981). There is also growing evidence that family relations are importantly linked with compliance. For example, in a study of 34 adolescents, general family conflict was associated with glucose testing compliance problems, and a measure of disease-specific nonsupportive behavior was associated with compliance problems with both glucose testing and diet (Schafer et al., 1983). Similarly, Kurtz and Delamater (1984) found low rates of disease-specific supportive behavior to be associated with glucose testing compliance problems. Bobrow, AvRuskin, and Siller (1985), in a study of mother–daughter interaction and regimen compliance, found that better compliance was associated with more effective communication and problem solving; poor compliance was associated with more emotionally charged, confrontative, and negative interactions.

Peers. Another important factor related to compliance of diabetic youths is peer pressure. Although this area has not been well studied, the available evidence suggests that the effects of peer pressure on compliance are significant, particularly for adolescents. In a study of situational factors related to dietary compliance problems (Delamater et al., 1988), adolescents reported compliance problems to be most frequent while at school, with friends, and at restaurants—all situations in which the effects of peer pressure are maximized. Furthermore, in this study significant relationships were observed between glycohemoglobin values and compliance at school and with friends. Social barriers to regimen compliance have been reported, especially in relation to the dietary and exercise regimen components (Glasgow, McCaul, & Schafer, 1986). Efforts to improve social coping skills of adolescents in high-risk situations have been explored, but their effects on regimen compliance have not yet been clearly determined (Follansbee, La Greca, & Citrin, 1983; Gross, Heimann, Shapiro, & Schultz, 1983; Gross, Johnson, Wildman, & Mullet, 1981).

Summary. Regimen compliance problems are common among diabetic youths. Studies indicate that compliance is more of a problem among older children and adolescents. Disease-specific knowledge and skills deficits are also common but are not clearly linked with compliance. Because increasing knowledge and skills does not necessarily lead to improved compliance, these factors appear to be necessary but not sufficient for performance of health behaviors. There is some evidence that health beliefs contribute to the performance of health behaviors, although these effects are likely significant only for older children and adolescents. There is stonger evidence that family relations are importantly linked with compliance. In particular, better compliance has been associated with less conflicted relationships, good communication and negotiation skills, and with disease-specific parental support and efficient problem solving. Peer pressure also appears to have effects on compliance, especially among adolescents.

COMPLIANCE INTERVENTION STUDIES

Single Case Designs

Several studies employing single case methodology have demonstrated improvement in compliance with the introduction of behavioral techniques. Stimulus control techniques and a parent-implemented point reinforcement system were utilized by Lowe and Lutzker (1979) in a study of a 9-year-old girl. Compliance improved dramatically to urine testing, diet, and foot care with the introduction of a memo and the point system, as demonstrated with a multiple baseline across behaviors design. The intervention period was 10 weeks and satisfactory compliance was maintained at 10-week follow up. Measures of metabolic control, however, were not provided in this report.

The effects of goal setting and behavioral contracts were studied by Schafer, Glasgow, and McCaul (1982). Three adolescents (16–18 years of age) were studied using a multiple baseline across behaviors design. Results showed that compliance improved to several aspects of the regimen (wearing I.D. bracelet, urine testing, exercise, insulin administration) with the introduction of goal setting alone; contracting provided an additional benefit in one patient for one target behavior. These effects were observed in two of the three patients, who also evidenced improvements in acute metabolic control; the third patient did not respond well to the the interventions, apparently due to family conflict. The intervention lasted 8 weeks and gains in compliance and metabolic control were maintained at follow-up 2 months later for the two patients who responded well. These findings demonstrate the value of goal setting and individual tailoring of the regimen to improve compliance among adolescents.

Gross (1982) used behavioral procedures to improve regimen compliance in four 10- to 12-year-old children. The patients met in a group self-management training class once each week for a 6-week period. Reinforcement, negotiation, and contracting were taught and related to diabetes situations and role played. Each of the children performed self-management programs related to their regimen. Contracts to increase urine testing were made and this intervention evaluated in a multiple baseline across subjects design. Results showed increased frequency of urine testing for each subject with the implementation of the contract. These gains were maintained at 2-week follow-up for all subjects, but only for two of the four at 4-week follow-up. Objective measures of metabolic control were not obtained.

Carney, Schechter, and Davis (1983) evaluated the effects of contingent parental praise and the use of a point-reinforcement system on compliance to blood glucose testing in three children, aged 10 to 14 years. A multiple baseline across subjects design was used. Frequency of testing increased significantly for each patient after the behavioral management procedures were implemented during the 5-week treatment, and these gains were maintained at 4-month follow-up. Furthermore, metabolic control as determined by measurement of glycosylated hemoglobin also showed significant clinical improvements.

Snyder (1987) reported a study of a 14-year-old boy with poor compliance and antisocial behavior. Behavioral analysis suggested that coercive family process was associated with noncompliance and behavioral problems. Behavioral family therapy was effective in sequentially treating noncompliance, antisocial behavior, family conflict, and school attendance, as demonstrated by multiple baseline across behaviors analysis. Self-monitoring and a reinforcement salary for compliance and punishment for noncompliance resulted in improved compliance; increased maternal monitoring, a behavioral contract, and communication and problem-solving skills training resulted in reductions in antisocial behavior and family conflict, as well as improved school behavior. Treatment occurred over a 21-week period, with gains maintained at 2-month follow-up.

Summary. Results from five studies using controlled single case methods provides support for the efficacy of behavioral approaches to improve health compliance behaviors in children from ages 9 to 18. These studies, summarized in Table 14.1, have shown that the use of techniques such as memos, goal setting, and parent-administered contingent praise and contracts may substantially improve compliance to various regimen component behaviors during fairly brief intervention periods. These gains have been maintained during follow-up periods lasting from 4 weeks to 4 months.

Randomized Group Designs

Relatively more compliance intervention studies are reported in the literature that have utilized randomized group designs. These studies have focused on improving regimen skills and compliance using a variety of interventions involving individual patients, families, and/or peer groups.

Individual Patient Interventions. Two controlled studies have investigated interventions to improve regimen skills. Epstein, Figueroa, Farkas, and Beck (1981) showed that children and adolescents could be trained to improve their urine glucose testing accuracy with informational feedback and reinforcement. Skill levels were assessed only once 20 minutes after the intervention, so maintenance effects in the natural environment were not evaluated. Gilbert et al. (1982) demonstrated that a peer modeling film helped 6- to 9-year-old children to self-inject insulin more accurately. These studies indicate that brief interventions may improve regimen skills; whether or not these effects persist remains to be demonstrated.

Two recent studies evaluated clinic-based individual interventions to improve compliance of adolescent patients. Marrero and colleagues (1989) randomized 29 patients to a 4-month intervention consisting of computer-assisted blood

TABLE 14.1
Compliance Intervention Studies in Diabetes: Single Case Multiple Baseline Designs

First Authors		N	Age	Targets	Intervention	PU	Outcomes Compl	MC
Lowe	(1979)	1	9	UT, D, Foot	Memo, Pt E-10 wk	10 wk	+	NA
Schafer	(1982)	3	16-18	UT, Ex, Ins	Goal Set -8 wk	2 mo	+	+
Gross	(1982)	4	10-12	UT	Contract-6 wk	4 wk	+	NA
Carney	(1983)	3	10-14	SMBG	Pt E-5 wk	4 mo	+	+
Snyder	(1987)	1	14	UT, D. Ins	Pt E, Contract, Pun, CST-21 wk	2 mo	+	NA

Note. UT = urine testing; D = diet; Ex = exercise; SMBG = self-monitoring of blood glucose; Pt E = point economy; Pun = punishment; CST = communication skills training; FU = follow-up; Compl = compliance; MC = metabolic control; + = improved; NA = not assessed.

glucose monitoring system involving a reflectance meter with memory and two visits with the physician to review blood glucose records; an additional 28 patients used reflectance meters without memory and reviewed blood glucose data with physicians two times (without computers) over the 4-month study period. Although there were no differences in groups on measures of metabolic control and self-reported regimen compliance, patients in the computer-assisted group reported significant improvements in their understanding of the treatment regimen, the importance of glucose monitoring, and their relationship with their physician.

Wysocki, Green, and Huxtable (1989) also evaluated a blood glucose monitoring intervention for adolescents. Thirty patients were randomized to interventions incorporating memory reflectance meters with or without a monetary contract targeting compliance with glucose testing at home. Patients returned to the clinic once a month for 4 months to receive computer-generated blood glucose feedback and monetary rewards contingent on their performance. Compliance of patients in the meter-alone condition got significantly worse over the course of the study, whereas patients in the meter plus contract group maintained acceptably high compliance over 4 months. Compliance to other aspects of the regimen was not affected by the intervention, demonstrating the specificity of the contract.

Combined Family and Peer Interventions. Epstein and colleagues (Epstein, Beck, et al., 1981) investigated the effects of a 12-week comprehensive education and behavior modification program for nineteen 8- to 12-year-old children and their parents. Behavioral contracts were negotiated between children and parents, and parents were taught to contingently reinforce target behaviors, including urine testing, diet, and exercise, using a point economy system. Although this approach was successful in improving percentage negative urine test results, improvements in metabolic control were not attained. Nevertheless, this was the first group study to provide support for the efficacy of family-based behavioral treatment for diabetic children.

Using a similar approach, Gross, Magalnick, and Richardson (1985) investigated the effects of a family-based behavioral self-management training program. Fourteen 9- to 14-year-old children were randomized to either the treatment group or an attention-placebo control group. Treatment consisted of weekly group sessions for 8 weeks, during which children and parents worked on specific behavior change projects designed to improve compliance to urine testing and/or rotation of insulin administration sites and reduce family conflict around regimen compliance. The results showed that patients in the self-management group improved regimen compliance and decreased family conflict relative to the control group; however, metabolic control was unaffected.

The use of peer groups and parent training in the treatment of young adolescents was evaluated by Anderson, Wolf, Burkhart, Cornell, and Bacon (1989).

Sixty patients were followed over 18 months. The treatment consisted of peer group problem solving and simultaneous parent groups focusing on negotiating appropriate levels of involvement in the regimen and reinforcing regimen compliance. Six sessions were held over the study period, each one occurring prior to the regular outpatient clinic visit. At the end of the study period, patients in the peer group/parent group intervention reported significantly more utilization of blood glucose testing data when they exercised and marginally significant improvements in compliance with insulin and diet based on blood glucose testing data. Furthermore, treated patients had significantly better metabolic control, suggesting that this type of intervention may prevent the worsening of metabolic control typically seen during early adolescence.

The effects of a 6-week multifamily group intervention and parent simulation of diabetes was investigated by Satin, La Greca, Zigo, and Skyler (1989) in a study of 32 adolescents. Patients were randomized to multifamily, multifamily plus parent simulation, and control groups. Patients in the multifamily plus parent simulation group showed significantly improved metabolic control compared with the untreated control group 6 weeks after the end of treatment, as well as at 6-month follow-up. Patients in the multifamily groups were rated by mothers as exhibiting improved regimen compliance; however, compliance was measured by only one retrospective global rating.

Delamater and colleagues (Delamater et al., 1991) used a peer group and family-based behavioral approach in a study of 13 adolescents with a history of compliance and metabolic control problems. Six patients were randomized to the treatment group and seven to a no-treatment control group. The intervention was designed to improve compliance with blood glucose testing and diet. Six group sessions were held over 2 months with a booster session 4 weeks later. Follow-up was conducted 4 months after the end of treatment. Families were trained in communication skills, goal setting with behavioral contracts, and problem-solving strategies; patients met with their peers during each treatment session for discussion and problem solving of difficult social situations related to regimen compliance. Compliance improved in treated patients but was only marginally significant, because patients in the control group also showed improvements over the course of the study. Improvements in metabolic control were not observed. Patients reported significant improvements in their relationships with parents, however.

Individual Family Interventions. In a study of family-based self-management training with 36 newly diagnosed patients, Delamater et al. (1990) found that patients who participated in self-management training had significantly better metabolic control 1 and 2 years postdiagnosis than patients who received standard outpatient treatment. The self-management training incorporated behavioral principles and emphasized utilization of blood glucose monitoring for solving daily diabetes management problems. Patients and their parents were seen in seven individual outpatient sessions during the first 4 months after diagnosis. Although self-management patients had better dietary compliance at 1-year postdiagnosis, there were no group differences in other measures of regimen compliance (i.e., number of glucose tests, injection–meal timing deviations) during the study period. The results of this study suggest that this type of intervention during the first few months after diagnosis may help prevent the deterioration in metabolic control commonly seen in children during the first 24 months after diagnosis.

Peer Group Interventions. The effects of a peer group intervention on compliance and metabolic control of adolescents were investigated by Kaplan, Chadwick, and Schimmel (1985). Twenty-one patients were randomized to either a social learning group or a control group. The social learning intervention focused on identifying social situations related to regimen noncompliance and problem solving to prevent noncompliance, whereas the control group was concerned with medical facts concerning diabetes and its treatment. The intervention was conducted in a summer school setting and the group met for 3 hours per day over 3 weeks. At 4-month follow-up patients in the social learning group had significantly better metabolic control and self-reported regimen compliance.

Peer group interventions have also been used in studies of the effects of exercise training programs on metabolic control. In a study of nineteen 5- to 11-year-old children, Campaigne Gilliam, Spencer, Lampman, and Schork (1984) found significantly improved metabolic control after 12 weeks of group exercise (held three times per week for 30 minutes each). Similarly, Stratton, Wilson, Endres, and Goldstein (1987) found benefical effects on metabolic control for 8 adolescent patients who participated in a group exercise program held three times per week (30–45 minutes each) over an 8-week period. These studies did not evaluate follow-up effects, however, to determine whether patients continued to exercise on their own and maintain improved glycemic control. In a recent study of 32 youths, a peer group exercise program did not improve metabolic control over 3 months; however, patients exercised only once per week (Huttunen, Lankelaa, Knip, Lautala, Kaar, Laasonen, Puukka, 1989).

Summary. Fourteen randomized group compliance intervention studies have been reported in the literature. Table 14.2 presents a summary of these studies in terms of number of subjects studied, age of subjects, target behaviors, types of interventions, and outcomes. The mean number of patients studied across these 14 studies was 30, with 14 per treatment group. The mean duration of treatment was 2.5 months, excluding one study that had 6 treatment sessions over 18 months and 2 studies that were 1-session interventions. Target behaviors have included exercise (3 studies), glucose testing (7 studies), overall compliance related to social situations (2 studies), and technical aspects of regimen skills (2 studies). Interventions with individual patients were used in 4 studies, individual

TABLE 14.2
Compliance Intervention Studies in Diabetes: Randomized Group Designs

First Authors		N	Age	Targets	Intervention	PU	Outcomes Compl	MC
Epstein	(1981)	35	6-16	UT skill	Feedback/Reinf.	NA	+	NA
Epstein	(1981)	19	8-12	UT	Educ, Pt E-12 wk	2 mo	+	NS
Gilbert	(1982)	28	6-9	Inj skill	Peer Model	NA	+	NA
Campaigne	(1984)	19	5-11	Exercise	Group Exer-12 wk	NA	NA	+
Gross	(1985)	14	9-14	UT, Ins	Contracts-8 wk	6 mo	+	NS
Kaplan	(1985)	21	13-18	Compl	Soc Sk Tr-3 wk	4 mo	+	+
Stratton	(1987)	16	13-17	Exercise	Group Exer-8 wk	NA	NA	+
Anderson	(1989)	60	11-14	SMBG util.	Peer PS/PT-18 mo	NA	+	+
Marrero	(1989)	57	10-18	SMBG	MD, Comp FB-2 mo	4 mo	+*	+*
Satin	(1989)	32	12-19	Fam funct	Fam-Par Sim-6 wk	6 mo	+	+
Wysocki	(1989)	30	13-17	SMBG	Contract-4 mo	NA	+	NS
Huttunen	(1989)	32	8-17	Exercise	Group Exer-3 mo	NA	NA	NS
Delamater	(1990)	36	3-16	SMBG util.	Fam. PS-6 mo	18 mo	NS	+
Delamater	(1991)	13	12-17	SMBG, Diet	Fam Contr-2 mo	4 mo	+*	NS

Note. Educ = education; Inj = injection; Ins = insulin use; Soc Sk Tr = social skills training; NA = not assessed; NS = not significant; PS = problem solving; PT = parent training; Comp FB = computer feedback; Par Sim = parent simulation; Contr = contracts; * = improved but NS from controls.

family intervention was used in 1 study, peer group interventions in 4 studies, and both family and peer interventions in 5 studies. Seven studies included follow-up evaluations; the mean follow-up period was 6.3 months. Twelve studies included measures of metabolic control; in 6 of these studies, patients in the compliance intervention groups exhibited significant improvements in metabolic control.

OTHER CHRONIC DISEASES

Selected compliance intervention studies for children with other chronic diseases are reviewed in this section. There are relatively few controlled intervention studies published in this area. The following representative chronic diseases for which one or more studies are available are considered: cystic fibrosis, renal disease, hemophilia, and myelomeningocele. (Compliance interventions for asthma and obesity, to the extent they are chronic diseases, are considered elsewhere in this volume.)

Cystic Fibrosis

Children with cystic fibrosis are expected to comply with a complex treatment regimen consisting of pancreatic enzyme and vitamin supplements, chest physiotherapy for postural drainage, and possibly antibiotics as well. Compliance with chest physiotherapy, usually prescribed two or more times per day, appears to be the most problematic aspect of the regimen (Passero, Remor, & Salomon, 1981). Very little controlled compliance intervention research has been reported in the literature in this area.

Stark, Miller, Plienes, and Drabman (1987) conducted a single case study of the effects of behavioral contracting to increase compliance with chest physiotherapy in an 11-year-old girl with cystic fibrosis. After a 3-week baseline period, a behavioral contract was instituted for a 4-week period, initially in the hospital for 1 week and then continued at home for an additional 3 weeks. The contract was gradually faded after the formal 4-week intervention. Follow-up was conducted 3, 6, and 9 weeks later. The primary dependent measure was self-reported frequency of chest physiotherapy, monitored daily by the patient. Reliability was acceptable, as assessed by independent reports from the mother.

Compliance improved from about once per day chest physiotherapy during baseline to the presribed three times per day immediately after the contract was initiated and was maintained throughout the follow-up period. In addition, the patient and mother reported a decrease in their arguments over compliance with this procedure. Despite the limitations of an A–B design, this study suggests that behavioral contracting targeting specific regimen behaviors may be helpful in improving compliance with chest physiotherapy for young patients with cystic fibrosis.

Renal Disease

Children with end-stage renal disease must have hemodialysis treatments several times each week in order to maintain their health. With the advent of new hemodialysis technology, this procedure can be performed at home. The procedure itself is fairly complex and must be performed carefully, so compliance depends on accurate performance. Besides regular hemodialysis, patients must follow a restrictive diet specifying limitations of potassium, sodium, protein, and fluids. Compliance with dietary prescriptions ensures adequate growth and development; noncompliance results in weight gain between hemodialysis treatments that may have acute health effects secondary to fluid retention and electrolyte imbalances.

Two studies have been reported in the literature with respect to hemodialysis and dietary compliance. Lira and Mlott (1976) examined the effects of a behavioral training program to improve home hemodialysis skills. Ten patients were randomized to either the behavioral training or to traditional training. The behavioral program was mastery based training in all the specific steps required in the procedure and incorporated modeling, rehearsal, feedback, and social reinforcement. Patients who received behavioral training required less time to reach criterion than did control patients, and they also reported increased participation and more confidence in the home dialysis program. The small number of patients studied and the lack of follow-up data limit the generality of these results but are consistent with the results of other studies utilizing behavioral approaches to skills acquisition.

Dietary compliance was targeted by Magrab and Papadopoulou (1977) in a study of four children. A token economy reinforcement system was developed for each patient, and the effects of weight gain between dialysis sessions evaluated in single case A–B–A reversal designs for each child. The intervention consisted of dietary instruction and token reinforcement contingent on meeting acceptable levels of weight gain, blood urea nitrogen, and serum potassium, all of which reflect dietary compliance. The 4-week intervention was successful in decreasing the weight gained between hemodialysis sessions for all four patients. During the reversal phase, weight gain increased to baseline levels, demonstrating the effectiveness of the compliance intervention.

Hemophilia

Hemophilia, characterized by bleeding episodes affecting joints and muscles, is managed by factor replacement therapy, consisting of intravenous administration of clotting factors from normal plasma. Because factor replacement therapy is most effective when initiated early in bleeding episodes, it is essential that parents learn to properly administer the treatment at home. Sergis-Deavenport and Varni (1983) evaluated the effects of behavioral skills training on proficiency of parents with factor replacement therapy. Parents of 12 young patients participated, with 5 in the treatment group who had no previous training compared with 7 others who had previous training. The intervention consisted of weekly training sessions over a 4- to 8-week period, during which the technique was practiced; modeling, rehearsal, feedback, and social reinforcement were used in the treatment sessions. Behavioral skills were measured at baseline and during follow-up evaluations conducted 2 and 19 weeks (on average) after patients were trained to criterion. Parents in the behavioral treatment group demonstrated significantly better skills by the end of the intervention and maintained their proficiency during the follow-up. Although this study is limited by the small sample size and lack of randomization, the results suggest that behavioral training in this procedure enhances parental compliance and may improve health care delivery for these children.

Besides helping the psychological and functional status of children with hemophilia, exercise may have beneficial effects on coagulation processes. In a study of 32 patients with hemophilia, Greene and Stickler (1983) found very low compliance with a simple daily exercise regimen. In an effort to improve compliance with therapeutic exercise, Greenan-Fowler, Powell, and Varni (in press) designed a 12-session group exercise program in which children were instructed in individualized therapeutic exercises and behavioral contracts were used to specify and reinforce specific exercise behaviors. Ten 8- to 15-year-old patients and their parents participated. Compliance with the exercise regimen improved substantially for these patients but decreased over a 9-month follow-up period.

Myelomeningocele

Because children with myelomeningocele have reduced active muscle tissue, lower basal metabolic rate, and limited mobility, they are at high risk for becoming obese. Killam, Apodaca, Manella, and Varni (1983) conducted a pilot study to evaluate the effects of a behavioral diet and exercise program for five children with myelomeningocele. The children and their parents participated in eight weekly sessions involving instruction and practice in diet and exercise. The standard "stop light diet" and behavioral approaches to eating regulation was used. Follow-up evaluation of weight was conducted several times during a 6-month follow-up period. Although a control group was not available, results showed that three children had reduced their weight from 7%–24% by 6 months; one of the other two stayed the same and the second gained 21%. However, four of the children were still significantly obese (greater than 25% overweight) at the 6-month follow-up evaluation. This report at least documents the feasibility of applying behavioral weight control techniques with this patient population. Further controlled research in this area is obviously needed.

FUTURE RESEARCH ISSUES

Compliance intervention research must be guided by an understanding of which health behaviors really matter. In diabetes, the question of treatment efficacy is addressed by studies of the relationship between regimen compliance and metabolic control. Notwithstanding significant methodological issues such as measurement of these variables, results from such studies inform interventionists about those regimen components most likely to improve metabolic control. For example, results from cross-sectional studies indicate that dietary noncompliance (Delamater et al., 1988; Lorenz, Christensen, & Pichert, 1985), exercise (Kuttner et al., 1990), and injection–meal timing deviations (Witt, White, & Santiago, 1983) are important regimen component behaviors to target; yet these specific health behaviors have been infrequently targeted in compliance intervention studies. Interventions targeting components such as frequency of glucose testing, wearing I.D. bracelets, foot care, or other behaviors not demonstrated to be significant correlates of metabolic control would not be expected to lead to improved health outcomes necessarily.

In this light, it is important to note that only 6 of 12 group studies and 2 single case studies that included measures of metabolic control demonstrated improvements in health outcomes. The intervention targets in these studies included exercise, utilization of data from self-monitoring of blood glucose, and situational factors related to noncompliance (i.e., peer and family influences). The interventions themselves incorporated use of peer groups for exercise or problem solving and family group problem solving and parent training in use of behavioral techniques such as contingent reinforcement and contracts. More studies are needed of interventions targeting behaviors shown to make a difference in metabolic control, particularly dietary compliance, exercise, and use of insulin. In addition, future research should study individual differences in compliance–health outcomes relationships, as well as developmental changes in these relationships. It is worth noting that only five single case studies are reported in the literature; more studies using this methodology are needed and would shed light on the question of individual differences in compliance–health outcome relationships and also be useful in the development and refinement of interventions for children of various ages.

One aspect of intervention programs associated with improved compliance and metabolic control is problem solving. Several interventions used this approach in the context of peer and family groups. Such an intervention focuses on the process of identification of situational factors related to compliance problems and alternative ways of handling such difficulties so as not to hinder performance of health compliance behaviors. Aside from these few intervention studies and some cross-sectional studies suggesting the role of psychological factors such as health beliefs and attributional styles, little is known about cognitive processing of regimen-related situations and behaviors. More research is needed in this area, particularly in developmental changes related to these variables.

Most of the compliance intervention studies reviewed here have intervened at the level of peer groups and families. Only two studies have intervened at the level of the individual health care provider–patient relationship (Marrero et al., 1989; Wysocki et al., 1989). In these studies, patients met individually with physicians to review the results of blood glucose monitoring records. Although these interventions were not associated with improved metabolic control, in one of the studies (Marrero et al., 1989) there were improvements in patient ratings of their relationship with their physician, their understanding of the treatment regimen, and the importance of glucose testing.

Few studies in the literature have addressed the health-care provider–patient relationship. In a study conducted in a child diabetes clinic, health care providers gave an average of seven regimen instructions, but patients and parents could recall only two of these when interviewed immediately after their outpatient visit (Page, Verstraete, Robb, & Etzwiler, 1981). Perrin and Perrin (1983) have shown that health care providers are inaccurate concerning what children can understand about their disease and its treatment. The affective quality of the relationship between health-care provider and patient is also significant. Research with general pediatric populations has shown that maternal satisfaction with the relationship is related to warmth and friendliness of the health-care provider and is associated with better compliance (Francis, Korsch, & Morris, 1969; Korsch, Gozzi, & Francis, 1968). Finally, Marteau, Johnston, Baum, and Bloch (1987) found significant differences between the treatment goals of parents and those of physicians treating diabetic children. The results of these studies indicate that interventions targeting the health-care provider–patient/family relationship would be a fruitful area to pursue. At this point, besides concluding that this is an important area for compliance intervention research, basic descriptive studies are needed to better understand the parameters of this relationship, the effects on compliance, and developmental changes associated with such relationships and their impact on compliance.

Whereas relatively more studies have concentrated on patient–family relationships, developmental changes in these relationships and their impacts on compliance have not been investigated. Given basic developmental effects in terms of more autonomy and peer group identification in early adolescence, the use of parent training approaches with young children and peer group approaches and family problem solving (i.e., communication, negotiation, contracts) with older children and adolescents is a rational strategy that has received some empirical support. However, more research is needed to understand how families negotiate responsibilities for performance and monitoring of health compliance behaviors throughout development.

Generally, intervention programs have been conducted independently of regularly scheduled outpatient follow-up care. Such programs are typically held at evening times over a relatively brief period (average of 2.5 months). Besides the scheduling difficulties, noncompliance with such protocols and eventual attrition makes such approaches impractical for widespread implementation, especially for patients with established histories of noncompliance and metabolic control problems. Two alternative strategies may be better in the long term and have already received some empirical support. One strategy is prevention: Intervene with patients before they develop problems. Delamater et al. (1990) have shown that patients participating in seven outpatient family-based self-management sessions in the first 4 months after diagnosis maintain significantly improved metabolic control 2 years after diagnosis than patients treated conventionally. The other strategy is to incorporate the compliance intervention into regular outpatient clinic procedures, as demonstrated by Anderson et al. (1989). In this approach, patients participated in psychoeducation group treatment sessions and parents participated in similar group sessions prior to patients' regularly scheduled quarterly outpatient follow-up visits. Patients who participated in the psychoeducational group treatment evidenced significantly better compliance and metabolic control than patients receiving standard treatment. Both of these intervention programs require modification of the health care system and provisions made for payment of such services. Further studies of the implementation of intervention programs shown to be efficacious are indicated.

SUMMARY AND CONCLUSIONS

Most controlled compliance intervention studies targeting children with chronic diseases have been conducted with diabetic samples. There is a paucity of controlled compliance intervention research in other chronic diseases of childhood (excluding asthma and obesity). Although the extant research is limited by small patient samples, results suggest that behavioral interventions may improve regimen skills and compliance in children with cystic fibrosis, renal disease, and hemophilia. More research of factors affecting compliance and controlled compliance intervention studies of children with various chronic diseases is needed.

Of those studies dealing with diabetes, five single case studies and 14 randomized group designs with fairly small sizes, mostly in the adolescent range, were identified. The results of these studies suggest that (a) regimen skills can be improved with brief interventions incorporating feedback or filmed models; (b) family-based programs that use behavioral interventions utilizing goal setting, contingency contracts, and parental reinforcement may improve compliance and metabolic control; (c) peer group interventions emphasizing exercise and social determinants of regimen noncompliance, as well as utilization of blood glucose and problem-solving techniques, may improve compliance and metabolic control; and (d) clinic-based interventions with individual patients that target glucose testing may improve compliance with targeted behaviors and relationships with health care staff. Because metabolic control has been shown to improve in only half of these studies, additional research is needed on behaviors that could impact on metabolic control more strongly, such as dietary compliance, exercise, and use of insulin.

Studies have not yet compared the relative benefits of various interventions with different age groups, but it seems reasonable to conclude that family-based interventions may be beneficial at all developmental levels, with appropriately different focus of treatment in younger versus older children. A promising approach with adolescents is a peer group format emphasizing skills and problem solving of compliance barriers, with a parallel parent group emphasizing communication and reinforcement skills. More research is needed to identify barriers to compliance at various developmental levels.

Family influences on compliance have been documented and family involvement in compliance intervention programs seems necessary. However, the mechanisms of change have not been well understood. For example, future research should answer questions such as how families negotiate responsibilities for performance and monitoring of health compliance behaviors over the course of child development. How much family involvement is needed, for which types of behaviors, at which points in development? Environmental control, such as contingency management procedures implemented by parents, would seem essential for younger children, but more internal mechanisms of change and psychological control, such as delay of gratification skills, may be appropriate for older children and adolescents. Research investigating cognitive processing of regimen demands is in a preliminary stage at present; cognitive interventions are unexplored but may be of benefit for some older children and adolescents. Mechanisms of change for short-term versus long-term compliance intervention strategies are probably quite different; research in this area should identify predictors of long-term maintenance of health behaviors.

Although research suggests that the relationship of patients and their parents with health care providers is a significant determinant of compliance, there are no controlled studies targeting this relationship to impact on patient compliance with pediatric chronic disease regimens. Interventions that focus on the health care provider in terms of education about developmental issues and training in relationship enhancement methods, providing regimen instructions, individual tailoring and gradual implementation of the regimen, and effective monitoring and reinforcement, would appear to be a very fruitful area for future research to pursue.

Most studies have been conducted with children who have been identified as having compliance problems. Very few compliance intervention studies have targeted children with newly diagnosed chronic disease. In the long term it would seem a cost-efficient method to intervene at early stages in the disease course in order to prevent compliance problems later on. Controlled work in this area should include measures of the cost of prevention-based intervention programs, as well as the expected savings related to predicted future health care costs.

In conclusion, education seems necessary but not sufficient to ensure compliance with chronic disease regimens. Regimen skills need to be retrained and reinforced; behavioral techniques such as modeling, rehearsal, feedback, and reinforcement have been shown to improve skills necessary for regimens to manage diabetes, renal disease, and hemophilia. Behavioral interventions facilitate short-term compliance to various regimen targets but may not generalize to other regimen behaviors or persist across time. Younger and older children are probably quite different with respect to compliance barriers, cognitive processing of the regimen, and responsiveness to different types of interventions involving peers and families. Health care provider–patient interactions seem to influence compliance, but the parameters of this relationship have not been well studied or tested in compliance intervention research. Finally, compliance interventions conducted early in the disease course may prevent later compliance problems and health complications; further work in this area should include cost analyses to demonstrate potential savings.

REFERENCES

Anderson, B. J., Miller, J. P., Auslander, W. F., & Santiago, J. V. (1981). Family characteristics of diabetic adolescents: Relationship to metabolic control. *Diabetes Care, 4,* 586–594.

Anderson, B. J., Wolf, R. M., Burkhart, M. T., Cornell, R. G., & Bacon, G. E. (1989). Effects of peer-group intervention on metabolic control of adolescents with IDDM: Randomized outpatient study. *Diabetes Care, 12,* 179–183.

Bobrow, E. S., AvRuskin, T. W., & Siller, J. (1985). Mother–daughter interaction and adherence to diabetes regimens. *Diabetes Care, 8,* 146–151.

Brownlee-Duffeck, M., Peterson, L., Simonds, J. F., Goldstein, D., Kilo, C., & Hoette, S. (1987). The role of health beliefs in the regimen adherence and metabolic control of adolescents and adults with diabetes mellitus. *Journal of Consulting and Clinical Psychology, 55*, 139–144.

Campaigne, B. N., Gilliam, T. B., Spencer, M. L., Lampman, R. M., & Schork, M. A. (1984). Effects of a physical activity program on metabolic control and cardiovascular fitness in children with IDDM. *Diabetes Care, 7*, 57–62.

Carney, R. M., Schechter, D., & Davis, T. (1983). Improving adherence to blood glucose testing in insulin-dependent diabetic children. *Behavior Therapy, 14*, 247–254.

Christensen, N. K., Terry, R. D., Wyatt, S., Pichert, J. W., & Lorenz, R. A. (1983). Quantitative assessment of dietary adherence in patients with insulin-dependent diabetes mellitus. *Diabetes Care, 6*, 245–250.

Delamater, A. M., Bubb, J., Davis, S. G., Smith, J. A., Schmidt, L., White, N. H., & Santiago, J. V. (1990). Randomized prospective study of self-management training with newly diagnosed diabetic children. *Diabetes Care, 13*, 492–498.

Delamater, A. M., Davis, S. G., Bubb, J., Smith, J. A., White, N. H., & Santiago, J. V. (1989). Self-monitoring of blood glucose by adolescents with diabetes: Technical skills and utilization of data. *The Diabetes Educator, 15*, 56–61.

Delamater, A. M., Smith, J. A., Bubb, J., Davis, S. G., Gamble, T., White, N. H., & Santiago, J. V. (1991). Family-based behavior therapy for diabetic adolescents. In J. H. Johnson & S. B. Johnson (Eds.), *Advances in child health psychology: Proceedings of the Florida Conference.* Gainesville: University of Florida Press.

Delamater, A. M., Smith, J. A., Kurtz, S. M., & White, N. H. (1988). Dietary skills and adherence in children with insulin-dependent diabetes mellitus. *The Diabetes Educator, 14*, 33–36.

Epstein, L. H., Beck, S., Figueroa, J., Farkas, G., Kazdin, A. E., Daneman, D., & Becker, D. (1981). The effects of targeting improvements in urine glucose on metabolic control in children with insulin dependent diabetes. *Journal of Applied Behavior Analysis, 14*, 365–375.

Epstein, L. H., Figueroa, J., Farkas, G. M., & Beck, S. (1981). The short-term effects of feedback on accuracy of urine glucose determinations in insulin dependent diabetic children. *Behavior Therapy, 12*, 560–564.

Etzwiler, D. D., & Robb, J. R. (1972). Evaluation of programmed education among juvenile diabetics and their families, *Diabetes, 21*, 967–971.

Follansbee, D. J., La Greca, A. M., & Citrin, W. S. (1983). Coping skills training for adolescents with diabetes. *Diabetes, 32* (Suppl. 1), 147.

Francis, V., Korsch, B. M., & Morris, M. J. (1969). Gaps in doctor–patient communication: Patients' response to medical advice. *New England Journal of Medicine, 280*, 535–540.

Gilbert, B. O., Johnson, S. B., Spillar, R., McCallum, M., Silverstein, J. H., & Rosenbloom, A. (1982). The effects of a peer-modeling film on children learning to self-inject insulin. *Behavior Therapy, 13*, 186–193.

Glasgow, R. E., McCaul, K. D., & Schafer, L. C. (1986). Barriers to regimen adherence among persons with insulin-dependent diabetes. *Journal of Behavioral Medicine, 9*, 65–77.

Greenan-Fowler, E., Powell, C., & Varni, J. W. (in press). Behavioral treatment of adherence to therapeutic exercise by children with hemophilia. *Archives of Physical Medicine and Rehabilitation.*

Greene, W. B., & Stickler, E. M. (1983). A modified isokinetic strengthening program for patients with severe hemophilia. *Developmental Medicine and Child Neurology, 25*, 189–196.

Gross, A. M. (1982). Self-management training and medication compliance in children with diabetes. *Child and Family Behavior Therapy, 4*, 47–55.

Gross, A. M., Heimann, L., Shapiro, R., & Schultz, R. (1983). Social skills training and hemoglobin A1c levels in children with diabetes. *Behavior Modification, 7*, 151–164.

Gross, A. M., Johnson, W. G., Wildman, H., & Mullet, N. (1981). Coping skills training with insulin dependent pre-adolescent diabetics. *Child Behavior Therapy, 3,* 141-153.

Gross, A. M., Magalnick, L. J., & Richardson, P. (1985). Self-management training with families of insulin-dependent diabetic children: A controlled long-term investigation. *Child and Family Behavior Therapy, 7,* 35-50.

Grossman, H. Y., Brink, S., & Hauser, S. T. (1987). Self-efficacy in adolescent girls and boys with insulin-dependent diabetes mellitus. *Diabetes Care, 10,* 324-329.

Hamburg, B. A., & Inoff, G. E. (1982). Relationships between behavioral factors and diabetic control in children and adolescents: A camp study. *Psychosomatic Medicine, 44,* 321-339.

Harkavy, J., Johnson, S. B., Silverstein, J., Spillar, R., McCallum, M., & Rosenbloom, A. (1983). Who learns what at diabetes summer camp. *Journal of Pediatric Psychology, 8,* 143-153.

Huttunen, N. P., Lankelaa, S. L., Knip, M., Lautala, P., Kaar, M. L., Laasonen, K., & Puukka, R. (1989). Effect of once-a-week training program on physical fitness and metabolic control in children with IDDM. *Diabetes Care, 12,* 737-739.

Ingersoll, G. M., Orr, D. P., Herrold, A. J., & Golden, M. P. (1986). *The Journal of Pediatrics, 108,* 620-623.

Johnson, S. B., Pollak, T., Silverstein, J. H., Rosenbloom, A., Spillar, R., McCallum, M., & Harkavy, J. (1982). Cognitive and behavioral knowledge about insulin-dependent diabetes among children and parents. *Pediatrics, 69,* 708-713.

Johnson, S. B., Silverstein, J., Rosenbloom, A., Carter, R., & Cunningham, W. (1986). Assessing daily management in childhood diabetes. *Health Psychology, 5,* 545-564.

Johnson, S. B., Tomer, A., Cunningham, W. R., & Henretta, J. C. (1990). Adherence in childhood diabetes: Results of a confirmatory factor analysis. *Health Psychology, 9,* 493-501.

Kaplan, R. M., Chadwick, M. W., & Schimmel, L. E. (1985). Social learning intervention to promote metabolic control in Type I diabetes mellitus: Pilot experimental results. *Diabetes Care, 8,* 152-155.

Killam, P. E., Apodaca, L., Manella, K. J., & Varni, J. W. (1983). Behavioral pediatric weight rehabilitation for children with myelomeningocele. *American Journal of Maternal Child Nursing, 8,* 280-286.

Korsch, B. M., Gozzi, E. K., & Francis, V. (1968). Gaps in doctor-patient communication: I. Doctor-patient interaction and patient satisfaction. *Pediatrics, 42,* 855-871.

Kurtz, S. M., & Delamater, A. M. (1984). Family interactions, adherence, and metabolic control in IDDM. *Diabetes, 33* (Suppl. 1), 78.

Kuttner, M. J., Delamater, A. M., & Santiago, J. V. (1990). Learned helplessness in diabetic youths. *Journal of Pediatric Psychology, 15,* 581-594.

Lira, F. T., & Mlott, S. R. (1976). A behavioral approach to hemodialysis training. *Journal of the American Association of Nephrology Nurses and Technicians, 3,* 180-188.

Lorenz, R. A., Christensen, N. K., & Pichert, J. W. (1985). Diet-related knowledge, skill, and adherence among children with insulin dependent diabetes mellitus. *Pediatrics, 75,* 872-876.

Lowe, K., & Lutzker, J. R. (1979). Increasing compliance to a medical regime with a juvenile diabetic. *Behavior Therapy, 10,* 57-64.

Magrab, P. R., & Papadopoulou, Z. L. (1977). The effect of a token economy on dietary compliance for children on hemodialysis. *Journal of Applied Behavior Analysis, 10,* 573-578.

Marrero, D. G., Kronz, K. K., Golden, M. P., Wright, J. C., Orr, D. P., Fineberg, N. S. (1989). Clinical evaluation of computer-assisted self-monitoring of blood glucose system. *Diabetes Care, 12,* 345-350.

Marteau, T. M., Johnston, M., Baum, J. D., & Bloch, S. (1987). Goals of treatment in diabetes: A comparison of doctors and parents of children with diabetes. *Journal of Behavioral Medicine, 10,* 33-48.

Page, P., Verstraete, D. G., Robb, J. R., & Etzwiler, D. D. (1981). Patient recall of self-care recommendations in diabetes. *Diabetes Care, 4*, 96–98.
Passero, M. A., Remor, B., & Salomon, J. (1981). Patient-reported compliance with cystic fibrosis therapy. *Clinical Pediatrics, 20*, 264–270.
Perrin, E. C., & Perrin, J. M. (1983). Clinicians' assessments of children's understanding of illness. *American Journal of Diseases of Children, 137*, 874–878.
Sanders, K., Mills, J., Martin, F., & Horne, D. J. (1975). Emotional attitudes in adult insulin-dependent diabetes. *Journal of Psychosomatic Research, 19*, 241–246.
Satin, W., La Greca, A. M., Zigo, M. A., & Skyler, J. S. (1989). Diabetes in adolescence: Effects of multifamily group intervention and parent simulation of diabetes. *Journal of Pediatric Psychology, 14*, 259–276.
Schafer, L. C., Glasgow, R. E., & McCaul, K. D. (1982). Increasing the adherence of diabetic adolescents. *Journal of Behavioral Medicine, 5*, 353–362.
Schafer, L. C., Glasgow, R. E., McCaul, K. D., & Dreher, M. (1983). Adherence to IDDM regimens: Relationship to psychosocial variables and metabolic control. *Diabetes Care, 6*, 493–498.
Sergis-Deavenport, E., & Varni, J. W. (1983). Behavioral assessment and management of adherence to factor replacement therapy in hemophilia. *Journal of Pediatric Psychology, 8*, 367–377.
Snyder, J. (1987). Behavioral analysis and treatment of poor diabetic self-care and antisocial behavior: A single-subject experimental study. *Behavior Therapy, 18*, 251–263.
Stark, L., Miller, S., Plienes, A., & Drabman, R. S. (1987). Behavioral contracting to increase chest physiotherapy: A case study of a young cystic fibrosis patient. *Behavior Modification, 11*, 75–86.
Stratton, R., Wilson, D. P., Endres, R. K., & Goldstein, D. E. (1987). Improved glycemic control after supervised 8-week exercise program in insulin-dependent diabetic adolescents. *Diabetes Care, 10*, 589–593.
Wing, R. R., Koeske, R., New, A., Lamparski, D., & Becker, D. (1986). Behavioral skills in self-monitoring of blood glucose: Relationship to accuracy. *Diabetes Care, 9*, 330–333.
Wing, R. R., Lamparski, D., Zaslow, S., Betschart, J., Siminerio, L., & Becker, D. (1985). Frequency and accuracy of self-monitoring of blood glucose in children: Relationship to glycemic control. *Diabetes Care, 8*, 214–218.
Witt, M., White, N. H., & Santiago, J. V. (1983). Roles of site and timing of the morning insulin injection in Type I diabetes. *Journal of Pediatrics, 103*, 528–533.
Wysocki, T., Green, L., & Huxtable, K. (1989). Blood glucose monitoring by diabetic adolescents: Compliance and metabolic control. *Health Psychology, 8*, 267–284.

Epilogue: Future Research Directions

Norman A. Krasnegor
National Institutes of Health

The preceding chapters attest to the fact that advances have been made in gaining an understanding of developmental aspects of health compliance behavior. Yet there is much to be learned in this field that is of interest to researchers, clinicians, and public health officials. This chapter provides an enumeration of research topics that should be pursued in the four main areas that comprise this volume: theory, measurement, prevention, and intervention.

THEORY

There are currently extant a number of theories that address the construct of health compliance behavior. The chapters by Iannotti and Bush, Anderson and Coyne, Leventhal, and that of Ewart, for example, each describe model systems within which to gain a metalevel understanding of compliance behavior. The availability of these theories should be taken advantage of to generate specific hypotheses that can be tested to determine whether the models help to better predict under what conditions health compliance can be achieved.

There is a great need to carry out theoretically based studies on health compliance behavior in the context of what is known about theories of development. Such studies could profitably be directed at questions concerning the determinants of short- and long-term compliance at different developmental stages. For example, investigations could be undertaken to determine the role of cognitive development in the appreciation of short- and long-term consequences associated with health compliance by children who have a chronic illness.

Another issue directly related to the interaction of developmental stage factors and health compliance behavior is: How does prospective memory relate to the capacity for children to be health compliant? A related question of theoretical relevance from both the health compliance and developmental perspectives is: How can the social context facilitate prospective memory?

Of theoretical relevance is the issue of whether cultural and ethnic factors influence health compliance behavior. Do children and their families dealing with the same chronic disease who are of different ethnic, cultural, or socioeconomic status behave similarly or differently with respect to the medical advice given to manage their condition?

A major issue that was raised by a number of the contributors to this volume relates to the interaction patterns between physician, families, and their children around the issue of health compliance. To the extent that studies can be undertaken on these interaction patterns, a vital data set can be accumulated that should provide information on this communication problem that has too long been ignored. Nested within such theoretical questions are the issues of: What are the roles of children in controlling their own treatment? How can health professionals be encouraged to communicate with children at a level that their developmental stage dictates? How can physicians be encouraged to enlist their patient's extended social network to enhance the child's health compliance behavior?

MEASUREMENT

The data presented by a number of the contributors to this book demonstrate that the measurement of compliance is not a simple task. Compliance is a multidimensional construct that requires multiple techniques and measures to accurately assess whether and to what degree it is occurring.

One need in the field of compliance research that would help get a better grasp on measurement is to encourage researchers to publish compliance rates in order that cross-study comparisons can more easily be made.

There is a need to conduct naturalistic-observational studies of how families negotiate changes in family treatment responsibilities across critical developmental stages (e.g., early childhood–elementary school age; middle childhood–adolescence; adolescence–young adulthood).

There is a need to investigate the claim that health status is related to health compliance behavior. Although physicians often come to this conclusion, a more careful analysis (e.g., glucose regulation in diabetic children) has demonstrated that there may be little correlation between the two measures. Therefore, more research is needed to determine under what conditions compliance and health status are synonymous and under what conditions this relationship is not safe to assume. The implications of such research have great importance for motivation and maintenance of health compliance behavior particularly in the case of the chronically ill child.

There is a need to undertake further research to validate the 24-hour recall method for assessing disease management (see Johnson, this volume) with children at different stages of development.

The responsibility of family members for the management of chronically ill children has not received sufficient attention. Additional research on this topic can help elucidate how family factors interact with health compliance behaviors of the affected children. This factor of family involvement is of crucial importance around the time of puberty when the ill child begins to assert his/her independence and, by extension, desires to take over the control of managing the medical regimen.

There is a need for more longitudinal research studies.

PREVENTION

Prevention is a topic of relevance at the public health level and for the individual child as well. Health compliance can be harnessed to promote behaviors that help avoid risks to well-being. In this regard there are two suggestions for future research. The first of these is that the range of topics relating to prevention needs to be expanded. Thus, diet, injury prevention, and immunization should be high priorities because these in the aggregate are so important for the public health of our nation. The second suggestion is to undertake prevention with individuals. Research should be carried out to determine how to best prevent compliance problems before such patterns begin. For example, if a child is diagnosed as being asthmatic, the physician and family should have sessions together to enhance self-management skills as soon as a diagnosis has been made and thereby decrease the chance of poor compliance and the attendant life-threatening breathing problems.

INTERVENTION

Effective intervention strategies to enhance compliance are, in effect, the bottom line in this whole genre of research. If health compliance behaviors can be promoted and maintained, the likelihood of a child living a more normal life, in spite of a chronic illness, is greatly increased.

There is a need to undertake research on the common principles among intervention strategies that could be of benefit to more than one disease.

There is a great need to study the compliance of health care providers in following up their patients (both acute and chronic diseases).

More intervention research is needed that employs experimental designs; that is, studies should be hypothesis driven and focused on identifying relevant independent measures of compliance that contribute significantly to the variance.

There is need to conduct additional research in which families are treated along with their children to determine whether this approach is more efficacious than treating the patient alone (see Epstein).

Other research should be carried out on decision-making skills to assist patients to optimize the self-management skills they can be taught.

More intervention research must be undertaken to target the education of the physician vis-à-vis the complexity of health compliance. Such research will help enhance the environmental conditions necessary to conduct investigations and manage medication research.

Author Index

A

Abelson, R. P., 257, 275
Abraham, S., 233, 247
Abramson, L. Y., 99, 101, 120
Adachi, J. D., 206, 209
Adams, G. R., 125, 149
Adebonojo, F. O., 31, 46
Ageton, S. S., 143, 147
Agras, W. S., 270, 277 287, 288, 291, 301, 311, 331
Ahmed, S., 202, 204, 212
Ajzen, I., 95, 121
Akehurst, M., 190, 208
Alderman, M. H., 93, 120
Alfredson, L. S., 198, 208
Allen, V. L., 130, 134, 149
Allison, J., 257, 280
Altman, D. G., 269, 280
Anderson, B. J., 34, 50, 78, 79, 81, 82, 88, 269, 275, 337, 341, 344, 349, 351
Anderson, C. A., 271, 275
Anderson, S., 197, 208
Andrasik, F., 234, 244, 245, 248
Andrian, C. A. G., 233, 234, 249
Apodaca, L., 33, 48, 347, 353
Aragano, J., 233, 234, 247
Archibald, E. H., 246, 247
Arnold, R. G., 31, 46
Ascione, F. J., 189, 190, 208
Atkins, E., 233, 249
Atkinson, J. W., 267, 276
Attie, I., 126, 129, 130, 131, 136, 142, 143, 144, 145, 147

Auslander, W. F., 269, 275, 337, 351
Averill, J. R., 259, 276
AvRuskin, T. W., 337, 351

B

Bachman, J. G., 118, 120
Backial, M., 311, 314, 324, 325, 326, 331
Bacon, G. E., 341, 344, 349, 351
Baer, D. M., 255, 257, 276, 280
Baer, J. S., 97, 98, 121
Baer, R. A., 33, 47
Bailey, J. S., 225, 231
Baker, E., 100, 120, 121
Baker, L., 77, 78, 81, 89, 270, 279
Baker, T. B., 96, 98, 99, 101, 122, 124
Bandura, A., 17, 24, 25, 63, 74, 94, 120, 137, 138, 145, 265, 267, 268, 276, 280, 290, 291, 301, 328, 331
Barber, P., 16, 25
Barglow, P., 32, 33, 46
Barnard, J. D., 227, 230
Barnes, K. E., 31, 46
Baron, R. A., 88
Barone, V. J., 223, 226, 228, 231
Barr, M., 190, 211
Barrett-Connor, E., 219, 230
Barrish, H. H., 228, 230
Barsky, A. K., 189, 208
Barton, C., 202, 204, 212
Bass, J. W., 31, 47
Battista, R. N., 100, 122
Baum, D., 35, 46, 305, 307, 331
Baum, J. D., 36, 49, 348, 353

Baumann, L. J., 105, 120, 264, 276
Baumrind, D., 68, 74, 136, 145
Bavry, J., 271, 278
Beck, D. E., 67, 68, 74
Beck, N. C., 197, 208
Beck, S., 33, 47, 48, 181, 182, 235, 248, 340, 341, 344, 352
Becker, D., 164, 181, 182, 336, 341, 344, 352, 354
Becker, M. H., 31, 32, 36, 40, 46, 49, 50, 63, 70, 74, 75, 76, 95, 120, 122, 132, 137, 138, 145, 148, 198, 207, 211, 212, 264, 278, 291, 301, 305, 332
Beckmann, J., 17, 26
Belmonte, M. M., 33, 47
Bennett-Johnson, S., 35, 47
Berenson, G., 142, 147
Bergman, A. B., 186, 208, 227, 230
Berndt, D., 32, 33, 46
Berndt, T. J., 134, 150
Berner, U., 207, 208
Bernholz, C. D., 200, 210
Bernstein, A. C., 133, 145
Berry, C. C., 186, 210
Berscheid, E., 258, 259, 260, 276
Best, J. A., 100, 120
Betschart, J., 336, 354
Beyth-Marom, R., 134, 147
Bianchi, B., 33, 48
Biglan, A., 271, 278
Bignell, C. J., 197, 208
Billy, J. O. G., 131, 151
Binik, Y. M., 162, 183
Binkoff, J. A., 246, 248
Bires, J. A., 227, 228, 231
Black, D. R., 263, 276
Blackwell, B., 93, 124, 286, 301
Blair, B., 195, 212
Blatter, M. M., 224, 227, 229, 231
Blechman, E. A., 271, 276
Bloch, S., 36, 49, 348, 353
Block, J. H., 135, 145
Blotcky, A. D., 35, 47

Blount, R. L., 33, 47
Bluming, A., 260, 279
Blyth, D. A., 125, 130, 134, 135, 145, 150
Bobrow, E. S., 337, 351
Bonduelle, D., 202, 204, 212
Borden, K. A., 35, 47
Botvin, E. M., 100, 120, 121
Botvin, G. J., 100, 120
Bowers, S. A., 219, 230
Boyer, C. B., 131, 141, 145
Bracs, P. U., 36, 50
Bradford, R. H., 291, 301
Brandon, T., 96, 98, 101, 122
Brekke, M. L., 100, 122
Breslau, N., 158, 184
Brief, E., 197, 208
Brink, S., 269, 278, 337, 353
Broadbent, D. N., 36, 51
Brody, D. S., 188, 199, 208
Brooks, P. H., 219, 231
Brooks-Gunn, J., 113, 123, 125, 126, 127, 128, 129, 130, 131, 132, 133, 134, 135, 136, 138, 139, 140, 141, 142, 143, 144, 145, 146, 147, 149, 150, 151
Brown, B. B., 134, 146
Brown, K. S., 100, 120
Brown, R. T., 35, 47
Brownell, K. D., 130, 146, 233, 244, 246, 247, 287, 301
Brownlee-Duffeck, M., 335, 337, 352
Bruch, H., 136, 146
Bruff, C. D., 226, 230
Brunswich, A. F., 142, 146
Bryan, C. K., 190, 209
Bubb, J., 342, 344, 349, 352
Buchanan, N., 32, 47, 48
Budd, J. R., 35, 48
Budd, K. S., 271, 276
Budlong-Springer, A. S., 32, 33, 46
Bugenthal, D. B., 15, 25
Burbach, D. J., 62, 74
Burdette, J. A., 191, 210

Burgeson, R., 131, 150
Burghen, G. A., 167, 183, 266, 278
Burish, T. G., 35, 48
Burkhart, M. T., 341, 344, 349, 351
Burnett, K. F., 270, 277, 287, 301
Burns, K. L., 311, 314, 323, 324, 325, 326, 331, 332
Burrow, C., 144, 145
Busemeyer, J. R., 16, 26, 328, 332
Bush, P. J., 64, 65, 67, 68, 69, 70, 74, 75, 76
Buss, A. H., 271, 277
Byrne, D., 133, 147
Byyny, R. L., 187, 192, 198, 200, 212

C

Cacioppo, J. T., 95, 123, 273, 279
Calder, D., 264, 277
Caldwell, H. S., 33, 48
Callas, E. R., 31, 46
Callas, J., 31, 46
Cameron, L., 59, 63, 75
Campaigne, B. N., 343, 344, 352
Canny, G. J., 330, 331
Carlton-Ford, S., 143, 146
Carmichael, C., 33, 48
Carney, R. M., 33, 47, 339, 340, 352
Caron, H. S., 199, 208, 286, 301
Carr, E. G., 246, 248
Carroll, M. S., 34, 50, 313, 320, 333
Carstenson, R., 33, 47
Carswell, F., 330, 331
Carte, E., 31, 46
Carter, R., 35, 47, 161, 162, 169, 170, 176, 178, 183, 336, 353
Carter, W. B., 195, 198, 210
Carver, C. S., 101, 121
Casey, R., 305, 333
Cassady, J., 233, 234, 247
Cassel, J. C., 191, 210
Cataldo, M. F., 219, 230
Cervone, D., 268, 276
Chacko, M. R., 177, 179, 182

Chadwick, M. W., 35, 48, 343, 344, 353
Chai, H., 319, 331
Chaiken, S., 111, 123
Chan, L. S., 195, 211
Charlop, M. H., 36, 49
Charney, E., 187, 188, 208, 236, 247, 248
Chassin, L., 115, 121
Chess, S., 271, 277
Chilman, C. S., 138, 146
Christensen, D. B., 59, 70, 74
Christensen, N. K., 336, 347, 352, 353
Christiaanse, M. E., 68, 74, 305, 331
Christophersen, E. R., 34, 36, 50, 219, 223, 224, 226, 227, 228, 229, 230, 231, 271, 276, 308, 309, 311, 332
Chrousos, G. P., 131, 151
Chudzik, G. M., 32, 47
Chwalow, J., 189, 210
Cioffi, D., 105, 121, 267, 276
Cipes, M. H., 35, 47
Citrin, W. S., 338, 352
Clark, L., 233, 234, 249, 263, 277, 278
Clark, N. M., 198, 212
Clark, S. D., Jr., 133, 152
Clark, V. A., 312, 332
Cleary, P. D., 96, 122
Clingerman, S. R., 35, 47
Cluss, P. A., 14, 25, 33, 47, 167, 182, 305, 308, 314, 331
Coates, T. J., 138, 139, 151
Cobliner, W. G., 133, 146
Coburn, P. C., 164, 182
Cohen, D. G., 35, 47, 207, 208
Cohen, E. A., 33, 47
Cohen, P., 190, 212
Cohen, S., 97, 121
Colcher, I. S., 31, 47
Coleman, V. R., 206, 208
Collins, G., 233, 247
Collins, W. A., 125, 135, 147, 150
Conaster, C., 35, 47
Contento, I. R., 265, 273, 279
Cook, T. D., 95, 121

Cooper, C. R., 135, 136, 147
Cooper, D., 187, 193, 201, 210
Cooper, K. H., 235, 248
Cornell, R. G., 341, 344, 349, 351
Correia, J., 313, 333
Costa, F. M., 266, 276
Cowan, P. A., 133, 145
Cox, D. J., 105, 106, 121
Coyne, J. C., 77, 78, 79, 80, 81, 82, 85, 88, 260, 276
Craig, O., 158, 182
Craighead, L. W., 98, 124
Cramer, J. A., 203, 205, 208
Creer, T. L., 18, 26, 35, 46, 303, 305, 307, 308, 309, 310, 311, 313, 314, 316, 318, 319, 320, 322, 323, 324, 326, 327, 328, 329, 331, 332, 333
Croft, R. D., 317, 324, 331
Crome, P., 190, 208
Cromer, B. A., 188, 189, 208
Croyle, R. T., 105, 115, 121
Cruickshanks, K. J., 159, 183
Csikszentmihalyi, M., 135, 146
Cummings, K. M., 61, 67, 68, 76, 177, 184
Cummings, M., 36, 50
Cummings, R., 24, 25
Cunningham, S., 274, 277
Cunningham, W., 35, 47, 161, 162, 169, 170, 176, 178, 183, 336, 353
Curb, J. D., 291, 301
Curry, S., 98, 99, 121
Cuskey, W. R., 34, 36, 49, 51, 314, 324, 325, 333
Cutler, G. B., 131, 151, 291, 301
Cvetkovich, G., 134, 146

D

D'Alessandra, D., 195, 212
d'Aquili, E. E., 129, 151
D'Avernas, J. R., 100, 120
D'Zarilla, R. J., 363, 276, 277
Dahlquist, L. M., 33, 47
Dalton, M., 204, 211

Damon, W., 133, 146
Daneman, D., 33, 47, 48, 181, 182, 341, 344, 352
Dantes, R., 195, 210
Dassel, S. W., 227, 230
Davidson, F. R., 65, 69, 74
Davies, J. G., 317, 332
Davies, M., 131, 149
Davis, J. B., 188, 210
Davis, S. G., 342, 344, 349, 352
Davis, T., 33, 47, 339, 340, 352
Dawson, D. A., 133, 137, 146
Dawson, K. P., 31, 47
DeAngelis, C., 35, 48
Deaton, A. V., 35, 47
DeBusk, R. F., 265, 277, 280
Deeds, S. G., 189, 210
DeFrieses, G. H., 100, 122
Delamater, A. M., 336, 337, 338, 342, 344, 347, 349, 352, 353
Delcher, H. K., 33, 48
Dershewitz, M. W., 219, 222, 224, 227, 229, 230
Des Jarlais, D. C., 139, 146
DeVellis, B. M., 63, 76
Devins, D., 190, 211
Dias, J. K., 67, 76
Dickey, F. F., 32, 47
Dickson, B., 233, 248
DiClemente, C. C., 100, 118, 123, 255, 276, 279
Dietz, W. H., 233, 246, 248
DiMatteo, M. R., 12, 17, 25
DiNicola, D. D., 12, 17, 25
Dirks, J. F., 303, 331, 192, 208
Doctors, S. R., 35, 47, 177, 179, 182
Dodd, D. K., 33, 47
Dohan, J. J., 195, 210
Dolan, T. F., 32, 49
Dolgin, M. J., 35, 47, 177, 179, 182
Donahue, M. J., 138, 146
Donnelly, J., 264, 277
Donovan, J. E., 266, 276
Dosik, G., 260, 279
Douglas, J. W. B., 233, 249

Drabman, R. S., 233, 234, 247, 345, 354
Drachman, R. H., 31, 32, 46, 47, 49, 50, 70, 74, 291, 301, 305, 332
Drash, A., 164, 182
Dreher, M., 34, 50, 162, 184, 337, 339, 354
Drexler, A., 34, 50
Drotar, D., 158, 183
Duback, U. C., 207, 208
Dubbert, P. M., 197, 208, 287, 301
Dubow, E., 32, 33, 46
Duke-Duncan, P., 131, 145
Dumas, J. E., 247, 249, 268, 280
Dunbar, J. M., 197, 208, 311, 331
Durant, R. H., 33, 47
Dusenbury, L., 100, 120

E

Ebbesen, E. B., 268, 279
Eckenrode, J., 271, 279
Edidin, D. V., 32, 33, 46
Edwards, M. M., 72, 75
Ehrhardt, A., 131, 145
Eichorn, D., 125, 129, 146
Eisen, M., 35, 47, 48, 138, 146
Eisen, S. A., 188, 201, 209
Eiser, R. J., 266, 277
Ekstrand, G., 69, 75
Ekstrand, L. J., 69, 75
Ellard, J. H., 260, 276
Elliott, D. S., 142, 143, 147
Elliott, G., 125, 147
Ellis, E. F., 303, 306, 307, 317, 320, 321, 332
Ellul-Micallef, R., 317, 332
Embry, L. H., 271, 276
Emery, R. E., 246, 248
Emmons, L., 168, 182
Emmons, R. A., 266, 277
Endres, R. K., 343, 344, 354
Eney, R. D., 32, 48, 303, 304, 305, 313, 332
Ensminger, M. E., 129, 147

Entyre, G. M., 168, 183
Epstein, L. H., 14, 25, 33, 47, 48, 106, 121, 164, 167, 181, 182, 233, 234, 235, 237, 239, 240, 244, 245, 247, 248, 249, 305, 308, 314, 331, 340, 341, 344, 352
Epstein, S., 33, 48
Eshelman, F. N., 190, 209
Etzwiler, D. D., 164, 183, 337, 348, 352, 354
Evans, E. E., 199, 209
Evans, H. E., 317, 332
Ewart, C. K., 251, 254, 256, 258, 262, 264, 265, 270, 271, 272, 274, 277, 278, 280
Ewing, L. B., 35, 48

F

Fairhurst, S. K., 255, 276
Falliers, C. J., 329, 332
Falvo, D., 164, 182
Farkas, G. M., 33, 47, 48, 181, 182, 340, 341, 344, 352
Faust, R., 116, 124
Fawcett, S. B., 219, 230
Fazio, R. H., 94, 121
Feely, M. P., 197, 208
Fehrenbach, A. M. B., 264, 277
Feinstein, A. R., 185, 196, 209
Feldman, C. H., 303, 315, 316, 318, 320, 321, 323, 325, 326, 329, 333
Feldman, D. E., 287, 301
Feldman, S. D., 125, 147
Felner, R. D., 139, 147
Felner, T. Y., 139, 147
Fennell, R. S., 67, 68, 74
Fenton, L. R., 36, 49
Fenton, T., 64, 76
Fernstrom, M. H., 247, 248
Fiese, B. H., 15, 25
Figueroa, J., 33, 47, 48, 181, 182, 340, 341, 344, 352
Fihn, S. D., 195, 199, 212
Filion, R. D. L., 129, 151

AUTHOR INDEX

Fine, R. N., 32, 48
Fineberg, N. S., 340, 344, 348, 353
Finkelstein, S. M., 35, 48
Finlay, J., 189, 210
Finnerty, F. A., 93, 121
Finney, J. W., 219, 224, 230, 269, 277
Fireman, P., 33, 47, 305, 308, 314, 331
Fischoff, B., 134, 147
Fishbein, M., 95, 121
Fisher, W., 133, 147
Fiske, V., 81, 82, 88
Fitz, A. E., 291, 301
FitzGerald, J. M., 330, 332
Fitzloff, J., 190, 209
Flagle, C. E., 190, 209
Flaherty, C., 112, 121
Flanagan, P. T., 195, 211
Flannery, E. M., 321, 333
Flay, B. R., 95, 98, 100, 120, 121
Fleming, R., 96, 98, 101, 115, 122
Fletcher, S. W., 198, 199, 209
Foch, T. T., 125, 149
Folkman, S., 101, 122
Follansbee, D. J., 136, 148, 338, 352
Ford, D. H., 16, 19, 20, 22, 24, 25, 261, 266, 277
Forehand, R., 34, 51
Forrest, J., 131, 139, 148
Fosarelli, P., 35, 48
Fox, G. L., 136, 148
Fox, S., 129, 151
Frame, 317, 333
Francis, V., 67, 75, 348, 352, 353
Frank, G. C., 142, 147
Frank, R. G., 197, 208
Frese, M., 271, 277
Freund, A., 163, 169, 170, 171, 172, 176, 177, 178, 181, 182, 183
Friday, G., 33, 47, 305, 308, 314, 331
Friedman, I. M., 35, 48, 67, 68, 75
Friedman, S. R., 139, 146
Frieman, J., 32, 48
Friman, P. C., 226, 231
Frohlich, E. D., 291, 301
Fry, D., 271, 278

Furby, L., 134, 147
Furstenberg, F. F., Jr., 126, 128, 129, 131, 133, 134, 138, 139, 142, 143, 145, 147

G

Gabriel, M., 190, 209
Gaddis, A., 140, 147
Gagnon, J. P., 190, 209
Gallagher, S. S., 226, 230
Galvis, S. A., 33, 47, 305, 308, 314, 331
Gamache, M., 197, 208
Gamble, T., 342, 344, 349, 352
Gardner, L., 188, 189, 208
Gardner, W., 134, 147
Garfield, E., 320, 332
Garfinkel, I., 132, 147
Garfinkel, P. E., 142, 147
Garguilo, J., 130, 134, 142, 146, 147
Garmezy, N., 126, 147
Garn, S. M., 233, 249
Garner, D. M., 142, 147
Geary, D., 67, 68, 74
Geden, E. A., 197, 208
Gelfand, D. M., 33, 47
Geller, E. S., 226, 230
Gentle, P., 266, 277
German, P. S., 189, 210
Gervasio, a. H., 86, 88
Gibson, E. S., 194, 200, 210, 212, 286, 301
Gilbert, B. O., 175, 182, 340, 344, 352
Gilbert, J. R., 199, 209
Gilbert, M., 134, 149
Gilliam, T. B., 343, 344, 352
Gillilan, R. E., 265, 277
Gillis, C. L., 81, 89
Glascow, R. E., 34, 49, 50, 160, 162, 167, 171, 180, 181, 182, 184, 264, 277, 336, 337, 338, 339, 340, 352, 354
Gleeson, J. G. A., 317, 332
Glenwick, D. S., 34, 51

Glynn, K., 115, 118, 121, 122
Goldberg, J., 187, 193, 201, 210
Golden, M. P., 336, 340, 344, 348, 353
Goldfried, M. R., 263, 277
Goldman, A. I., 291, 301
Goldman, J. D., 133, 147
Goldman, N., 131, 139, 148
Goldman, R. J., 133, 147
Goldsmith, C. H., 186, 196, 209
Goldsmith, H. H., 271, 277
Goldstein, D. E., 343, 344, 354
Goldstein, D., 335, 337, 352
Goldstein, E. O., 32, 48, 303, 304, 305, 313, 332
Gonder-Frederick, L. A., 105, 106, 121
Gonso, J., 269, 277
Gonthier, M., 33, 47
Gooding, W., 235, 236, 237, 240, 248
Goodman, H. C., 236, 247, 248
Gordis, L., 13, 25, 186, 209
Gordon, J. R., 98, 99, 100, 121, 123, 246, 249
Gordon, M., 187, 193, 199, 201, 210
Gortmaker, S. L., 158, 183, 184, 233, 248
Gottman, J. M., 258, 277
Gotzsche, P. C., 195, 209
Gozzi, E. K., 67, 75, 348, 353
Graves, T., 233, 234, 249, 263, 277, 278
Gray, A. S., 31, 46
Green, L. W., 139, 147, 189, 190, 209, 210, 211, 341, 344, 348, 354
Greenan-Fowler, E., 346, 352
Greene, D., 264, 278
Greene, J. Y., 188, 209
Greene, S. H., 35, 48
Greene, W. B., 346, 352
Greger, J. L., 168, 183
Griner, P. F., 188, 211
Groff, T. R., 131, 151
Gross, A. M., 33, 35, 48, 162, 168, 183, 337, 338, 339, 340, 341, 344, 352, 353
Grossman, R. M., 271, 280

Grote, B., 134, 146
Grotevant, H. D., 135, 136, 147
Gullotta, T. P., 125, 149
Gunn, T., 33, 47
Gunnar, M. R., 125, 147
Gunther, D., 31, 46
Guttmann, M., 13, 18, 24, 26, 59, 63, 75, 92, 93, 96, 104, 105, 122, 123, 254, 255, 268, 278, 279
Guyatt, G. H., 206, 209
Guyer, B., 226, 230

H

Hackett, B. C., 286, 301
Haddon, W., 222, 230
Haefner, D. P., 32, 46
Hall, J., 93, 122
Halper, L. V., 245, 249
Halverson, D., 35, 48
Hamberg, B. A., 33, 48, 64, 75, 337, 353
Hann, D. M., 268, 280
Hanna, K. J., 264, 270, 271, 274, 278
Hansen, C. A., 163, 178, 181, 183
Hanson, C. L., 167, 183, 266, 278
Hanson, E. A., 135, 149
Hardy, R. J., 291, 301
Hargreave, F. E., 330, 332
Harkavy, J., 164, 175, 183, 336, 353
Harper, S. J., 198, 199, 209
Harris, E. S., 233, 249, 269, 278
Harris, J. E., 61, 75
Harris, M. B., 33, 48
Harrison, J. E., 246, 247
Hart, D., 133, 146
Harter, S., 133, 147
Hartup, W. W., 134, 135, 148
Hassanein, R. S., 223, 227, 228, 231
Hatcher, M. E., 190, 209
Hauser, A., 34, 50
Hauser, S. T., 68, 75, 136, 143, 148, 150, 177, 183
Hauser, S. T., 269, 278, 337, 353
Hawkins, C. M., 291, 301

Hayes, C. D., 128, 129, 134, 139, 142, 148
Hayes, M., 168, 182
Haynes, R. B., 12, 17, 25, 92, 95, 124, 158, 160, 183, 185, 186, 188, 189, 193, 194, 195, 199, 200, 209, 210, 211, 212, 229, 230, 286, 301, 303, 315, 316, 318, 320, 321, 323, 325, 326, 329, 333
Healy, R., 330, 331
Heckhausen, H., 17, 25
Hefner, D. P., 70, 74
Heimann, L., 338, 352
Hein, K., 131, 141, 145, 147
Heinonen, O. P., 197, 200, 211
Hellmuth, G. A., 196, 210
Hendeles, L., 306, 307, 332
Henderson, H. R., 190, 211
Henderson, T., 93, 122
Henggeler, S. W., 167, 183, 266, 278
Henretta, J. C., 161, 183, 336, 353
Henry, R. L., 317, 332
Henshaw, S., 131, 139, 148
Henson, R., 35, 48
Herbison, G. P., 321, 333
Herrold, A. J., 336, 353
Hershey, J. C., 188, 210
Herskowitz, R. D., 68, 75, 177, 183
Hidinger, K. C., 317, 332
Hill, J. P., 135, 136, 141, 148, 151
Himmelsbach, C. K., 93, 121
Hinde, R. A., 271, 277
Hindi-Alexander, M., 303, 315, 316, 318, 320, 321, 323, 325, 326, 329, 333
Hirschman, R. S., 115, 118, 121, 122, 123
Hochbaum, G. M., 95, 122, 124
Hoette, S., 335, 337, 352
Hoff, C., 138, 139, 151
Hofferth, S. L., 128, 129, 134, 136, 137, 138, 139, 142, 148
Holcomb, R., 291, 301
Holland, J. H., 16, 26
Hollander, M. A., 92, 124

Hollingshead, A. B., 236, 249
Holroyd, K. A., 18, 26
Holtgrave, D. R., 64, 76
Holtzman, D., 35, 48
Holyoak, K. J., 16, 26
Holzworth-Munroe, A., 269, 278
Hong, H., Jr., 312, 332
Horne, D. J., 337, 354
Houlihan, J., 68, 75, 177, 183
Houts, A. C., 246, 248
Hovland, C. I., 95, 122
Howard, G. S., 11, 26
Howard, M., 138, 148
Huizinga, D., 143, 147
Hulka, B. S., 188, 191, 210
Hunt, W. A., 97, 122
Hunter, P., 226, 230
Huttunen, N. P., 343, 344, 353
Huxtable, K., 341, 344, 348, 354
Hyland, M. E., 19, 26, 267, 278

I

Iannotti, R. J., 64, 65, 67, 68, 70, 74, 75
Inazu, J. K., 136, 148
Inbar-Saban, N. I., 266, 280
Ingersoll, G. M., 336, 353
Inhelder, B., 61, 62, 75, 133, 148
Inoff, G. E., 33, 48, 64, 75, 337, 353
Inoff-Germain, G., 131, 151
Inui, T. S., 195, 198, 199, 207, 210, 212
Irwin, C. E., 132, 148
Isles, A., 313, 333
Israel, A. C., 233, 234, 249
Izard, C. E., 131. 150

J

Jacobson, A. M., 68, 75, 136, 148, 177, 183, 269, 278
Jacobson, N. S., 269, 278
Jaechke, R., 206, 209
Jamison, A., 31, 47
Jamison, R. N., 35, 48

Janis, I. L., 95, 122, 229, 230
Janz, N. K., 95, 122, 132, 138, 148, 264, 278
Jarvis, I. L., 273, 278
Javela, K., 197, 211
Jay, M. S., 33, 47
Jay, S., 36, 49
Jeffery, R. J., 243, 244, 249, 278
Jeffery, R. W., 244, 246, 247
Jelliffe, D. B., 236, 249
Jemmott, J. B., 105, 115, 121
Jensen, J., 33, 47
Jerin, M. J., 188, 209
Jerome, A., 303, 307, 308, 309, 310, 311, 313, 316, 318, 319, 324, 329, 332
Jessor, R., 129, 136, 148, 266, 276
Job, R. F. S., 137, 148
Johansen, W. J., 186, 210
John, E. C., 222, 231
Johnson, A. L., 188, 194, 210, 212, 286, 301
Johnson, C. A., 100, 123
Johnson, S. B., 161, 162, 163, 164, 169, 170, 171, 172, 173, 174, 175, 176, 177, 178, 181, 182, 183, 184, 336, 340, 344, 352, 353
Johnson, W. G., 338, 353
Johnston, G. D., 188, 212
Johnston, L. D., 118, 120
Johnston, M., 36, 49, 348, 353
Jones, E., 131, 139, 148
Jones, F. A., 33, 48
Jones, J. B., 133, 148
Jones, P. K., 72, 75
Jones, S. L., 72, 75
Jones, S., 99, 123
Jordan, I., 31, 46
Joyce, C. R. B., 204, 210
Jurs, S. G., 72, 76

K

Kaar, M. L., 343, 344, 353
Kadlec, G. J., 32, 50

Kadlec, G. J., 304, 305, 315, 316, 325, 329, 333
Kahneman, D., 111, 122
Kandel, D. B., 116, 124, 131, 142, 149
Kanfer, F. H., 16, 18, 26, 101, 122, 267, 278, 327, 328, 332
Kanter, J. F., 129, 133, 152
Kaplan, R. M., 35, 48, 343, 344, 353
Karibo, J. M., 32, 50, 304, 305, 315, 316, 325, 329, 333
Karmarck, T. W., 97, 121
Karoly, P., 14, 15, 16, 17, 18, 19, 24, 26, 59, 75
Kass, M. A., 187, 193, 199, 201, 210
Kaszuba, A., 35, 48
Katchadourian, H., 127, 149
Katz, E. R., 35, 47 177, 179, 182
Katz, J., 72, 75
Katz, R. M., 198, 212
Kaufman, E. M., 33, 48
Kay, D. R., 197, 208
Kazdin, A. E., 33, 48, 181, 182 257, 258, 278, 341, 344, 352
Keating, D. P., 132, 149
Keesey, R. E., 106, 122
Keet, J., 190, 208
Kegeles, S. S., 34, 49
Kelemen, M. D., 265, 277
Kelemen, M. H., 265, 277
Kelleher, K., 195, 212
Keller, J. L., 206, 209
Kelley, H. H., 95, 122
Kelly, A. B., 223, 230
Kelly, H. W., 307, 332
Kennedy, M. C., 195, 212
Kersell, M. W., 100, 120
Kessen, W., 17, 26
Killam, P. E., 33, 48, 347, 353
Kilner, L., 143, 150
Kilo, C., 335, 337, 352
King, A. C., 197, 208, 269, 280
King, D. R., 35, 48
Kingsolver, K., 97, 121

Kinsman, R. A., 192, 198, 208, 212, 303, 315, 316, 318, 320, 321, 323, 325, 326, 329, 331, 333
Kirby, D., 137, 149
Kirschenbaum, D. S., 108, 122, 233, 249, 268, 278
Kirscht, J. P., 31, 32, 46, 47, 70, 74, 189, 208, 291, 301
Kirson, D., 259, 280
Klauber, M. R., 219, 230
Klein, M. A., 189, 210
Klinger, E., 257, 278
Klopovitch, P., 35, 47
Kniker, W. T., 305, 332
Knip, M., 343, 344, 353
Kniskern, J., 271, 278
Koepsell, T. D., 195, 199, 212
Koeske, R., 106, 121, 234, 235, 236, 237, 240, 244, 245, 248, 336, 354
Koff, E., 140, 149
Kog, E., 270, 278
Kogan, K., 271, 276
Kohn, M. L., 271, 278
Kolski, G. B., 333
Korsch, B. M., 31, 32, 48, 67, 75, 348, 352, 353
Kotok, D., 36, 51
Kotses, H., 314, 326, 328, 331, 333
Kottke, T. E., 100, 122
Kraemer, C., 35, 48
Kraemer, H. A., 270, 277
Kress, M. J., 233, 234, 249
Kristeller, J. L., 255, 278
Kronz, K. K., 340, 344, 348, 353
Kruger, S., 33, 48
Kucynski, L., 68, 75
Kuhl, J., 17, 26
Kujawa, S. J., 35, 48
Kupper, L. L., 191, 210
Kurtz, S. M., 336, 337, 338, 347, 352, 353
Kuttner, M. J., 336, 337, 347, 353
Kwiterovich, P. O., Jr., 264, 270, 271, 274, 278

L

Laasonen, K., 343, 344, 353
LaGreca, A. M., 338, 342, 344, 352, 354
Lake, D. C., 321, 333
Lake, M., 197, 208
Lamparski, D., 336, 354
Lampman, R. M., 343, 344, 352
Lancelot, C., 129, 149
Landman, G., 64, 76
Langlie, J. K., 115, 122
Lankelaa, S. L., 343, 344, 353
LaPorte, R. E., 159, 183
Larsen, F. J., 195, 211
Larsen, R. J., 24, 26
Larsen, V. L., 140, 149
Larson, R., 135, 146
Lasagna, L., 188, 211
Latiolais, C. J., 186, 210
Launier, R., 101, 122
Laursen, B., 135, 150
Lautala, P., 343, 344, 353
Lavelle, M., 233, 249
Laventurier, M. F., 195, 211
Lavigne, J. V., 68, 74, 305, 331
Lawrence, R. A., 36, 51
Lazarus, R. S., 101, 122
Leake, H. C., 227, 230
LeBaron, S., 305, 332
LeClaire, S., 223, 230
Lee, H., 317, 332
Lehman, D. R., 77, 79, 80, 85, 88 271, 278
Leibowitz, R., 260, 279
Leirer, V. O., 201, 210
Leistyna, J., 312, 332
Lempert, R. O., 271, 278
Lepper, M. R., 264, 278
Lerner, C. V., 68, 74, 305, 331
Lerner, R. M., 125, 130, 149
Leung, P., 311, 314, 324, 325, 326, 331
Leupker, R. V., 100, 123
Levenson, R. W., 258, 277

Leventhal, H., 13, 18, 24, 26, 59, 63, 75, 92, 93, 94, 95, 96, 98, 99, 101, 104, 105, 115, 116, 118, 120, 121, 122, 123, 124, 189, 210, 254, 255, 264, 268, 276, 278, 279
Levin, R. A., 36, 50
Levine, D. M., 189, 190, 209, 210
Levine, M. D., 64, 76
Levison, H., 313, 330, 331, 333
Levy, R. L., 60, 75, 190, 211
Lewin, K., 109, 123
Lewis, C. C., 134, 149
Lewis, C. E., 65, 75, 303, 315, 316, 318, 320, 321, 323, 325, 326, 329, 333
Lewis, M. A., 65, 75
Lewis, P. S., 314, 326, 333
Lewis, S., 35, 48
Ley, P., 36, 50, 60, 75, 94, 123, 189, 211, 269, 278
Li, Q., 321, 333
Libow, L. S., 188, 212
Lichtenstein, E., 97, 121, 244, 246, 247, 271, 278, 287, 301
Lichtman, R., 260, 279
Lilienfeld, A. M., 186, 209
Lincoln, R., 131, 139, 148
Lindaman, F. C., 220, 231
Linder, C. W., 33, 47
Lindsley, C. B., 34, 36, 50
Liptak, G. S., 36, 40, 49, 70, 72, 75, 207, 211
Lipton, T., 93, 122
Lira, F. T., 345, 353
Lisk, D. R., 35, 48
Litt, I. F., 33, 34, 35, 36, 47, 48, 49, 67, 68, 75
Little, B. R., 266, 279
Locke, E. A., 94, 123
Loftus, G. R., 60, 75
Logan, A. G., 195, 211
Logan, J. A., 142, 149
LoGerfo, J. P., 195, 199, 212
Long, N., 228, 230
Lorenz, R. A., 336, 347, 352, 353

Loriaux, D. L., 131. 151
Losch, M., 287, 301
Lovato, C. Y., 139, 147
LoVerde, M. E., 187, 192, 198, 200, 212
Lowe, J., 178, 184
Lowe, K., 167, 183, 338, 340, 353
Lowman, J. T., 32, 50
Lucas, M. K., 321, 333
Ludwig, W. W., 246, 249
Lund, A. K., 34, 49
Lutzker, J. F., 167, 183
Lutzker, J. R., 338, 340, 353
Lynch, M. E., 135, 148
Lyon, B., 236, 247, 248
Lyon, G., 204, 211

M

Macaulay, J., 312, 332
MacLeod, S., 313, 333
Maenpaa, H., 197, 200, 211
Magalnick, L. J., 35, 48, 341, 344, 353
Magnusson, D., 130, 134, 149, 151
Magrab, P. R., 32, 49, 346, 353
Mahoney, M. J., 267, 276
Maiman, L. A., 32, 36, 40, 46, 49, 51, 70, 72, 74, 75, 95, 120, 207, 211
Malkonen, M., 197, 211
Mallon, J., 177, 184
Mallon, M., 36, 50, 61, 67, 68, 76
Malone, J., 163, 178, 181, 183
Malott, J. M., 267, 279
Mamin, J. J., 188, 209
Mandler, G., 17, 26
Manella, K. J., 33, 48, 347, 353
Manley, J. D., 265
Manne, S. L., 260, 279
Manninen, V., 197, 200, 211
Marion, R. J., 311, 314, 324, 325, 326, 331, 332
Markello, J., 32, 49
Markowitz, M., 196, 209
Marks, B., 247, 247
Marksman, H., 269, 277

AUTHOR INDEX

Marlatt, G. A., 18, 26, 98, 99, 100, 121, 123, 244, 246, 247, 249, 287, 301
Maronde, R. F., 195, 211
Marquis, K. H., 168, 183
Marrero, D. G., 340, 344, 348, 353
Marshall, G., 192, 198, 200, 212, 291, 301
Marshall, L. F., 219, 230
Marsiglio, W., 137, 149
Marteau, T. M., 36, 49, 348, 353
Martin, E. M., 99, 124
Martin, F., 337, 354
Martin, J. E., 197, 208
Mashigo, S., 32, 47
Masten, A. S., 126, 147
Matarazzo, J., 97, 122
Mathews, J. R., 226, 231
Mattar, M. E., 32, 47, 49
Matthews, L. W., 158, 183
Mattson, R. H., 203, 205, 208
Mawhinney, H., 198, 212
Mazzullo, J. M., 188, 211
McAdoo, W. G., 246, 249
McAlister, A. L., 35, 47, 48, 138, 146
McBride, M., 236, 247, 248
McCall, R. B., 271, 277
McCallum, M., 164, 175, 182, 183, 336, 344, 352, 353
McCann, K. L., 246, 249
McCaul, K. D., 34, 49, 50, 160, 162, 167, 171, 180, 181, 182, 184, 267, 279, 336, 337, 338, 339, 340, 352, 354
McClelland, D. C., 267, 279
McCollum, A., 85, 89
McCord, J., 143, 149
McCormick, M. C., 305, 333
McCubbin, H. I., 77, 89
McCubbin, M. A., 77, 89
McCurley, J., 239, 247, 248
McDevitt, D. G., 188, 212
McGrath, P., 190, 212
McGrew, J., 115, 121
McGuire, W. J., 94, 123
McHugh, R., 196, 211

McKenney, J. M., 190, 211
McKenzie, T. L., 247, 249
McKinley, R., 72, 76
McLanahan, S., 132, 147
McLean, J. C., 34, 49
McLorie, G. A., 34, 49
McPhee, S. J., 189, 210
MeSweeney, F. K., 271, 280
Meachem, J. A., 61, 76
Meichenbaum, D., 17, 26
Meltzer, D. W., 187, 193, 199, 201, 210
Menendez, R. A., 303, 315, 316, 318, 320, 321, 322, 323, 325, 326, 329, 333
Mermelstein, R., 97, 121
Messeri, P., 142, 146
Mewborn, R., 269, 277
Meyer, D., 93, 122, 104, 105, 123, 264, 268, 278, 279
Meyerowitz, B. E., 111, 123
Meyers, A. W., 233, 234, 249, 263, 277, 278
Meyers, A., 32, 49
Michela, J. L., 265, 273, 279
Michelson, J., 233, 248
Miklich, D. R., 311, 314, 324, 325, 326, 331
Miller, A. T., 265, 271, 273, 279
Miller, B. C., 137, 138, 148
Miller, D. K., 188, 201, 209
Miller, D. R., 158, 183
Miller, H. G., 133, 137, 151
Miller, J. P., 269, 275, 337, 351
Miller, K. A., 304, 305, 332
Miller, L. P., 158, 183
Miller, L., 204, 211
Miller, N. E., 157, 183
Miller, N. H., 265, 280
Miller, P. H., 23, 26
Miller, R. E., 224, 227, 229, 231
Miller, S., 345, 354
Milley, J. E., 68, 75, 177, 183
Mills, J., 337, 354
Millstein, S. G., 132, 148

AUTHOR INDEX 371

Milne, B. J., 195, 211
Milner, A. D., 317, 332
Minuchin, P., 136, 149
Minuchin, S., 77, 78, 81, 89, 270, 279
Miraglia, M., 35, 47
Mischel, W., 18, 26, 268, 279
Mitchell, W. D., 192, 197, 198, 200, 202, 212
Mittelmark, M. B., 100, 123
Mlott, S. R., 345, 353
Montemayor, R., 125, 135, 149
Montgomery, S. B., 72, 75
Moore, K. A., 134, 147
Moore, M. C., 142, 147
Moos, R., 269, 277
Moran, M. G., 316, 318, 332
Moren, F., 317, 332
Morgan, S. P., 126, 129, 138, 142, 143, 147
Morrill, C., 311, 314, 324, 325, 326, 331
Morris, M. J., 348, 352
Morris, N. M., 131, 151
Morrison, D. M., 133, 138, 149
Morrow, D. G., 201, 210
Morton, B. G., 188, 210
Mosbach, P., 116, 123
Moses, L. E., 133, 137
Mott, F., 137, 149
Moulding, T. S., 201, 211, 297, 301
Mucklow, J. C., 199, 212
Mueller, D., 32, 49
Mukherjee, J., 200, 210
Mulcahy, F. M., 197, 208
Mullen, P. D., 190, 211
Mullet, N., 338, 353
Murray, D. M., 100, 123
Myers, P. R., 11, 26

N

Nadelman, S., 245, 248
Nader, P. R., 247, 249, 271, 280
Nathanson, C. A., 32, 46, 47

Nazarian, L. F., 36, 40, 49, 70, 72, 75, 207, 211
Neel, E. U., 36, 49
Neely, E., 186, 211
Negrete, V. F., 31, 32, 48
Nelson, E. C., 188, 211
Nerenz, D., 264, 278
Neutra, R. R., 188, 211
New, A., 336, 354
Newcomb, R. W., 319, 331
Newcomer, S. F., 134, 149
Newhouse, M. T., 206, 209
Newman, R., 190, 212
Newth, C., 313, 333
Nezu, A. M., 246, 249, 263, 279
Nicholls, J. G., 265, 271, 273, 279
Nierenberg, D. W., 197, 211
Nimmer, J. G., 226, 230
Nisbett, R. E., 16, 26, 271, 278
Noam, G. G., 136, 148
Nordsieck, M., 233, 247
Norell, S. E., 197, 198, 199, 201, 208, 211
Norman, D. C., 190, 213
Notarius, C., 269, 277
Nottelmann, E. D., 131, 151

O

O'Brien, R. O., 98, 124
O'Brien, R. W., 64, 76
O'Connell, J. K., 72, 76
O'Connor, C., 259, 280
O'Grady, L. F., 33, 47
O'Leary, K. D., 271, 276
O'Malley, P. M., 118, 120
Ockene, J. K., 100, 123
Oldridge, N. B., 265, 279
O'Leary, A., 63, 76
Omoto, A. M., 258, 260, 276
Ooms, T., 136, 149
Orme, C. M., 162, 183
Orr, D. P., 336, 340, 344, 348, 353
Osborn, L. M., 227, 231
Osnes, P. G., 255, 280

Ossip, D. J., 234, 235, 244, 245, 248

P

Page, E. G., 34, 50, 313, 320, 333
Page, P., 164, 183, 348, 354
Paige, K. E., 140, 149, 150
Paikoff, R. L., 113, 123, 126, 127, 128, 131, 132, 133, 134, 135, 138, 140, 141, 143, 144, 145, 146, 150
Palta, M., 196, 211
Pantell, R. H., 67, 76
Papadopoulou, Z. L., 32, 49, 346, 353
Pappius, E. M., 198, 199, 209
Parcel, G. S., 64, 74, 76
Pariante, G. M., 201, 210
Parker, J. C., 197, 208
Parks, G. A., 18, 26
Parrish, J. M., 36, 49
Patrick, M. L., 186, 211
Patsy, B. M., 195, 199, 212
Patterson, G. R., 84, 89, 258, 269, 279
Patterson, J. M., 79, 89
Patterson, T. L., 247, 249, 271, 280
Patti, E. T., 246, 249
Peaker, S., 197, 208
Pearlman, R. A., 195, 210
Pecoraro, R. C., 195, 198, 210
Pedersen, S., 317, 332
Pederson, L. L., 100, 123
Pencharz, P. B., 246, 247
Pendelton, D., 286, 301
Penick, S. B., 246, 249
Pennebaker, J. W., 105, 123, 271, 280
Penner, B. C., 233, 234, 249
Pepper, S. C., 18, 26
Perfetto, G., 36, 50
Perkins, J. G., 204, 211
Perkins, K. A., 247, 248
Perri, M. G., 246, 249
Perri, M. G., 263, 279
Perrin, E. C., 175, 183 348, 354
Perrin, J. M., 175, 183, 348, 354
Perry, C. L., 100, 120
Perry, H. M., 291, 301

Persinger, G. S., 190, 211
Pervin, L. A., 24, 26
Petersen, A. C., 125, 126, 129, 131, 133, 136, 145, 146, 150
Peterson, C., 63, 76
Peterson, J. L., 134, 147
Peterson, L., 62, 74, 264, 277, 335, 337, 352
Petrou, C., 330, 331
Petty, R. E., 95, 123, 273, 279
Philliber, S., 133, 148
Phillips, R., 32, 33, 46
Phillips, S. A., 177, 179, 182
Piaget, J., 61, 62, 75, 133, 148
Pichert, J. W., 336, 347, 352, 353
Pikkarinen, J., 197, 211
Pinkerton, P., 77, 78, 89
Pinski, R. B., 271, 280
Pitkanen-Pulkkinen, L., 68, 76
Pitman, K. J., 137, 151
Plaut, T. F., 319, 321, 332
Pless, I. B., 77, 78, 89, 222, 231
Plienes, A., 345, 354
Plomin, R., 271, 277
Podgainy, H. J., 222, 231
Pollak, T., 164, 175, 183, 336, 353
Pollard, S. J., 32, 50, 304, 305, 315, 316, 325, 329, 333
Porter, A. M. W., 186, 211
Powell, C., 346, 352
Powers, S. I., 136, 143, 148, 150
Powers, W. T., 19, 24, 26, 101, 123
Prasada-Rao, P., 198, 212
Pratt, L., 68, 76
Pratt, R., 236, 247, 248
Prentis, S., 142, 147
Presson, C. C., 115, 121
Price, J. F., 317, 332
Price, J. H., 72, 76
Print, C. G., 321, 333
Prochaska, J. O., 100, 118, 123, 255, 276, 279
Prohaska, T. R., 115, 123
Prudharm, D., 199, 212
Przybeck, T. R., 188, 201, 209

Pullar, T., 197, 208
Purviance, M. R., 36, 50
Puukka, R., 343, 344, 353

R

Rachelsfsky, G. S., 198, 212
Rachlin, H., 111, 123
Radius, S. M., 32, 47, 49, 50 305, 332
Raj, M. N., 131, 151
Ransom, D. C., 78, 89
Rapoff, M. A., 34, 36, 50, 308, 309, 311, 332
Rapp, S. R., 197, 208
Rappaport, L., 64, 76
Ratner, P., 305, 332
Raveis, V. H., 131, 149
Rawlins, P., 33, 48
Read, P. B., 131, 150
Rebuck, A. S, 330, 331
Reed, C. E., 304, 307, 321, 332, 333
Reef, M. J., 131, 150
Reese, L. B., 265, 277
Reichgott, M. J., 188, 210
Reid, J. B., 84, 89
Reisinger, K. S., 222, 224, 227, 228, 229, 231
Reisman, J., 330, 331
Reiter, E. O., 128, 129, 140, 146
Relles, D. A., 168, 183
Renick, N. L., 100, 121
Renne, C. M., 305, 308, 323, 333
Reynolds, L. A., 172, 173, 184
Richards, G. A., 67, 68, 74
Richards, M., 36, 50, 61, 67, 68, 76, 177, 184
Richardson, P., 35, 48, 341, 344, 353
Riddle, M., 264, 277
Rierdan, J., 140, 149
Riley, D., 271, 279
Riley, W., 169, 170, 173, 174, 184
Riner, L. S., 271, 276
Robb, J. R., 164, 183, 337, 348, 352, 354
Roberts, M. C., 219, 225, 231

Roberts, R. S., 188, 194, 210, 212, 286, 301
Roberts, S. M., 72, 76
Roberts, T. R., 222, 231
Robinson, J. D., 67, 68, 74
Rodin, J., 130, 150, 255, 278
Rodriguez, M. L., 268, 279
Rogel, M. J., 133, 150
Rogers, J. P., 36, 50
Rogers, R. J., 322, 333
Rogers, R. W., 264, 279
Rohr, A. S., 198, 212
Rokeach, M., 266, 279
Rosen, D., 32, 50
Rosen, T. J., 99, 123
Rosenberg, A., 34, 49
Rosenbloom, A. L., 35, 47, 161, 162, 164, 169, 170, 175, 176, 178, 182, 183, 336, 340, 344, 352, 353
Rosenbloom, D., 206, 209
Rosenstock, I. M., 32, 47, 49, 50, 63, 69, 76, 95, 124, 305, 332
Rosenthal, B. L., 271, 280
Rosman, B. L., 77, 78, 81, 89, 270, 279
Rosoff, J., 131, 139, 148
Ross, A. W., 67, 76
Ross, L. V., 226, 231
Rossi, J. S., 255, 276
Rosso, J., 142, 146
Roth, H. P., 197, 199, 208, 212, 286, 301
Rothbart, M. K., 271, 277
Rounds, K. A., 36, 40, 49, 70, 72, 75, 207, 211
Rozin, R., 113, 124
Ruble, D. N., 135, 140, 150
Rudd, P., 187, 192, 197, 198, 200, 202, 204, 212
Rudd, S., 34, 49
Ruehlman, L. S., 260, 266, 280
Russell, G., 317, 333
Russell, M. L., 197, 212
Russell, R. P., 189, 210
Rutter, M., 126, 131, 147, 150
Ryan, K. B., 100, 120

S

Sabbath, B., 81, 88
Sackett, D. L., 12, 25, 92, 93, 95, 124, 158, 160, 183, 185, 187, 188, 193, 194, 198, 200, 210, 212, 229, 230, 286, 301
Sallis, J. F., 129, 131, 150, 247, 249, 271, 280
Sameroff, A. J., 15, 25
Samson, G., 162, 183
Samuelson, G., 168, 184
Sanders, K. M., 245, 249, 337, 354
Sanders, S., 162, 183
Santiago, J. V., 269, 275, 336, 337, 342, 344, 347, 349, 351, 352, 353, 354
Sappenfield, W., 158, 183
Satin, W., 342, 344, 354
Savin-Williams, R. C., 134, 150
Sbrbaro, J. A., 303, 315, 316, 318, 320, 321, 323, 325, 326, 329, 333
Schafer, L. C., 34, 50, 162, 167, 171, 180, 181, 182, 184, 336, 337, 338, 339, 340, 352, 354
Schawartz, N. L., 34, 50
Schberth, K. C., 32, 47
Schechter, D., 33, 47, 339, 340, 352
Scheier, M. F., 101, 121
Scherba, D. S., 263, 276
Scheyer, R. D., 203, 205, 208
Schimmel, L. E., 35, 48, 343, 344, 353
Schmidt, L., 342, 344, 349, 352
Schnaper, H. W., 291, 301
Schoenbaum, E., 93, 120
Schooler, C., 271, 278
Schork, M. A., 343, 344, 352
Schuberth, K. C., 32, 49, 50, 305, 332
Schultz, R., 338, 352
Schunk, D. H., 267, 276
Schwartz, C., 330, 331
Schwartz, G. E., 18, 27, 253, 280
Schwartz, J., 259, 280
Schwartz, S. H., 266, 280

Scott, P., 313, 333
Searle, J. P., 34, 36, 50, 305, 333
Sears, M. R., 321, 333
Seekins, T., 219, 230
Seeman, J., 253, 280
Seligman, M. E. P., 99, 101, 120
Selman, R. L., 133, 150
Senediak, C., 233, 249
Sergis-Davenport, E., 34, 50, 164, 184, 346, 354
Shafer, M., 131, 145
Shainess, N., 140, 150
Shannon, B., 188, 189, 208
Shapiro, R. M., 246, 249
Shapiro, R., 338, 352
Sharp, J. P., 233, 249
Shaver, P., 259, 280
Shaw, J., 34, 36, 50, 305, 333
Shaw, L. W., 93, 121
Sheikh, J. I., 201, 210
Sheingold, K., 140, 149
Shelton, M., 133, 150
Shendel, R. J., 36, 50
Shennum, W. A., 15, 25
Sherman, F. T., 188, 212
Sherman, S. J., 115, 121
Shimp, L. A., 189, 190, 208
Shivvers, N., 197, 208
Shmarak, K. L., 31, 50
Shoda, Y., 268, 279
Shoffitt, T., 33, 47
Shope, J. T., 34, 50
Siegel, S. C., 198, 212
Siegel, S. E., 35, 47, 177, 179, 182
Silberstein, L. R., 130, 150
Siller, J., 337, 351
Silverman, J., 131, 148
Silverman, W. K., 233, 249
Silverstein, J. H., 35, 47, 161, 162, 163, 164, 169, 170, 171, 172, 173, 175, 176, 177, 178, 181, 182, 183, 184, 336, 340, 344, 352, 353
Siminerio, L., 33, 47, 164, 182, 336, 354
Simmons, M. S., 312, 332

AUTHOR INDEX

Simmons, R. G., 125, 130, 131, 134, 135, 145, 150
Simon, L. G., 233, 249
Simonds, J. F., 335, 337, 352
Singer, R., 99, 123
Single, E., 116, 124
Skyler, J. S., 342, 344, 354
Slater, M. D., 268, 280
Slining, J. D., 190, 211
Smetana, J. G., 135, 150, 151
Smith, A., 199, 212
Smith, C. S., 189, 210
Smith, C., 162, 183
Smith, D. A. F., 81, 82, 88, 260, 276
Smith, E. A., 134, 151
Smith, E. O., 291, 301
Smith, E., 197, 208
Smith, J. A., 336, 338, 342, 344, 347, 349, 352
Smith, L., 36, 50, 61, 67, 68, 76, 177, 184
Smith, N. A., 34, 36, 50, 305, 333
Smith, R. S., 126, 151
Smith, S. D., 32, 50
Smyth-Struch, K., 158, 184
Snitzer, J., 33, 48
Snow, J. C., 93, 95, 124
Snyder, J., 339, 340, 354
Snyder, M., 258, 260, 276
Solomon, H. S., 188, 211
Sonenstein, F. L., 137, 142, 151
Sorauf, T., 186, 210
Sosland-Edelman, D., 223, 230
Souter, B. R., 195, 212
Sowers-Hoag, K. M., 225, 231
Spangler, D. L., 34, 50, 313, 320, 333
Spector, R., 190, 212
Spector, S. L., 198, 212, 303, 312, 315, 316, 318, 319, 320, 321, 322, 324, 325, 326, 329, 333
Speigel, C. N., 220, 231
Spence, S. H., 233, 249
Spencer, M. L., 343, 344, 352

Spevack, M., 169, 170, 173, 174, 184
Spillar, R., 164, 175, 182, 183, 336, 353, 336, 340, 344, 352, 353
Spitznagel, E., 188, 201, 209
Squires, S., 235, 244, 248
Stall, R. D., 138, 139, 151
Stark, L., 345, 354
Stark, O., 233, 249
Stason, W. B., 188, 211
Stattin, H., 130, 149, 151
Steckel, S. B., 190, 212
Stein, M. T., 227, 231
Steinberg, K., 188, 189, 208
Steinberg, L., 116, 124, 135, 136, 151
Steiner, J. F., 195, 199, 212
Steranchak, L., 233, 248
Sternberg, R. J., 14, 22, 25, 27
Stewart, K. J., 265, 277
Stewart, T. J., 67, 76
Stickler, E. M., 346, 352
Stimson, G. V., 92, 124
Stokes, T. F., 255, 280
Stolmaker, L., 233, 234, 249
Strandberg, L. R., 195, 211
Stratton, R., 343, 344, 354
Strecher, V. J., 63, 76, 198, 212
Striegel-Moore, R., 130, 150
Strunk, R. C., 322, 333
Stunkard, A. J., 63, 76, 98, 124, 129, 151, 168, 184 246, 249
Sublett, J. L., 32, 50, 304, 305, 315, 316, 325, 329, 333
Sullivan, S. R., 195, 211
Summey, P., 32, 50
Sumner, J. Y., 32, 49
Susman, E. J., 131. 151
Susser, I. S., 34, 50
Sutton, M., 33, 48
Sutton, S. R., 118, 124, 137, 151
Svarstad, B., 59, 76
Swain, M. A., 190, 212
Szasz, T., 92, 124
Szefler, S. J., 322, 333
Szykula, S., 271, 276

T

Tabachnik, E., 313, 333
Taggart, A. J., 188, 212
Tajima, N., 159, 183
Talbert, T., 131, 151
Taplin, P. S., 311, 314, 324, 325, 326, 331
Tashkin, D. P., 312, 332
Tattersall, R. B., 178, 184
Taylor, C. B., 265, 270, 277, 280, 287, 301
Taylor, D. W., 12, 25, 158, 160, 183, 188, 194, 200, 210, 212, 229, 230, 286, 301, 321, 333
Taylor, S., 260, 279
Teasdale, J., 99, 101, 120
Tebbi, C. K., 36, 50, 61, 67, 68, 76, 177, 184
Teets, K. C., 32, 47, 49, 50, 305, 332
Tellegen, A., 126, 147
Terry, N. S., 99, 123
Terry, R. D., 336, 352
Thagard, P. R., 16, 26
Thomas, A., 271, 277
Thomas, J., 169, 170, 171, 172, 176, 177, 182
Thomas, K. A., 223, 227, 231
Thornton, D., 188, 189, 208
Thyer, B. A., 225, 231
Tiffany, S. T., 98, 99, 124
Timberlake, W., 257, 280
Tinkelman, D. G., 34, 50, 313, 320, 333
Tinsley, B. J., 64, 76
Tippy, P., 164, 182
Titus, C., 187, 192, 198, 200, 212
Tobin-Richards, M., 133, 150
Tomarken, A. J., 108, 122, 233, 249, 269, 278
Tomer, A., 131, 148, 161, 183, 336, 353
Toobert, D. J., 264, 277
Tortu, S., 100, 120
Towson, S. M. J., 100, 120

Trostle, J. A., 34, 50
Trueworthy, R. C., 32, 50
Tucker, J. A., 109, 124
Tugwell, P., 193, 194, 199, 209, 212
Turk, D. C., 17, 26
Turner, C. F., 133, 137, 151
Turner, C., 33, 47
Turner, D. S., 225, 231
Tversky, A., 111, 122
Twentyman, C. T., 246, 249

U

Udry, J. R., 130, 131, 134, 149, 151
Ullman, S., 311, 314, 324, 325, 326, 331
Uretsky, N., 190, 212

V

Valenti, S. A., 265, 277
Valoski, A., 106, 121, 233, 234, 235, 236, 237, 239, 240, 245, 247, 248
Vandereyken, W., 270, 278
Vanderpool, G. E., 34, 50, 313, 320, 333
Varni, J. W., 33, 34, 48, 50, 164, 184, 346, 352, 353, 354
Vaughan, R., 115, 124
Velasquez, M. M., 255, 276
Velicer, W. F., 255, 276
Verstraete, D. G., 164, 183, 348, 354
Vertommen, H., 270, 278
Vestal, R., 204, 211
Voss, H. L., 142, 143, 147
Voyles, J. B., 303, 318, 320, 321, 322, 326, 329, 333
Vuchinic, R., 109, 124

W

Wadden, T. A., 130, 146, 233, 246, 247, 249
Wagner, E. D., 195, 199, 212

Wahler, R. G., 247, 249, 268, 271, 276, 280
Walsh, D. C., 60, 76
Wandless, I., 199, 212
Warach, J. D., 188, 212
Ware, J. E., Jr., 168, 183
Warner, E. E., 126, 151
Warren, M. P., 129, 130, 131, 134, 142, 143, 144, 145, 146, 147, 149, 150, 151
Warren-Boulton, E., 34, 50
Warwick, W. J., 35, 48
Waszak, L., 36, 50
Watson, D. W., 271, 280
Watson, D., 105, 123
Watt, E., 68, 75., 177, 183
Watts, J. C., 99, 123
Waxman, M., 168, 184
Webb, S., 36, 51
Wedgewood, R. J., 227, 230
Weinberger, M., 188, 209, 306, 307, 332, 333
Weinstein, A. G., 34, 36, 51
Weinstein, A. M., 314, 318, 324, 325, 333
Weinstein, N. D., 110, 116, 124, 132, 151, 268, 280
Weiss, B., 136, 148
Weissman, M. M., 143, 151, 158, 184
Weisz, J. R., 265, 280
Wells, J. F., 222, 231
Wells, P., 67, 76
Wells, R. D., 177, 179, 182
Wentworth, S., 269, 278
Werner, R. J., 186, 208
Wertlieb, D., 68, 75, 177, 183
Wertlieb, E., 269, 278
Westoff, C., 131, 139, 148
Wetterlin, K., 317, 332
Whalen, C. K., 267, 276
White, L., 133, 147
White, N. H., 336, 338, 342, 344, 347, 349, 352, 354
Whiting, B., 69, 76
Whiting, J. W. M., 69, 76

Wielinski, C. L., 35, 48
Wigal, J. K., 303, 307, 308, 309, 310, 311, 313, 314, 316, 318, 319, 324, 326, 329, 332, 333
Wildman, H., 338, 353
Williams, A. F., 221, 222, 231
Williams, C. A., 34, 51
Williams, G. E., 223, 228, 231
Williams, G. H., 189, 213
Williams, M. H., Jr., 319, 320, 333
Williams, R. L., 36, 51
Williamson, J. W., 207, 210, 222, 227, 230
Wills, T. A., 115, 124
Wilson, A. L., 139, 147
Wilson, D. P., 343, 344, 354
Wilson, G. T., 244, 246, 247, 287, 301
Wilson, W., 160, 182
Winder, J. A., 327, 331
Windham, C. A., 201, 209
Winett, R. A., 269, 280
Wing, R. R., 106, 121, 233, 234, 235, 236, 237, 239, 340, 244, 245, 247, 248, 249, 336, 354
Winget, C., 93, 124
Winter, L., 133, 151
Witt, M., 347, 354
Wolchik, S. A., 260, 266, 280
Wolf, R. M., 341, 344, 349, 351
Wolfe, R. R., 246, 248
Wolff, O. H., 233, 249
Wolfsdord, J. I., 68, 75, 177, 183
Wong, B. S. M., 190, 213
Wood, J., 260, 279
Wood, P. R., 305, 333
Woodall, K., 233, 234, 249
Woodward, R. S., 188, 201, 209
Wooley, S. C., 93, 124
Wortman, C. B., 77, 79, 80, 85, 88
Wright, J. C., 340, 344, 348, 353
Wucher, F., 224, 227, 229, 231
Wulf, D., 131, 139, 148
Wuori, D., 33, 47
Wyatt, S., 336, 352
Wysocki, T., 341, 344, 348, 354

Y

Yaffe, J., 32, 49
Yates, D. M., 321, 333
Yokley, J. M., 34, 51
Yost, R. L., 67, 68, 74
Youniss, J., 135, 151
Yourtee, E. L., 207, 210

Z

Zabin, L. S., 133, 152
Zachary, V., 202, 204, 212
Zahaykevich, M., 136, 146
Zakin, D. F., 134, 145
Zaslow, S., 336, 354
Zautra, A. J., 260, 279
Zeiss, A. R., 268, 279
Zellman, G. L., 35, 47, 48, 138, 146
Zelnik, M., 129, 133, 152
Zeltzer, L. K., 305, 332
Zevon, M. A., 36, 50, 61, 67, 68, 76, 177, 184
Zifferblatt, S. M., 190, 213
Zigo, M. A., 342, 344, 354
Zimmerman, R., 13, 18, 24, 26, 59, 63, 75, 92, 96, 123, 254, 255, 278
Zuehlke, M. E., 133, 150

Subject Index

A

Action State model, 258, 261, *see* Health promotion
Addictive disorders, 18, 19, *see* Substance abuse
Adherence, 92, 93, 94, 158
   adolescents and, 114-120, 127, 177-179
   appraising outcomes, 103
   as multidimensional, 96
   assessment of, 179
   chronically ill children, 283
   clinical outcome, 288
   compliance/noncompliance, 93
   counselors and, 291, 292
   failures in, 97, 99
   fear-arousal techniques, 137, 138
   group cohesiveness and, 282
   interaction system, 102
   interpreting stimuli, 102
   intervention and, 137-139, 282, 283
   long-term, 97, 111
   measurement, 180, 181
   models of, 290, 291, *see* Compliance
   motivation for, 109-111
   multidimensional nature of, 130
   multilevel, 285, 286
   operant behavior models, parents as factors in, 135
   physician ratings of, 166, 167
   promoting preference behavior, 108
   school-based programs, 137
   self-regulation framework, 101-104, 107, 108
   self-report, 167
   situational hypotheses, 93
   target goals, 103
   see also Compliance; Coronary Primary Prevention Trial
Adherence models
   behavior cues, 93
   cognitive decision models, 94, 95
   communication and, 94
   social learning and, 94
Adherence research, acute vs. chronic illness, 96
Adolescence,
   adherence, 114-120, 127, 177-179, 180, 296
   barriers to the study of, 139-141
   compliance behavior and, 8, 53, 55, 56
   decreasing compliance in, 68
   health promotion and, 44, 56, 125-145, 273, 274
   nutrition, 56
   pregnancy, 43, 131, 132, 133
   risk behavior, 100
   sexual behavior and, 56
   see also Childhood chronic illness; Obesity,
Age
   compliance and, 44, 336
   health behavior and, 129
   intervention and, 350

379

Age-related developmental issues, 175-178
Age-related
  adherence, 295, 296
  medication and, 206, 207
AIDS, 128, 141, 252
Air bags, 212, 222
Alcohol, 2, see Substance abuse
Allergy, medication and, 66
Alzheimer's disease, 80
Anorexia, 78
Arthritis, 8, 260
Assessment strategies, developmental issues, 180
Asthma, 8, 20, 38, 66, 78
  altering treatment, 318-322
  biochemical indicators, 304-307
  education for medication, 314-317
  medication compliance, 68, 282-284, 303, 304
  monitoring, 313
  observational procedures, 308
  self-reports, 309-311
Autonomy, 55, 80, 82-84, 175
  family perspective on, 68, 78-81
  medication and, 66, 67
  miscarried helping, 55
  responsibility and, 64, 65
  self-care and, 54

B

Blame, failed treatment and, 85, 86
Breastfeeding, 44

C

Cardiovascular disease, 1, 95, 252
Caretaking, compliance and, 12
Child Health Belief Model, 64
Childhood chronic disease
  family and, 77-83, 158
  interactional/situational approaches, 86
  physician/patient interaction, 158, 164
  survival rate, 158
  under/overinvolvement, 79-82
  see Asthma, Diabetes
Childhood compliance framework
  causality, 60-63
  personal control, 60-63
Childhood compliance, cultural differences 68, 69
Children's Health Belief Model (CHBM), 53, 60, 61, 70-72
Cholesterol, 205, 281, 282, 293
  efficacy of cholestyremine, 282
  medication for, 289, 290
  see Coronary Primary Prevention Trial
Chronic illness, see Childhood chronic illness, Clinic performance, 291, 291
Clinic/patient relationship, 292, 348
  family relations and, 348, 349
  see Counselors
Cognition, 175, 355
  adherence and, 291
  health beliefs and, 336, 337
  minimizing health threats, 105
  regimen and, 350
Cognitive processes, 57, 60-63, 126, 131, 132, 154
Cognitive-behavioral analysis, 94
Communication, for compliance, 356
Complex medical regimens
  assessment of, 179
  multiple behaviors and, 179
Compliance assessment strategies
  behavioral observation techniques, 167
  recall interviews, 168-174
  self-reports, 166
Compliance/noncompliance, 303, 304, 313, 316, see Medication
Coronary Primary Prevention Trial (CPPT), 285, 286, 289-292
Counselor training, 292

SUBJECT INDEX

Compliance
  adolescents and, 53, 57, 111
  as a concept, 12-14
  as adaptive process, 21
  as multidimensional, 1, 3, 4, 56, 153, 336
  as multivariate, 55
  as nondevelopmental, 16
  awareness and, 15
  behavior deficiencies of, 13-17
  biopsychosocial framework, 56
  causal relationships, 54
  clinics and, 348, 349
  cognitive development and, 355
  componential model, 22, 23
  construct of, 11, 15
  contextual model, 23, 24
  cultural factors, 53, 60, 67, 69, 73, 356
    Indian children, 69
    Swedish children, 69
  defined, 1, 3, 12, 13, 18, 185, 186, 251
  determinism/nondeterminism, 11
  developmental aspects of, 53, 60-63, 175, 288, 355
  experiential model, 24
  factors in, 53
  family size and, 68
  feedback/feedforward systems, 22
  framework for, 18-21
  framing and, 113, 114
  health professionals and, 14, 15, 357, 358
  health status and, 165, 166, 180, 181
  health threats and, 215, 216, 217
  historical perspective, 1
  impact on family, 86
  influences on, 72-74
  intelligence and, 14, 22, 23
  interventions, 1-3, 281-284, 348, 349
  life-span view, 60
  measurement of, 1, 3, 356
  medication and, 65, 66, 185-207, 314-317
  memory and causality in 53
  negative aspects of, 92
  nonagentic mechanism, 11, 12
  personal control and, 53
  predictors and determinants of, 155, 156
  psychotherapy and, 87, 88
  randomized group designs, 284
  reinforcement, 288
  reward and, 339
  self-protecting capabilities, 275
  single-case design approach, 284
  social factors, 53
  submodels, 22-25
  target groups, 285-287
  theory, 1, 3
  to a regimen, 158, 159, 161, 164, 165, 284
  see also Asthma; Diabetes; Childhood chronic illness; Health promotion; Childhood compliance; Developmental processes; Injury control; Pediatrics
Compliance behavior
  appraisal of outcomes, 99
  as variable, 45, 46
  developmental theory of, 54
  engendering desired, 55
  interactive process, 80
  motivational variables, 98
  priorities, 43, 44
  puberty, 55, 56
Compliance literature, overview of, 154
Compliance research, history of, 91
  psychological/sociological theory, 92
Compliance assessment strategies, physician ratings of adherence, 166, 167
  health status indicators, 166
Compliance/noncompliance, 11-13, 61, 93, 161, 164, 165, 179, 303, 304, 313, 316

diabetes, 337, 339
financial reward and, 336, 339
see physician/patient interaction;
Medication
Continuing Education for Parents
Program, 228
Contraception, 43, 127, 129, 131
Control systems model, 12
Control theory
as a framework, 18, 19, 21
dynamic equilibrium and, 19
inside-out/outside-in models, 22
negative feedback loop, 19, 20
self-regulation and, 21, 22
Coronary Primary Prevention Trial
(CPPT), 285, 286, 289-296
basic problems in, 293, 294
clinic organization 291, 292
counselor training, 292, 293
family, 295, 296
final-lap campaign, 298, 299
newsletter, 296
NIH involvement, 300
results, 299, 300
staff performance, 297
theoretical model, 290, 291
see Compliance; Interventions
Cystic fibrosis, 158, 344, 345

D

Decision-making skills, 131, 134
Delayed gratification, 132, 268
Dental, compliance, 38, 43, 112, 113, 115
Despair/guilt, abstinence violation effect and, 98
Developmental issues, assessment of, 180
Developmental processes
commitment, 61
memory, 60, 61
understanding causality, 61

Diabetes, 8, 20, 21, 38, 78, 81, 84-87, 153, 154, 157, 159, 161, 164, 165, 283, 284
diet and, 346
family and, 337
glucose testing, 337
intervention studies, 338-349
lack of adherence and, 180, 181
locus of control, 54, 60, 64, 65, 67
metabolic control and, 347, 348
peers and, 337, 338, 340
problem-solving skills, 264, 265
recall interventions, 168-179
self-regulation and, 105-107
Diet, 56, 131, 132, 143, 158, 357
adolescents, and, 336
chronic disease and, 346, 347
diabetes and, 346
renal disease, 345, 346
Dietary studies, 38, 39
Disease prevention, *see* Health promotion
Disease, control of, 43, 44

E

Eating disorders, *see* Adolescents
Exercise, 2, 129

F

Family Adjustment and Adaptation
Response Model, 77, 79
Family interaction, 54
dysfunctional, 78, 79
involvement, 356, 357
health care provider and, 348, 349
intervention and, 350
Framing concept
automation of behavior, 111
incentives, 112, 113
health threats and, 56
preferential behavior, 113, 114

SUBJECT INDEX 383

G

Gender, 63, 70
Goodness-of-fit, compliance and, 12, 22
Guidelines for future research, 179-182

H

Health Belief Model (HBM), 63, 69, 70
Health care provider/patient, relationship, 348
   compliance and, 357, 358
Health care
   established relationships and, 44
   medication and, 44, 45
Health compliance behavior
   future research, 3
   theories of, 3
Health compliance research, 3, 7
Health compliance
   acute illness and, 8
   as a construct, 7, 8
   assessment of, 4
   definition of, 7
   measurement and, 4
   medication and, 3-5
   model of, 7, 8
   normal cognitive development and, 3, 4
Health education 229
Health promotion model
   goal appraisal, 266
   motivation, 264
   problem solving for health gains, 261-269
   self-efficacy, 265
   social interaction, 269
Health promotion
   a social action conception, 251, 252
   adherence, 273
   behavior chains, 257
   biological/social constraints, 271
   compliance, 253, 254
   contextual determinants, 270, 271
   contextual model, 255
   integration/reinforcement value, 257, 258
   intervention, 253
   maturation and, 270
   process models, 255
   social interdependence, 258-260
   state model of self-protective action, 256
   see Prevention
Health regimes, *see* Adolescents
Health status, compliance and, 180, 181
Health statutes, psychologists and, 179
Health, targets for change, 56
Hemodialysis, 345
Hemophilia, 346, 351
Hypertension, 99, 104-107, 189
Hypertension Detection and Followup Study (HDFP), 291

I

Illness, conceptions of, 62
Illness-as-relationship problem, 54
Immunization, 43, 220, 357
Income, 44, 53
Independence, compliance and, 55
Infant car seats, 212
Injury control prevention,
   parents and, 215, 216, 219-229
Injury control
   active vs. passive measures, 221, 222
   compliance and, 219-229
   group education approaches, 227
   health education for, 222, 223, 225, 226
   legislation, 220
   Media as resource, 223, 224
Injury prevention, 357
Integrated Model of Adjustment, 77, 78
Intelligence, 60, 61
   compliance and, 14, 22, 23
Interactional/situational approach, 80, 86

Interactive cycle, 83
Interactive processes, 80
Intervention, 53, 57
    across life span, 356, 357
    adherence and, 137-139
    as preventive measure, 349
    chronic illness and, 55
    cultural differences, 69
    during illness, 100
    for compliance, 348
    health promotion and, 274, 275
    medication taking and, 189, 190
    multifamily groups, 343
    need for early, 351
    psychotherapy for, 87, 88
    organizational levels, 285
    social interaction models, 274, 275
    strategies in, 285-289
    trageting behaviors, 343
    see also Coronary Primary Prevention Trial; Health promotion; Pediatrics; Childhood chronic disease

L

Leukemia, 158
Life span
    adherence, 295, 296
    compliance, 274
    intervention, 356, 357
    self-protective activities, 274
Literature, 296
    on compliance, 154, 158, 186
Locus of control, 54, 60, 64, 65, 67
    causality in, 64
    diabetes, 64
    internal, 64
    personal control and, 63, 64
    socioeconomic influences, 64

M

Measurement, 153-155, 288
    adherence, 180, 181
    assessing the health compliance construct, 153
    compliance and, 53
    methods of, 155
    technology for, 155
    time-related data, 176
    see Compliance
Measuring compliance, 154
Media, as resource, 223, 224
Medication Event Monitoring System (MEMS), 202, 205
    see Measurement
Medication assessment
    instruments for, 312
    monitoring, 319
Medication compliance
    age related, 206, 207
    epidemiology of, 186-188
    self-monitoring and, 197-205
Medication
    access to, 66, 286, 289, 290
    adherence measures and, 168, 293, 294
    allergy and, 66
    asthma, 303-307, 309-312, 316, 317, 319, 323-329
    dispensing methods, 297
    health care and, 44, 45
    long-term, 198
    management, 20, 154, 158, 198-204
    pediatrics and, 38
    peer influences and, 72
    placebo, 282
    school use, 66, 67
    self-regulation and, 104
    side effects of, 297, 298, 320
    stratification for compliance, 314-317, 322-329
Memory, 164,
    compliance and, 53, 311, 356
    see Physician/patient interaction
Metabolic control, compliance and, 335-337, 342, 343
    diabetes and, 347, 348
Miscarried helping

adequate medical care, 86
age-related factors, 84, 85
coercive control, 84
defined, 79, 80, 81
developmental factors, 84
evolution of, 82
failed treatment, 85, 86
see Autonomy
Miscarried Helping Model, 77, 80
Miscarried helping theory, 55, 78-81, 84
Miscommunication, 154
Motivation, 55, 56
compliance and, 17, 54
framing the message, 111
health promotion and, 63
sources of, 54
sustained, 100
Multidimensional nature of compliance, 56, 153, 336, 356
Multilevel approach, *see* Adherence; Intervention; Pediatrics; Coronary Primary Prevention Trial
Myelomeningocele, diet and, 347

N

NIH involvement, 300
Noncompliance
family conflict and, 68
personal control and, 63
see Compliance/noncompliance
Nutrition, 44, 106, 115, 129, 131, 132, 143, *see* Diet

O

Obesity, 56, 142, 144, 216, 217, 286, 287
behavior modification, 235
compliance and, 233, 234, 243-245
long-term results, 236, 237, 240-242
parent-child study, 235, 245-247
self-regulation, 244
treatment variability, 239

Organizational levels, compliance and, 285, 286

P

Parent/child dyad, 55
Parental health beliefs, children and, 67
Parental style
compliance and, 68, 71, 72
family size and, 68
Parenting, *see* Childhood chronic illness
Parents
as factors in adherence, 135, 285
as influences, 135, 136
injury control prevention, 215, 216
Pediatric compliance research, 30-46
dietary studies, 38, 39
illness areas, 37, 38
intervention studies, 40, 41
measurement of, 39, 40
Pediatric populations, 29
dental, 38, 43
Pediatrics, 2-4, 8, 9, 287, 288
acute/chronic illness, 42, 43
care by physician and, 44, 45
medication and, 38
outpatient surgery 38
prevention interentions, 43, 44
see immunization; Injury control
Peer influences, 72
compliance and, 68
medication use and, 65, 66
Peers, 67, 113-115
cognitive processes, 57
conformity to, 134
diabetes and, 337, 338, 340
family and, 341, 342, 343, 347
health promotion and, 274
medication and, 72
risk behavior, 127, 129, 130
Personal control, 54
locus of control 63, 64
self-efficacy and, 63
Phenylketonuria (PKU), 264